Females Are Mosaics

Females Are Mosaics

X Inactivation and Sex Differences in Disease

SECOND EDITION

BARBARA R. MIGEON

OXFORD
UNIVERSITY PRESS

Oxford University Press is a department of the University of Oxford.
It furthers the University's objective of excellence in research, scholarship,
and education by publishing worldwide.

Oxford   New York
Auckland   Cape Town   Dar es Salaam   Hong Kong   Karachi
Kuala Lumpur   Madrid   Melbourne   Mexico City   Nairobi
New Delhi   Shanghai   Taipei   Toronto

With offices in
Argentina   Austria   Brazil   Chile   Czech Republic   France   Greece
Guatemala   Hungary   Italy   Japan   Poland   Portugal   Singapore
South Korea   Switzerland   Thailand   Turkey   Ukraine   Vietnam

Oxford is a registered trademark of Oxford University Press
in the UK and certain other countries.

Published in the United States of America by
Oxford University Press
198 Madison Avenue, New York, NY 10016

© Oxford University Press 2014

Library of Congress Cataloging-in-Publication Data
Migeon, Barbara R.
Females are mosaics : X inactivation and sex differences in disease / Barbara R. Migeon.— 2nd ed.
   p. ; cm.
Includes bibliographical references and index.
ISBN 978-0-19-992753-1 (alk. paper)
I. Title.
[DNLM: 1. Mosaicism.   2. X Chromosome Inactivation—physiology.   3. Genetic Diseases,
X-Linked.   4. Sex Factors. QS 677]
QH600.5
616′.042—dc23   2013017154

For Sara, Sheila, Nicole, Mary, Sophie, Meghan, Colette,
and all the other mosaic females.

CONTENTS

ACKNOWLEDGMENTS

I am indebted to many.

To my teachers: Barton Childs, for being a lifelong mentor, role model, and friend, for showing me the power of genetics as an investigative tool and introducing me to X inactivation. Mary Lindley, an editor of *Nature*, who taught me how to cut a paper by half. Her admonitions about how not to write for a scientific journal are always with me. And her joy in writing was contagious. Donald D. Brown, for the challenging sabbatical year in his laboratory at the Carnegie Institution's Department of Embryology that helped change the focus of my research from cytogenetics to molecular cytogenetics. Mary Lyon, for her brilliant hypothesis that has been the focus of my research.

My colleagues: Patricia Jacobs, at the University of Southampton, my longtime collaborator and friend. Gail Stetten, Roger Reeves, and Iain McIntosh at Johns Hopkins, who were always willing to contribute their expertise to our joint explorations.

My students: Scott Gilbert, Cheryl Corsaro, Stan Wolf, David Kaslow, Daniel Driscoll, Ethylin Jabs, and Mihir Jani, who have taught me as much, and perhaps more, than they have learned from me.

My husband, Claude Migeon: for his enthusiastic and enabling support of everything I wanted to do.

Those who helped me in the preparation of this book: I am most grateful to Scott Gilbert, Barton Childs, Nathaniel Comfort, Patricia Jacobs, Kara Pappas, Hans Bjornsson, Jennifer Marshall Graves, and Claude Migeon for their helpful suggestions for the chapters that they have read. I very much appreciate the help of Andrew Wilkie, Stephen Robertson, Robert Desnick, Christine Desteche and Ethylin Jabs with interpretations of model diseases. I am also grateful to Peter Jeppesen, Ahmad Khalil, Dan Driscoll, Christine Clemson, Marco Novelli, and Rob Willemsen, who provided original photomicrographs for this book, and to Michael Schmid for the portrait of Susumu Ohno. With regard to the illustrations, I have benefited tremendously from the advice and assistance of Rick Tracey in the department of pathology. I also acknowledge Chester Reather for the cover photograph of my collage of the mosaic female.

I must also acknowledge the National Institutes of Health and the National Library of Medicine for supporting my research and the writing of this book, respectively. I had the good fortune to have the Oxford University Press as publisher. I thank editors Emily Perry and Chad Zimmerman for their contributions to the creation of this second edition.

Finally, I am grateful to Dr. Susumu Ohno, biologist extraordinaire, whose writings and personal discussions of X inactivation have influenced my thoughts. During the writing of this book I have thought so many times of the Arabian proverb he related in the Preface of his monograph, *Sex Chromosomes and Sex-Linked Genes* [1]. The proverb suggests that while the magnificent Arabian steed and the ungainly camel were made of the same material, the horse was created by one god, whereas the camel was the creation of a committee. I have much admired the elegance with which he told his story and hope that my story has coherence not possible in a multi-authored work.

The word *mosaic*, according to the *Oxford English Dictionary*, is a form or work of art in which pictures are produced by joining together minute pieces of glass, stone, and other materials of different colors. Biologists use the word to describe the hybrids, or chimeras, that result from mixing one embryo with another, or cells of one species with another, referring to the composite nature of such organisms. Mosaicism may also result from the abnormal behavior of chromosomes during cell division in the fetus, such that some cells, but not all of them, have an extra chromosome, or lose a chromosome. In this case, both kinds of cells—the normal ones and the abnormal ones—intermingle during fetal development. Yet, not all mosaicism is the result of manipulation or accident, because a form of mosaicism is part of the developmental program for females of our species.

A female is mosaic because she consists of a mixture of two kinds of cells—each with different functional X chromosomes. The developmental program responsible for this mosaicism—referred to as *X chromosome inactivation*, or *X inactivation*—is an evolutionary solution to the age-old 1X:2X problem. Because XY males have a single X chromosome, whereas XX females have two of them, some kind of adjustment is needed. In our species, the problem is solved by turning off the activity of one of the two X chromosomes in females. Survival *in utero* depends on this, as we know of no one with two *intact* X chromosomes that does not inactivate one of them. Occasionally, we see girls who express a *few* genes from both X chromosomes. Not surprisingly, such girls suffer from developmental anomalies; they are mentally retarded and have severe birth defects.

Because of X inactivation, most women are natural mosaics. Although all their cells have the same two X chromosomes—one from each parent—the mother's copy works in some cells, whereas the father's works in the others. The two kinds of cells often function differently, especially if one of the X chromosomes carries a defective gene.

You may ask, "But isn't this true of most cells in the body?" All cells of an individual have the same genes, but only some of them are used in each cell. A liver cell differs from a kidney cell by virtue of the fact that each expresses different subsets of genes and not the whole repertoire. The answer is that the differential expression of tissue-specific genes is not mosaicism, because each specialized cell within a single tissue expresses the identical subset of such tissue-specific genes. The mosaicism that characterizes normal females is unique because within each and every tissue, cells differ regarding which of their two X chromosomes is expressed—that is, which copy of each pair of genes (*alleles*) is expressed.

Not all mammalian females are mosaics. Laboratory mice are inbred to such a degree that the genes on their maternal and paternal chromosomes are identical. However, because we humans are such a remarkably outbred species, our maternal alleles differ a great deal from our paternal alleles. Therefore, human females in fact have a mixture of cells that often differ in their ability to carry out cellular functions. This sets up the possibility for interactions between them, ranging from sharing of gene products to elimination of mosaic cells of one parental type or the other. It is the outcome of such interactions that determine if a woman is healthy—or ill.

Much has been written about the Y chromosome and its role in inducing maleness. Less has been said about the blueprints for female development, or about the role of biological factors, other than hormones, as the cause of sex differences in human disease. What is usually ignored is the contributions of the X chromosomes and X inactivation to female phenotypes and to sex-specific manifestations of disease. The X chromosome is extraordinary, because it is the only chromosome subject to programmed inactivation of this kind. Abnormalities in numbers of X chromosomes are responsible for the abnormal development of the gonads in the syndromes described by Turner (45,X syndrome) and Klinefelter (47,XXY syndrome). And the chromosome carries genes that, when mutated, are responsible for well-known genetic diseases such as hemophilia, muscular dystrophy, Lesch Nyhan syndrome, adrenoleukodystrophy (Lorenzo's oil disease), colorblindness, lysosomal storage diseases such as Hunter syndrome and Fabry disease, and a variety of endocrine disorders, including dysfunction of the parathyroid, thyroid, and adrenal glands, premature ovarian failure, and the inability to develop as a male. In addition, the X chromosome bears many genes whose mutant alleles produce syndromes of mental retardation, including the fragile X syndrome, the most common of them all. These diseases mainly affect males because any defective copy is their only copy of the relevant gene. In contrast, females with a single copy of the same mutant allele are usually protected to a large extent by their cellular mosaicism, because cells expressing the normal copy of the gene carry out at least part of the function, and often more.

The fact that females are mosaics is not common knowledge, even among scientists, medical researchers, physicians, science writers, and especially women. This is not because such information is inaccessible. A search of the recent scientific literature on PubMed for relevant terms reveals 10,900 citations for mosaicism, 2,536 for X chromosome inactivation, and 3,741 for X inactivation. Therefore, whereas the subject is well represented in the scientific literature, the content of these papers is usually discussed only by the investigators who are involved in this research. At best, textbooks of biology, mammalian development, or genetics devote a few pages to the subject—in most, less than a half page with little mention of the mosaicism that results. Many biologists who work in this field do not realize the clinical implications because they work with *inbred* animals whose maternal and paternal X chromosomes are genetically identical. In these species, both kinds of cells in the mosaic female usually make the very same proteins—unlike human females.

In fact, I am surprised by the relatively small impact this subject has had in medicine, despite its role as a determinant of women's health. The conclusions drawn from most clinical studies of women do not consider the role of cellular mosaicism. Sex differences in disease are usually attributed merely to differences in body size, hormones, or occupational hazards. Unquestionably, after puberty the sex hormones have an enormous effect on sex differences in how we express our genes. Many genes on autosomes are transcribed more in one sex than the other, and this is correlated with sex differences in binding sites for these hormones in the genes that are differentially expressed. Yet, the X chromosome, the underappreciated contributor to sex differences in disease, is present from shortly after conception, at a time when all fetuses live within an estrogen-dominated milieu. X inactivation may not account for all the sex differences, but it does contribute heavily to determining health status: The single active X in males makes them susceptible to a host of diseases not usually seen in females. The single active X in females is coupled with cellular mosaicism, thereby conferring on them an extraordinary biological advantage. In most cases, the mosaicism mitigates the manifestations of X-linked mutations. However, for one of a number of reasons discussed in this book, the patterns of X inactivation in some individuals may eliminate this biological advantage, and as a consequence, they manifest diseases usually seen only in males. Clearly, X inactivation is directly relevant to the health of female fetuses, children, and adults.

For all of these reasons, it seemed appropriate to put this information together in a single place, so that physicians, medical students, graduate students, genetic counselors, nurses, and other health professionals, as well as medical scientists and other biologists, and all those interested in knowing more about the determinants of femaleness, might learn about it. Having investigated this subject for more than 40 years, as both scientist and clinician, I want to communicate what I have learned. It is not an easy subject, which may explain why those who write about science for lay publications have not taken it on. But it is fascinating human biology and worth the effort to learn about it. It is time that a wider audience was privy to this information.

I discuss what is known about X inactivation—not only about the underlying molecular mechanisms but also about the role it plays in determining the biological characteristics of females of our species.

Part I builds a bridge between X inactivation and sex-specific diseases. It provides the evidence that many of these disorders have their basis in X chromosome biology. Also included is an introduction to the concepts of X dosage compensation and the single active X, compensatory mechanisms in other organisms, and experimental models for studies of X inactivation.

Chapter 1 introduces the subject of sex differences in diseases, and the evidence that males are biologically more vulnerable than are females at most stages of their lives. This chapter also introduces genetic diseases that are sex specific—that is, affecting mainly males or affecting mostly females. I argue that the X chromosome plays a role in sex differences in disease susceptibility and that sex-specific diseases are attributable to the single active X chromosome in males and the cellular mosaicism in females.

Chapter 2 is concerned with the evolution of our sex chromosomes, a process that deconstructed the Y chromosome. The Y has fewer genes than any other chromosome and has lost huge regions of DNA—thus creating the 1X:2X problem. Also considered is the gene content of our X chromosome and evidence that the original mammalian X has been maintained relatively more intact during its evolution than other chromosomes.

Chapter 3 provides a brief overview of X chromosome dosage compensation, summarizing the various means that have evolved to equalize the expression of X-linked genes in other organisms with the 1X:2X problem. Although there are striking similarities among mechanisms used by worms, flies, and mammals, each of these organisms has its own inimitable way to compensate for sex differences in expression of X-linked genes.

Chapter 4 is concerned with X inactivation—our version of X dosage compensation—and how it was discovered. The circumstances leading up to this discovery remind us that novel breakthroughs such as this are not made *de novo*. Instead, they are built upon prior revelations that illuminate the problem and provide the means to resolve it.

Chapter 5 describes the experimental models that have been used to gain insights into this developmental process in mammals.

Part II presents the two major themes of X inactivation in mammals: the choice of active X and *cis* inactivation of the other(s). Also included are the major variations on these themes during the evolution of mammals.

Chapters 6 and 7 are concerned with those features of X inactivation common to most mammals. As might be expected, X inactivation itself, like most biological processes, is subject to changes during mammalian evolution. However, the essential features of this developmental pathway are the ones that remain unchanged. This common, or basic, theme of X inactivation has to do with maintaining the single active X during embryogenesis. What are the events occurring during early embryonic development that choose an X chromosome to be protected from inactivation, and what is the pathway that inactivates all the others? The steps that initiate the process are considered in chapter 6, and subsequent steps in chapter 7.

Chapters 8, 9, and 10 deal with the variations on the basic theme: species differences brought about by evolutionary tinkering that does not interfere with the process. In fact, many of the variations reinforce it. These include mechanisms that stabilize X inactivation after it occurs, transferring memory of which X has been silenced to the cell's progeny. Stability, discussed in chapter 9, seems to be more important for some mammals than for others and is a prominent feature of X inactivation in our species. Also variable is the choice of which parental X chromosome remains active. The preference in the choice process, which is referred to as *imprinted* or paternal X inactivation, is discussed in chapter 10. Underlying some of the variable features are the changes within the X inactivation center itself, which are discussed in chapter 8. These changes provide unique insights into how developmental processes as this one evolve.

Part III deals with the genetic and clinical consequences of the single active X, especially the creation of cellular mosaicism in females. The biological advantages of mosaicism are discussed in relation to genetic diseases and the enhanced variability afforded to mosaic females.

Chapter 11 deals with the clinical importance of the single active X chromosome in both sexes. All the other chromosomes in our genome (the *autosomes*) occur in pairs and provide two sets of genes, both copies working in each cell. Having a single active X chromosome means that any cell—whether male or female—has only one set of functional X-linked genes. This chapter concerns chromosomal abnormalities involving the X chromosome, including Turner syndrome and Klinefelter syndrome. Considered are questions such as how we cope with an X monosomy, why the single X is detrimental in Turner syndrome, and what genetic and clinical outcomes are associated with extra copies of the X chromosome.

Chapter 12 considers the other aftermath of X inactivation—the effect of cellular mosaicism in normal women, as well as the medical consequences for those who carry defective copies of X-linked genes. Every female starts out with a mixture of cells; some cells express only the X chromosome alleles inherited from her father, whereas other cells express only the ones inherited from her mother. Interactions between these mosaic cell populations have a large influence on her ultimate health status. Sequencing the human genome has revealed that many of us—males and females alike—may be mosaic for other cell populations as well. The discussion of interactions between mixed cell lineages has relevance for mosaic populations wherever they occur.

New to this edition is chapter 13, entitled "Epimutations, Chromatin Disorders, and Sex Differences in Phenotype." I thought it was time to discuss the effect of other epigenetic phenomena on sex differences in disease. We are increasingly aware of mutations in genes, which affect the nature of chromatin and therefore have an important role in regulating the function of many genes. The possibility of transmitting epimutations to offspring is also considered.

It is now chapter 14 that summarizes the determinants of the female phenotype relevant to X inactivation, and the dynamic way that mosaic cell populations and stochastic factors interact to achieve this. Also considered is the contribution of cellular mosaicism to phenotypic diversity.

I have added more figures and tables throughout the book to clarify the points I wish to make. I hope that my readers who teach biology and genetics will find them useful teaching aids. There are now three appendixes, which supplement information about specific X-linked disorders: *Appendix A*, which is concerned with inborn errors of single-gene origin; *Appendix B*, which considers chromosomal aneuploidy; and the new *Appendix C*, which summarizes phenotypic differences in male and female manifestations of disease. *Appendix C* also provides information about the role of skewing of X inactivation and cell selection in determining the sex differences in expression of the disorders.

Seven years have passed since the publication of the first edition of this book. This new edition reflects the research advances that have occurred since then. We have learned a great deal more about how the inactive X chromosome is silenced and kept silent. We have also been made more aware of the species differences in the process of mammalian X inactivation, and the ways that evolution tinkers with developmental processes. This edition also includes much more about the medical consequences in both sexes of having a single active X.

Despite all the new discoveries included in this edition, much is not yet known. Whereas the pace of science as measured by publications and headlines in *The New York Times* may be incredibly fast, the answers to important questions come slowly. Hopefully, this book will stimulate young scientists to complete the story, and tell us, among other things, how the single active X chromosome is chosen and kept active.

As before, my intention is to make this book accessible not only to graduate students studying molecular biology and genetics, and to clinicians, but also to those who enjoy reading *Scientific American* or have had a college class in biology but have had little prior knowledge of X inactivation and who want to learn about this fascinating topic. Therefore, many terms are defined when first used in the text, and terms not easily explained within the text can be found in the glossary. Those with less knowledge of molecular biology are advised to read through some of the more detailed passages without getting bogged down in the details. Hopefully, the ideas that I wish to convey will become clear enough as the book proceeds. Although I hope the reader will look at the book as a whole, it is written in such a way that many chapters can stand alone. This necessitates a bit of repetition, but I have been told that a little repetition is a good thing.

Females Are Mosaics

PART ONE

Background

Sex Differences in Disease

Ever since 1662, when John Graunt—the father of demography—noticed fewer women than men among deaths reported in London,[1] it has been recognized that females outlive males by a significant number of years. Insurance companies use this biological fact as a basis for determining their rates. The sex difference in mortality is seen throughout the world, irrespective of economic or political factors. The reasons for the greater longevity of women are complex, because many factors are involved [3]. Much has been attributed to the differences in lifestyle, especially with regard to occupational risks—perhaps less valid now than when women spent all their time at home. Risky behavior, such as smoking—which was more characteristic of men at that time—might have contributed to the greater incidence of premature deaths from cancer or heart disease in males. Yet, careful scrutiny picks up another significant component of sex differences in mortality: the biological differences between the sexes. Certainly, gonadal and hormonal differences—testosterone in men and estrogen in women—are responsible for a good deal of sex differences in disease. Breast cancer and the delayed onset of schizophrenia in females, and prostate cancer and the higher incidence of heart disease in males, can be attributed to a combination of environmental and hormonal factors. Yet, even when environmental and hormonal differences between the sexes are not prominent, it is clear that mortality and morbidity are greater in males.

1.1. MALES MORE VULNERABLE AT EVERY AGE

Tables 1-1 and 1-2 show that more males than females die in the infancy and preschool periods. Infant mortality is greater in males irrespective of the length of gestation (averaging about 20% greater). The greater loss of males is also observed *in utero*, based on studies of recognized fetal loss. Needless to say, the sexing of embryos—and, for that matter, even the sexing of newborns—is subject to errors. Even karyotypes of fetal specimens may be misleading because of contaminating maternal tissue. Yet, well-executed studies of chromosomes in newborn populations tell us that the male-to-female (M:F) sex ratio at birth is about 1.05:1.

1. Among his conclusions were that "physicians have two women patients to one man, and yet more men die than women" [2].

Table 1-1. SEX RATIOS FOR INFANT MORTALITY IN THE UNITED STATES FOR 2008.
(TOTAL DEATHS THAT YEAR WERE 28,039)

Age	Males:Females
Under 1 day	1.24:1
1–6 days	1.38:1
7–27 days	1.18:1
28–333 days	1.28:1
Total	1.26:1

Data from Demographic Yearbook 2009–2010 United Nations, Table 16. Available at http://
unstats.un.org/unsd/demographic/products/dyb/dyb 2009–2010.htm. [Accessed September
13, 2012.]

Because of cytogenetic surveys, we also know something about the sex ratio of
fetuses with sex chromosome abnormalities. While some survive the nine-month
gestation, many more fail to implant into the uterus, fail to form a placenta, or fail
to properly form the heart or another essential organ and are not fit enough to
endure the demands of subsequent developmental stages. In their study of fetuses
spontaneously aborted in the first trimester (those embryos and fetuses that die
from natural causes), Hassold et al. [4] found that the sex ratio varied with the
age of the fetus and whether or not the chromosomes were abnormal. The most
common chromosomal abnormality is *trisomy*—that is, three copies of a particular chromosome instead of two. Except for Down syndrome, where the presence
of a Y chromosome seems to predispose some male germ cells to gain an extra
chromosome 21 [5], the occurrence of most trisomies is not usually influenced

Table 1-2. SEX RATIOS FOR DEATH AT VARIOUS AGES IN THE UNITED STATES FOR 2008
(TOTAL DEATHS = 2,473,018)

Age (years)	Males:Females	Age (years)	Males:Females
0–1	1.26:1	40–49	1.56:1
1–4	1.32:1	50–59	1.63:1
5–9	1.26:1	60–69	1.34:1
10–14	1.49:1	70–79	1.15:1
15–19	2.62:1	80–84	0.89:1
20–29	2.87:1	85+	0.54:1
30–39	1.92:1		

Data from Demographic Tables 2000–2009, United Nations, Table 19. Available at http://
unstats.un.org/unsd/demographic/products/dyb/dyb2009–2010.htm. [Accessed September 13,
2012.]

by the sex of the fetus. Yet, for chromosomal trisomies 13 and 18—abnormalities with no sex bias in causation [6, 7]—the M:F ratios are 0.88:1 and 0.90:1, respectively, which are significantly different from the 1.07:1 sex ratio in the nontrisomic population undergoing prenatal testing.[2] This indicates that male fetuses trisomic for chromosomes 13 or 18 do not survive as well as female fetuses with these abnormalities. In addition, the females that are born live longer than their male counterparts [8].

Not all prenatal loss is due to chromosomal abnormalities. Fetuses are lost for many reasons, including maternal–placental disorders, metabolic diseases and other developmental abnormalities incompatible with intrauterine survival. The M:F ratio in these chromosomally normal fetuses (1.3:1) is higher than at birth (1.05:1), again consistent with the poorer survival of males [4].

Paradoxically, the greater number of male births, despite the greater loss of males in the prenatal period, has led to the assumption that there is even more of an excess of males at conception. Yet, there is little evidence to support this. Although it is difficult to measure the sex ratio at that time, none of the available evidence suggests that it differs from 1:1. The ratio of X- to Y-bearing sperm does not differ significantly from 1:1, eliminating the possibility of bias at the time of sperm production. Further, there is no difference in the ability of either kind of sperm to swim, or the rate at which they swim [9]. Therefore, there is little to suggest a biased primary sex ratio during spermatogenesis or at the time of conception, and the best evidence suggests that the greater number of males at birth reflects sex differences in intrauterine survival [9]. If this is true, then it means that more females must die *in utero*, yet the data obtained from recognizable pregnancies is not compatible with excessive female loss *in utero*.

How can the excess of males at birth be reconciled with the excess of males among recognized miscarriages? Charles Boklage has suggested that the secondary sex ratio depends on differential survival of embryos prior to implantation [9], and this is the likeliest explanation. We know from the elegant prospective studies carried out in England by Miller et al. [10] that the recognized miscarriages are a relatively small proportion of those that actually occur before the time when pregnancies become recognizable.[3] Their studies of women who were trying to become pregnant revealed that many of those with positive pregnancy tests never show clinical evidence of pregnancy. Such prospective studies indicate that the miscarriage rate is in fact 43% of all conceptions instead of the 10–15% of recognized miscarriages usually cited. Therefore, we must conclude that the numbers of human fetuses lost *prior to* implantation far exceed those lost *after* implantation.

Because it is not possible to study embryos that abort before implantation, we can only imagine the reasons that they are lost based on our knowledge of those lost subsequently. Recognizable miscarriages during the first trimester

2. The estimated ratios in prenatal controls were 1.06 ($N = 49,427$) for amniocenteses (at >15 weeks).
3. Most fetal deaths in clinically recognized pregnancies occur prior to 8–9 weeks (fetal age), being retained *in utero* 2–3 weeks prior to expulsion.

are predominantly due to chromosome abnormalities; about one in three of them are *aneuploid*, that is, having too many or too few chromosomes. Among the chromosomal abnormalities are individuals with three copies of a chromosome (*trisomy*) or even three sets of chromosomes (*triploidy*), instead of the two parental sets expected. Missing from this group are individuals with *monosomies*—that is, having only one copy of a chromosome instead of two of them (See *Appendix B*). A few individuals with X chromosome monosomy do survive gestation, but monosomies of *autosomes* (any chromosome except a sex chromosome) have not been observed in newborns or among recognizable miscarriages. The absence of monosomies is surprising because errors in chromosome segregation should produce monosomies as often as trisomies. Therefore, autosomal monosomies of both sexes must be among those lost prior to implantation. Yet, this would not be expected to alter the sex ratio, as both sexes are equally affected. One explanation for early female loss is that more females are lost prior to implantation because they do not successfully carry out X inactivation. More about this possibility later in this chapter and section 6.7, Choosing the Active X Chromosome. In any case, the evidence from abnormal fetuses that are aborted after the time of implantation, tells us that males are at higher risk of miscarriage than females.

The greater loss of males at all stages of postnatal development is in part explained by their greater susceptibility to infectious diseases. Males are more susceptible to respiratory distress in the immediate postnatal period and to septicemia and meningitis as newborns [11]. But not all the greater susceptibility has a direct relationship to infection. A 10-year follow-up study of all children born in Finland in 1987 ($N = 60,284$) showed that boys had 20% higher risk of distress at birth and 11% greater chance of being premature [12]. And later on, boys had a 64% higher incidence of asthma, 43% more intellectual disability, and 22% greater mortality. A study of almost 5,000 opposite-sex twins born in Florida showed that boys have a 29% higher risk of birth defects than do girls despite the shared environments [13]. Boys also had a 2- to 3-fold risk of having delayed development, postponed school starts, and need for special education [12]. The preponderance of girls among infants with the salt-losing form of congenital adrenal hyperplasia is attributable to the death of males with this disorder immediately following birth [14]. And among children 0–9 years of age with malignancies affecting their blood cells, males are far more susceptible than females; for example, in the case of Hodgkin's lymphoma, the M:F sex ratio ranges from 4.8:1 to 7.5:1 [15].

Clearly, boys seem to be more vulnerable than girls even when sex differences in their environment (hormonal and activity related) are minimal. And this increase in vulnerability must be due to biological differences. Sex differences due to differences in physiological processes are likely to persist into adulthood. However, by that time they may be obscured by sex differences in experiences and the hormonal milieu.

1.2. VULNERABILITY OF MALES LEADS TO SEX-SPECIFIC DISEASE

What, then, is responsible for the greater biological vulnerability of males? I believe that much of it is due to the differences in the nature of the sex chromosomes—the chromosomes responsible for the sexual differentiation of gonads and body characteristics of males and females. The sex chromosomes in females consist of a pair of X chromosomes, whereas in males, they consist of a single X paired with a Y chromosome. As I describe in chapter 2, the Y chromosome is unique to males, and it carries the critical determinants of maleness. However, it carries little else. Recent studies have led to estimates that about 1,000 genes are located on the X chromosome (*X-linked genes*). In contrast, the Y chromosome carries very few functional genes (probably <100) and lacks working copies of most of the genes that reside on the X chromosome. A good deal of the sex differences in disease is attributable to the sex differences in the numbers of X chromosomes. Having only one copy of their X-linked genes (one allele) makes males more vulnerable to deleterious mutations that adversely affect the function encoded by these genes—certainly more vulnerable than the female, who has two copies of them (two alleles). If his mutated allele no longer functions, a male can be in big trouble because he no longer can carry out the function encoded by that gene. However, the same mutated allele in the female is usually less problematic, because she has a normal backup copy (on the other X) that can do the job. This explains why so many *male-only* diseases are attributable to defective genes on the X chromosome.

A brief description of some conditions due to genes residing on the X chromosome is given in *Appendix A*, in alphabetical order. The list is not exhaustive, and it is biased because I chose them to illustrate points I will make throughout the book. Nonetheless, the diseases described in *Appendix A* are a sample of the large number of mutations in X-linked genes that give rise to *inborn errors of metabolism*, that is, abnormalities present at birth that affect normal physiological function. Readers are encouraged to refer frequently to it as they read about these diseases in subsequent chapters.

As described in *Appendix A*, Bruton agammaglobulinemia and the Wiskott Aldrich syndrome are two conditions caused by X-linked mutations that interfere with the ability to make antibodies—those proteins that protect us against infections. Clearly, mutations in these genes contribute to the sex differences in the incidence of septicemia and meningitis of the newborn. Any male with a defect in one or another of these genes would have a deficiency of immunoglobulins as he relies on his single copy of the gene for synthesis of these proteins. In contrast, a female with the same mutation is protected by the normal copy of the gene on her other X chromosome. Therefore, it is not be surprising that most of the victims of such immunodeficiencies are male. The inability to respond to bacterial invasions by producing antibodies makes males singularly prone to severe infections not only in childhood but also as adults. Mutations leading to a severe deficiency of antibodies may not permit survival past childhood, but a less severe reduction in the levels of immunoglobulins could increase susceptibility to bacterial infections. The greater incidence of tuberculosis in males of all ages is likely to be due to sex differences in resistance to infections.

Mutations that produce immunodeficiencies are not the only ones responsible for greater male mortality. Table 1–3 and *Appendix C* show that for many diseases caused by X-linked mutations, males have a more severe form of the disease than do females. Males are the ones to have the clinical manifestations of such diseases as Duchenne muscular dystrophy, hemophilia, and Lesch Nyhan syndrome, and they are the ones to die *in utero* or in early infancy from such diseases as hyperammonemia and incontinentia pigmenti. In contrast, females with the same mutations in one of their two copies of the gene may have no recognizable clinical abnormalities (e.g., females who carry Lesch Nyhan syndrome or muscular dystrophy mutations); alternatively, they may have milder symptoms than their male relatives (e.g., female carriers of hyperammonemia and incontinentia pigmenti). Clearly, this advantage is due to their having a normal copy of the gene in addition to the mutant one.

The opportunity to carry two alleles at the same locus provides a significant advantage for females. If both of her alleles—the normal one (called *wild type*) along with the mutant one—were expressed within a single cell, each cell would have at least 50% of the normal activity. In most cases, half normal activity is enough for normal function. But in the case of X-linked genes, both alleles do not function in the same cell. In fact, like males, females have only one working copy in each cell. Therefore, the fact that females benefit from having two alleles may seem somewhat surprising. However, the active X in each cell is chosen randomly, so either chromosome has a chance to be the working X. As a consequence, women are mosaics, having some cells with an active maternal X, and others with an active paternal X. In the case of human females, cellular mosaicism is not merely an abstract concept. Because many of her X-linked genes come in various forms, her parental alleles are likely to differ from one another in some way. Because they may encode proteins with varying abilities to carry out their functions, some of these differences may be significant ones. The heterozygous female with a mutation in one of her X-linked genes expresses her normal copy in at least some of her cells; she will therefore benefit from having some cells to carry out the function that has been compromised by the mutation.

It would be misleading to suggest that females never have diseases attributable to their X chromosomes. First of all, women are susceptible to these X-linked genetic diseases if they carry two mutant alleles, one on each X chromosome. Such women are said to be *homozygous* for the mutation. Although having one mutant allele may be enough to produce a disease, almost invariably that disease will be less severe than in males. For example, if the same mutation on the male X is lethal to the male embryo, females may be abnormal, but they will survive because their normal copy of the gene can ameliorate some of the deleterious effects of the mutation (table 1-3). Some examples of *female-only* diseases that are almost always lethal in males are incontinentia pigmenti and Rett syndrome

Table 1-3. SEX DIFFERENCES IN CLINICAL MANIFESTATIONS OF X-LINKED DISEASES[a]

Disease	Mutant Gene	Males[b]	Females[b]
Bruton agammaglobulinemia	BTK	Severe immunodeficiency; no mature B cells	Unaffected; no mutant B cells
Duchenne muscular dystrophy	DMD	Gradual destruction of muscles; death in teens	Unaffected
Fabry disease	αGLA	Episodic pain; renal & heart failure; premature death	Milder disease, if any
Fragile X syndrome	FMR1	Severe mental retardation	Milder retardation
Hemophilia A	F8	Bruising; prolonged bleeding with trauma	Unaffected
Hunter syndrome	IDS	Dwarfing; abnormal bones; mental retardation	Unaffected
Hyperammonemia	OTC	Severe hyperammonemia	Mild or moderate hyperammonemia
Incontinentia pigmenti	NEMO	Death *in utero*	Abnormalities of skin, hair, teeth
Lesch Nyhan syndrome	HPRT	Gout; cerebral palsy; mental retardation; self-mutilation	Unaffected
Rett syndrome	MECP2	Death in infancy	Hand wringing; ataxia; progressive dementia
Wiskott Aldrich syndrome	WAS	Severe immunodeficiency; lack of T-cells & platelets	Unaffected
X-linked hemolytic anemia	G6PD	Severe hemolytic anemia	Unaffected
X-linked ichthyosis	STS	Congenital skin rash	Uneffected

[a] See *Appendix A*.
[b] Males and females are *hemizygotes* and *heterozygotes*, respectively. In each case the common manifestations are indicated.

(table 1-3 and *Appendix A*). Therefore, one consequence of sex differences in numbers of X chromosomes is the existence of sex-specific diseases. More about sex-specific diseases can be found in chapters 11–13.

In addition, women may be uniquely susceptible to mutations that interfere with the X inactivation process. All normal females must inactivate one of their X chromosomes in order to survive. Even girls who express a small subset of genes from both X chromosomes will be mentally retarded and congenitally malformed and may even be miscarried during embryogenesis (see "Ring X Chromosomes" in section 11.5). And the process of X inactivation may be perilous for 46,XX[4] female embryos; most likely females who cannot complete the process of *dosage compensation* account for some of the preimplantation loss of female embryos. A significant loss of females at the time of X inactivation would explain at least part of the excess of males found at birth that is erroneously attributed to a distorted primary sex ratio at conception. In any case, it seems that those females who survive preimplantation are less vulnerable than are males to developmental abnormalities *in utero* and to severe health problems thereafter.

Therefore, both males and females are subject to the adverse effects of mutations affecting the functions encoded by their X-linked genes (table 1-3). However, an X-linked disease in females tends to be less severe than the same disease in males. The following chapters discuss why this is true and how X inactivation serves to attenuate many manifestations of X-linked diseases in females. As you will see, the possession of two X chromosomes and the process of X chromosome inactivation contribute significantly to the sex differences in the pathogenesis of disease.

1.3. SUMMARY AND SPECULATIONS

Like most vertebrates, we use sexual reproduction as the means to ensure survival of our species, because it enables genetic recombination and the creation of individuals with combinations of genes that differ from their parents'. Such novelty is an advantage when new environments require changes in the genetic blueprint. Sexual reproduction necessitated the evolution of special sex-determining chromosomes, usually called X and Y, containing the genes needed for this sexual differentiation. The decision made at the time of fertilization as to whether the zygote will be XX or XY initiates a cascade of subsequent biological events that differentiate one sex from the other. As pointed out by Barton Childs [11], "differences between the sexes are thus created, which sometimes appear to be unrelated to reproductive functions, but which are traceable ultimately to them, and some of these differences might represent a hazard to one or other sex" (p. 809). As described in the following chapters, the fact that males have had to give up one of their X chromosomes in order to carry out their reproductive functions has put them at a decided disadvantage regarding other physiological functions. Having two X chromosomes clearly provides females with a biological advantage. One might ask why a system that causes loss of males has been tolerated through evolution. We must conclude that the advantages of new combinations of genes afforded by sexual reproduction for our species far outweigh the disadvantage of the reduced viability in individual males.

---

4. By convention, the chromosome content of a cell is represented by a number giving the total number of chromosomes in each cell followed by the sex chromosomes present. Thus, 46,XY is the karyotype for a normal male, and 46,XX for a normal female; 45,X is a girl with Turner syndrome, and 47,XXY is a boy with Klinefelter syndrome.

2

Evolution of the Human Sex Chromosomes and a Portrait of the Human X

Aside from self-preservation, the most pressing issue for an organism is to reproduce itself. Reproduction can be as simple as cleaving one cell into two; in this case, the daughter cells produced are exact copies of the cell from which they were derived. However, reproduction of most organisms involves contributions from two nonidentical gametes, the egg and sperm—each supplies different genetic attributes to the progeny of their mating. Sexual reproduction of this kind provides infinite numbers of new combinations of the parental genes. Some of these may specify novel traits that enable the offspring to better adapt to a changing ecological niche than could their parents. Therefore, sexual reproduction usually has been favored during evolution because it provides a "fittest" to survive.

2.1. CHROMOSOMAL BASIS OF SEX DETERMINATION

Although some organisms can differentiate into one sex or the other in response to chemical or thermal differences in their environment,[1] sexual reproduction usually requires a few sex-specific genes—the ones responsible for the sexual differences between males and females. It was the acquisition of such genes that led to the evolution of sex chromosomes. The sex chromosomes are designated X and Y in many species that have them, distinguishing them from the rest of the chromosomes (called autosomes). The X and Y chromosomes usually evolve from a homologous pair of autosomal chromosomes (figure 2-1), after one of them starts to accumulate genes essential for determination of one sex or the other. To keep these genes from recombining during meiosis, one of the pair of autosomes has to be modified so that it no longer exchanges the relevant genetic content

---

1. For example, incubation temperature of eggs determines sex of the gonad in crocodiles, turtles, and some lizards. Higher temperatures promote male development in crocodiles but female development in many species of turtles.

Evolution of the Human Sex Chromosomes

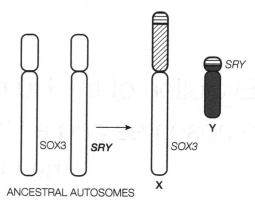

Figure 2-1. Diagram showing ancestral autosomes and the evolution of the human X and Y, initiated after SRY became a testes determinant and other male determining genes accumulated on the future Y chromosome. The extent of the conserved region of the human X (in white) is controversial (see footnote 5). The Y-specific region is black, the region added to the X chromosome during mammalian evolution has diagonal stripes, and the shared pairing region has horizontal stripes. A second, smaller shared region at the bottom of both X and Y is not shown (see figure 2-5).

with its pairing partner. Recombination can be suppressed by a series of deletions and inversions that disrupt the linear arrangement of genes on one chromosome, making it unlike that of its pairing partner, thus interfering with the pairing process needed for recombination. As a result, the sex-determining genes are not swapped between X and Y chromosomes.

The mammalian genes that are essential for maleness reside on the Y chromosome. To ensure that they remain in males, the mammalian Y chromosome has undergone extensive remodeling during its evolution. In the process of becoming the essential determinant of maleness our Y chromosome has lost most of the genes carried on the X chromosome. This essentially is the same as losing an X chromosome. In contrast to the Y, relatively few genes on the gene-rich X chromosome are needed for reproductive functions; the majority of them are required for the metabolic and regulatory functions of the somatic cells. Therefore, X chromosomes are not disposable, and both males and females need at least one of them. Males have only one set of X-linked genes, because their second sex chromosome is the Y chromosome. The mammalian Y is a potent male determinant: all individuals with a Y, irrespective of the number of X chromosomes, have a male body plan, whereas those who lack the Y have a female body plan. Based on studies of individuals with 45,X Turner syndrome (see *Appendix B*), who are females despite having only one X chromosome, it is clear that a single X chromosome is a sufficient blueprint for the female body plan. On the other hand, two X chromosomes are needed for her fertility. Apparently, double doses of one or more genes on the X chromosome are essential to maintain normal oocytes and ovarian function (discussed further in section 11.4, "Turner Syndrome").

In many organisms with sex chromosomes including mammals, the male is the one with two different sex chromosomes, that is, the X and Y (he is *heterogametic*), while the female has two of the same sex chromosome, that is, XX (she is *homogametic*). However, this is not true of birds, where females are heterogametic, having Z and W sex chromosomes, and males are homogametic with two Z chromosomes. Further, because the Y chromosome is subject to continual change and is a rather unstable chromosome, some species have lost their Y-linked, sex-determining genes and even the Y chromosome. Although flies have a Y chromosome, this small chromosome lacks a sex-determining gene, and instead, flies use the ratio of X chromosomes to autosomes as the primary signal for sexual differentiation. Grasshoppers have lost the Y altogether and have an XX/X sex-determining mechanism.

2.2. THE HUMAN SEX CHROMOSOMES EVOLVED FROM AVIAN AUTOSOMES

As a consequence of the degradation of the Y chromosome, the human X and Y chromosomes are readily distinguishable; in fact, they in no way resemble each other (figure 2-2). The Y chromosome is less than one-third the size of the X chromosome and has less than 1% of its genes, yet this pair of sex chromosomes has long been thought to originate from the same ancestral chromosome. The biologist Susumu Ohno, in his prophetic 1967 monograph *Sex Chromosomes and Sex-Linked Genes* [1], was among the first to suggest that the X and the Y of mammals were originally an homologous pair of autosomes (figures 2-1 and 2-3). His evidence was based on observations of some snakes with a chromosomal sex-determining mechanism. He noted that their two opposing sex-determining chromosomes, although almost entirely homologous to each other, had acquired enough differences that the vital sex-determining genes were exchanged only rarely. Ohno reasoned that any evolutionary changes in this pair of sex chromosomes that prevented the exchange of the sex determinants would be favored during evolution. He predicted that such chromosomes would consist of both homologous and nonhomologous segments. Reasoning that changes on the Y could trigger the cascade leading to its effective isolation, he suggested that the first step in creating such morphological differences was an inversion of part of the Y chromosome to discourage recombination. Inversions result when a fragment, created by two breaks in the chromosome, flips while reattaching to the chromosome such that it is in the reverse head-to-tail orientation; hence, the order of the genes on the chromosome is inverted. If the inversion occurs in a Y chromosome, then the genes within the fragment can no longer pair with their mates on the X chromosome.

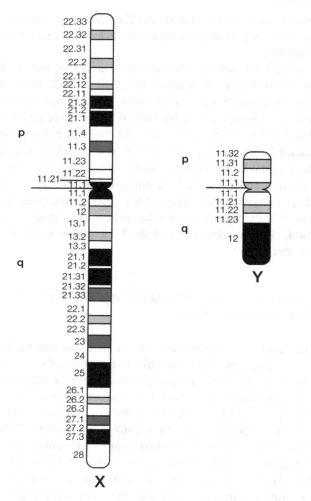

Figure 2-2. Ideogram showing X and Y chromosomes at high resolution (850 bands). Adapted from Shaffer and Tommerup [16].

The validity of Ohno's predictions has been shown by the sequencing of the human sex chromosomes. Our X and Y originated in mammals,[2] and in fact, they evolved from a pair of avian autosomes. From the DNA sequence, it is clear that, even today, some genes are common to both our sex chromosomes and that the Y chromosome contains many relics of genes that still function on the X chromosome.

The Y chromosome has been subject to greater changes and specialization than any other mammalian chromosome; it has lost many of the genes that were

2. Gene mapping and sequence data tell us that bird sex chromosomes retain similarities to mammalian autosomes but not to the sex chromosomes. Because there is no homology between chick and human sex chromosomes, each must have evolved independently from a different autosome. That the homologue of the therian X is an autosome in monotremes, but a sex chromosome in marsupials, implies that our X and Y arose in a common ancestor to therian mammals, sometime after diverging from monotremes, but before we diverged from marsupials [17].

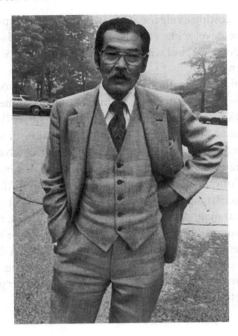

Figure 2-3. Dr. Susumu Ohno. Photo courtesy of Dr. Michael Schmidt.

originally present, and that have remained on its partner, the X chromosome. The DNA sequence reveals the series of inversions and deletions that created our present Y chromosome and has provided insights into when these changes occurred during mammalian evolution. David Page, a geneticist who studies the human Y chromosome, compared the Y chromosome of several mammals ranging from monotremes[3] to humans. He interpreted his observations to indicate that there were at least four major inversions on the Y chromosome [18] (five, based on DNA sequence data). The first event that marked the beginnings of X–Y divergence occurred after the separation of marsupials and monotremes. As one might expect, among the few genes remaining on the eutherian Y chromosome is the major male-determining gene, *SRY* (*sex region Y*), which triggers the cascade of events that induce the bipotential primordial gonad to become a testis rather than an ovary. Encoding a DNA-binding protein, *SRY* is the key gene in this pivotal step in sex determination, acting either as a classic transcription factor or regulating transcription in other ways so as to induce differentiation of the testicular sertoli cells.

In fact, *SRY* is located in the very first segment of the Y chromosome that was prevented from recombining with the X. Even now, *SRY* has a homologue on the X chromosome—*SOX3*—that is transcribed mainly in the developing central

3. Mammals evolved about 300 million years ago. The three major extant mammal groups are the Eutheria, the Metatheria (marsupials), and the Prototheria (monotremes). The monotremes were the first to diverge.

nervous system, suggesting a role for *SOX3* in neural development. Also expressed in the region of the developing gonads, *SOX3* protein binds to the same DNA sequence motif as does *SRY*, but with different affinities, and *SOX3* is not required for male sex differentiation.

The prevailing thought is that an ordinary pair of autosomes, sometimes referred to as *proto-sex chromosomes,* became sex chromosomes when a mutation in one allele of *SOX3* created the male-sex determinant, *SRY* (figure 2-1). This was followed by the accumulation of genes that function in spermatogenesis in the region of the proto-sex chromosome close to SRY. A chance inversion that prevented any exchange between the region with the male sex determining genes was favored in evolution—hence becoming the first step in the formation of the Y chromosome. Consistent with its putative mammalian origin is the fact that *SRY* is not the critical male sex determinant in all vertebrates, and not even in the most primitive mammals, the monotremes. Therefore, while the components of the pathway that determines sex seem to be conserved, the Y-linked master gene is not the same in all vertebrates. The DNA sequence of the Y chromosome in humans and other mammals also shows that it is enriched for genes that function only during spermatogenesis.

2.3. DEGENERATION OF THE Y CHROMOSOME

Clearly, the Y-linked genes have borne the brunt of the evolutionary changes, and few of them are fully homologous to X-linked genes; most are no longer functional, or even homologous at all. I do not mean to imply that the only changes in the Y chromosome are those that eliminate X-linked genes. During mammalian evolution, the Y chromosome has expanded and contracted due to the addition and deletion of repeated sequences, with the result that among human males, the Y chromosome is more variable in size than any other chromosome. The DNA sequence shows an accumulation of repetitive DNA sequences unique to the Y that lend bulk to the chromosome—presumably facilitating proper chromosome segregation. Such palindromic reduplications within the chromosome may be needed to maintain the presence of a chromosome large enough to pair with the X chromosome during *meiosis* [19].

The expected outcome of isolating the Y chromosomes from a pairing partner is the accumulation of genes beneficial for male specific function. Therefore it is not surprising that the only Y-linked protein-coding genes that are male specific— that is, genes known to be transcribed *only* from the Y chromosome—are either testes determinants or fertility factors that influence the motility and effectiveness of sperm. And so, up to now, all of the known Y-specific genes have to do with sexual functions, and none that have been found have been identified as candidates for those genes postulated to convey male-specific cognitive traits.

Paradoxically, a relatively recent inversion in the human Y chromosome has placed the *SRY* gene (which is on the long arm of the Y in lemurs and sheep [20]) onto the short arm of the human Y, dangerously close to the homologous region of X and Y chromosomes at the tip of the short arms (see discussion of the pseudoautosomal region, section 2.5). As a result, the *SRY* gene is occasionally transferred from Y to the tip of the X chromosome, a region where recombination still occurs; these infrequent exchanges account for rare occurrences of XX males (having gained *SRY*) and XY females (having lost *SRY*). It is clear that the human X and Y chromosomes continue to be subject to modification, and the evolution of our sex chromosomes is a dynamic process with no end in sight.

2.4. OHNO'S LAW AND THE CONSERVATION OF THE ORIGINAL X

It was also Ohno who pointed out that, while the Y sheds its ancestral genes, these genes were conserved by the X. He presented evidence that the amount of functional X chromosome relative to the total genome was similar from one mammal to another [1, 21]. He found that the X comprised about 5% of the functional genome in all the mammals he studied. Interpreting this to mean that the original X had been conserved, he predicted that the gene content of these regions would be the same in all placental mammals. Ohno referred to this hypothesis as *homology of the X-linked genes in placental mammals*, and it became known as *Ohno's law* by others.

Although at that time there were only a few examples of genes on the X in more than one species to support this hypothesis (only *G6PD* and *hemophilia* were known to be X-linked in several mammals), the bulk of subsequent experimental evidence has proven over and over again the validity of Ohno's law. All the genes on the long arm and regions close to the centromere of the human X chromosome are found on the X of our most distantly related mammals, the marsupials that diverged from eutherian mammals about 160 mya.[4] Therefore, this region of our X chromosome represents the original mammalian X[5] that has been conserved for at least 160 million years, perhaps for as long as 320 million years (figure 2-5). Yet, the X chromosome has also acquired additional autosomal genes, presumably by X-autosome translocations during its evolution. Most of the genes on the distal short arm of our X chromosome reside on autosomes in marsupials and monotremes. (See XAR in figure 2-4). The recognized exceptions to Ohno's law (reviewed in Graves [22]) reflect these additions to the X chromosomes after the divergence of marsupials from eutherians, by evolutionary translocations of autosomal segments to the X chromosome [24].

---

4. Mammals have been divided into the two subclasses: (1) Theria, the metatherian (marsupial) and eutherian lineages, and (2) Prototheria, represented only by the egg-laying monotremes. Monotremes are the earliest offshoot of the mammalian lineage, having reptilian as well as mammalian features.

5. There is some controversy about whether the proximal short arm of the X is included in the X conserved region (XCR). Because some of the genes on the human X short arm (Xcen–Xp 11.3) are on the long arm of marsupials, and elephants, Graves believes that the proximal X short arm should be part of the XCR. [23]. However, based on DNA sequence, Ross et al. believe that the proximal short arm (Xcen–Xp11.3) should no longer be considered part of the XCR [30].

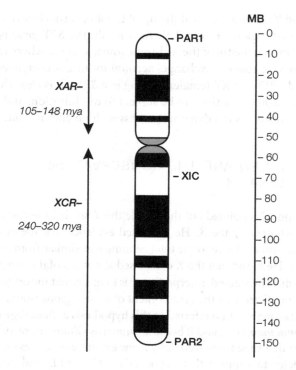

Figure 2-4. The human X chromosome consists of approximately 155 megabases (MB) of DNA. The X conserved region (XCR) is the original X, containing the X inactivation center (XIC). The X added region (XAR), evolutionary additions to the X chromosome, includes pseudoautosomal region 1 (PAR1). PAR2 is the pseudoautosomal region added most recently, 4–7 million years ago (mya). (Dates are merely reasonable estimates.)

2.5. RESIDUAL HOMOLOGY AND THE PSEUDOAUTOSOMAL REGIONS

Only a couple of small regions of our X and Y chromosomes are still able to recombine; these are called pseudoautosomal regions (PAR). In these regions, there is as much as a 50% chance that the copy on the Y chromosome of the father will end up on the X chromosome that he transmits to his daughter. I used to think that these regions at the tips of both chromosomes were remnants of their original autosomal progenitor, but recent evidence indicates that this is not the case. The small (~2.7 MB) pseudoautosomal region at the end of the short arms of both X and Y chromosomes, called PAR1 (see tables 2-1 and 2-2 and figure 2-5)—where genes are still swapped during every meiosis—was added to both chromosomes along with the X added region (XAR) 105–148 mya. Although present on most mammalian sex chromosomes, the pseudoautosomal

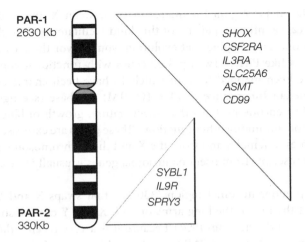

Figure 2-5. The human X chromosome, showing the PAR1 and PAR2 regions of X and Y chromosomes. Also shown are some important genes that recombine (50% recombination for PAR1, 8% for PAR2). Only genes whose function is given in OMIM are shown; see Table 2.2 for the others. *SHOX,* short stature homeobox; *CSF2RA,* colony stimulating factor 2; *IL3RA,* interleukin-3 receptor; *SLC25A6,* solute carrier family 25, member A6; *ASMT,* acetylserotonin methyltransferase; *CD99* (*MIC2*); *SPRY3,* homolog of sprouty; *SYBL1,* vesicle-associated membrane protein 7; *1L9R,* interleukin-9 receptor. Note: all genes from PAR1 are expressed from all sex chromosomes, but only *IL9R* is jointly expressed from PAR2 [28].

regions' content tends to vary to some extent among mammals. In fact, the mouse PAR1 has lost 9 kilobases (kb) of the XAR, which include almost all of the human PAR1 genes. DNA sequence data suggest that exon duplication, exon shuffling, and gene fusion are frequent events in the evolution of PAR 1 (see table 2-1).

Table 2-1. HOMOLOGOUS GENES ON X AND Y CHROMOSOMES

Region of X	Megabases[a]	Origin (estimated Mya)	No. XY Genes
PAR1[b]	0.1–02.7	105–148	24[c]
X Added (*XAR*)	3.6–44.6	105–148	15[c]
X Conserved (*XCR*)	60.0–148.6	240–320	7[d]
X Transposed (*XTR*)	88.5–91.3	4–7	3[d]
PAR 2	154.6–54–9	4–7	5

[a] Distance from Xpter, the tip of the X short arm in megabases (MB).
[b] PAR1 is considered part of the XAR
[c] These genes descend from another autosome pair (homologous to chick chromosome 1) that were added later to X and Y later.
[d] These genes descend from the autosome pair that gave rise to the original mammalian sex chromosomes (homologous to chick chromosome 4).

PAR1 is the major region for interchanges between X and Y during male meiosis.—Because intimate pairing of this kind facilitates proper chromosome segregation—one can imagine that evolution would favor the creation of small pairing regions like PAR1. Twenty-four genes with functional copies on both X and Y have been mapped to it, of which 13 have been characterized in the Online Mendelian Inheritance in Man (OMIM) database (see figure 2-5 and table 2-2). They encode proteins that affect stature, growth of blood cells, and energy metabolism, among other functions. These genes are expressed from both X chromosomes in females and from the X and the Y chromosome in males, so the dose of transcripts from pseudoautosomal genes is usually the same in both sexes.

A second pseudoautosomal region (330 kb) that swaps X and Y genes has been found at the tips of the long arms of both X and Y chromosomes. Called PAR2, this region differs from PAR1 because it is a very recent addition to the Y chromosome; the Y copy of PAR2 was derived from the X chromosome since the divergence of the human and chimpanzee lineages about 4 to 7 mya. Unlike PAR1, PAR2 does not function to hold the X and Y chromosomes together during meiosis, and only one of its three genes characterized by OMIM is expressed from both sex chromosomes [25] (Table 2-2). Recent evidence suggests that there is a recombination hotspot in PAR2, close to the SPRTY3 gene. Yet, the frequency of exchanges in this region is variable and significantly less than that at PAR1 [26]. That the crossover frequency between X and Y at PAR2 of males is only 8% means that the long arm of the male X has no stable pairing partner, and explains its frequent flipping to pair with itself [27] (see "Hemophilia A" in section 12.5).

Tables 2-1 and 2-2 and figure 2-6 show the location of genes in PAR1, PAR 2, and elsewhere on the sex chromosomes that are still jointly transcribed from both X and Y chromosome. Whereas some Y genes have acquired divergent functions, the few remaining homologous XY genes retain similar functions. One wonders why these genes persisted on both sex chromosomes. Most likely, the double dose of their gene product was advantageous and continues to be advantageous at this time.

2.6. GENETIC PORTRAIT OF THE HUMAN X

The X chromosome is indeed a unique chromosome. In males it has no pairing partner, and so any exchange of genes with the Y chromosome is limited to the pseudoautosomal regions. In addition, only the X chromosome is targeted for sex dosage compensation. The unique biology of the X chromosome has its origins in the evolution of our sex chromosomes. Until recently, our ideas about the genetic content and evolutionary history of the X chromosome were based on snapshot-like glimpses; now, however, with the complete DNA sequence of the X chromosome known, we have been given an extraordinary portrait of our X chromosome.

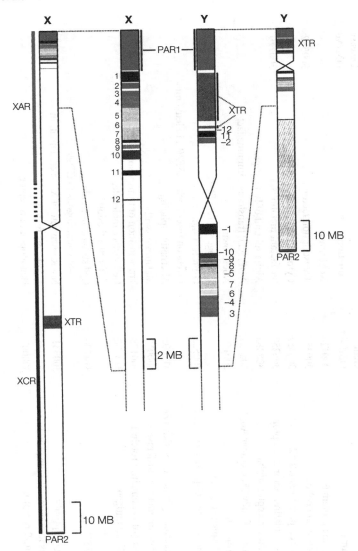

Figure 2-6. The human X and Y chromosomes, showing the location of homologous genes.
The entire X and Y are shown using the same scale on the right and left sides of the figure, with expanded views in the center. The colored segments on X and Y show the position of homologous genes on the two sex chromosomes. The red numbers along the Y chromosome indicate that the segment is inverted with respect to the X. Adapted from Ross et al. [30], figure 6, with permission. [See color plate.]

The "finished" DNA sequence of the human X chromosome[6] was published in March 2005 [30] and is updated regularly. It provides information about the genetic content, as well as the linear order of genes and other structural features

6. The "finished" sequence represents 99.3% of the chromosome, excluding the centromere, with gaps representing a total of <1%.

Table 2-2. GENES IN PAR1 AND PAR2. ALL GENES ARE CO-EXPRESSED FROM X, Y, AND THE INACTIVE X, UNLESS OTHERWISE INDICATED[a]

Distance from Xpter (in MB)	Gene Symbol	Gene Name	Gene OMIM#	Function	Disease OMIM#
0.17	GTPBP6	GTP binding protein 6	300124	Not known	
0.57	SHOX	Short stature homeobox	300357	Transcription factor	300582
1.31	CRLF2	Cytokine receptor-like factor 2	300357	Cytokine receptor for CD4+T cells	
1.38	CSF2RA	Colony-stimulating factor 2 receptor	306250	Surfactant metabolism	300770
1.52	IL3RA	Interleukin-3 receptor, alpha	308385	Alpha subunit of IL3 receptor	
1.55	SLC25A6	Solute carrier family 25, member A6	300151	ADP/ATP translocase, immune factor	
1.59	ASMTL	Acetylserotonin methyltransferase-like	300162	Not known.	
1.66	P2RY8	Purinergic receptor, G-protein coupled	300525	Pseudogene of *ASTM*? G-protein signaling. Inversion fuses it with *CSF2RA* in leukemia	
1.76	AKAP17A	Splicing factor, arginine/serine rich 17A	312095	Alternative splicing	
1.79	ASMT	Acetylserotonin methyltransferase	300015	Melatonin synthesis	
2.41	ZBED1	Zinc finger (BED domain) protein 1	300178	Transposition of transposons	
2.63	CD99	CD99 (MIC2) antigen	313470	Cell surface molecule, T-cell adhesion	
2.63	XG	XG blood group	314700	Cell surface molecule 48% homologous to CD99	
154.57[a]	SPRY3	Homolog of sprouty	300531	Not known; site of XY recombination	
154.71[a]	SYBL1	Vesicle associated membrane protein 7	300053	Membrane fusion	
154.81	IL9R	Interleukin-9 receptor	300007	Hematopoetin receptor	

[a] Silent on inactive X and Y [25].

along the chromosome. The sequence was assembled by a large group of molecular biologists, who identified many genes and their order on the chromosome. That these putative genes are in fact genes has been confirmed by searching databases and the literature for reports about X chromosome genes and X-linked diseases. This confirmation process is referred to as *annotation*. Comparing the DNA sequence of our X chromosome to that of the Y chromosome and several human autosomes and annotating it with sequence data from X chromosomes from other species has painted an excellent picture of this extraordinary chromosome. This portrait also tells us about how our X has evolved. Yet, remember that the portrait is also evolving, so what we have on hand is more like an unfinished portrait of the X chromosome. Although the resemblance is good, and the major features are characteristic of the X, some of the details may change with further studies, especially with further annotation.

The human X chromosome is about 155 megabases (MB)[7] in length, consisting of approximately 51 MB of genes—somewhat less gene-dense than other chromosomes of its size, but denser than the larger chromosome 4. The rest of the chromosome consists of interspersed DNA sequences that are not unique to the X because they occur as repeats all over our genome. There are 826 protein coding genes on the X chromosome, only slightly less than the 878 genes on chromosome 7, which is essentially the same size. The largest gene is the 2.2 MB Duchenne muscular dystrophy gene, whereas the shortest consists of a mere 114 base pairs. The structure of these X-linked genes is similar to that of autosomal ones regarding the size and numbers of exons and introns.

Forty-nine percent of the known genes include CpG islands. These are 0.5–2 kilobase (kb) clusters of CG (cytosine–guanine) dinucleotides in the promoter region of genes that are widely expressed, on the X and throughout the genome. There are more than 8,000 X-linked CpG islands that occur all along the chromosome, with a frequency of 5.2 islands per MB of DNA. The clustered CpGs that are within or near to genes have a role in the regulation of those genes (considered in section 7.2, "Maintaining Inactivation by DNA Methylation of CpG Islands"). All chromosomes have CpG islands similar to these, but those on the X chromosome have been adopted by the X dosage compensation mechanisms as the means to maintain silence of the inactive X (see section 7.2).

The mammalian X chromosome is truly unique because its genetic content is not found in X chromosomes of nonmammalian species. The X conserved region (XCR) that has been maintained through mammalian evolution as the long arm of our X chromosome is homologous to one found at the end of chick chromosome 4, whereas the distal short arm of the X (including PAR1) referred to as the X added region (XAR; see figure 2-4) is homologous to a region of chick chromosome 1. Therefore, it seems that the long arm of our X was derived from one autosome pair, whereas the short arm was added later and was contributed by another autosome.

Comparing the X sequence to that of the human Y chromosome reveals the ancient relationship between our sex chromosomes and the extensive remodeling

---

7. One megabase equals a million nucleotides, or a thousand kilobases (kb).

of the Y chromosome during mammalian evolution. Of the 54 genes that are homologous on X and Y, 24 of them are conserved in the pairing region (pseudo-autosomal region) at the top of the X and Y chromosomes. Another five genes are in PAR2, but only three are characterized in OMIM. There is also spotty homology between X and Y at other regions of these chromosomes: The remaining 26 homologous genes are widely distributed with 15 in the XAR and 3 in the region called XTR (X transposed region), because it arose by duplication of a piece of the X chromosome that was transposed to the Y quite recently—about 4-7 mya (figure 2-6).[8] Whether or not all of these genes are functional remains to be seen. Of interest, there are a few protein-coding genes on the Y chromosome with no obvious homologues on the X, and most of them constitute genes expressed in the testes that have accumulated on the Y in more recent times. Similarly, some female fertility factors have accumulated on the X. There seem to be several X-linked genes that influence the survival of oocytes in the ovary.

One needs to remember that changes in the X and Y chromosomes are not static and that these chromosomes are still in the process of evolution, so many of the genes present on the Y may be relatively new additions. Table 2-1 lists some of the known genes in various regions. Like the XTR, the 330 kb pseudoautosomal pairing region at the bottom of the X and Y (PAR2) was created by duplication of material from X and transposition to Y since the divergence of humans and chimps. Although some recombination occurs between X and Y in this region, PAR2 is not a very good pairing segment in males, accounting for the tendency of the male X to pair with itself at other homologous segments [27].

The portrait provided by annotation of the DNA sequence gives us the first credible estimate of the degree to which females are heterozygous for their X-linked genes. In the DNA making up this 155 MB chromosome, more than 153,000 nucleotides (~0.1%) are not the same on all X chromosomes. Because many of these single nucleotide differences occur with a frequency of at least 1 per 100 individuals, these sites are said to be *polymorphic*, and they are called single nucleotide polymorphisms, or SNPs (pronounced "snips"). One of these SNPs can be found in every kilobase of DNA along the X chromosome. Most of them are not detrimental, and in fact, some may provide advantages, but in either case, they do furnish variation for evolution to work on. Not only do they provide a measure of heterozygosity for X-linked genes, but they are also genetic markers for mapping genetic diseases in families. The SNP frequency on the X chromosome is about half that on the autosomes, reflecting the fact that males have only one X chromosome. Also, because there was no normal allele to balance it, any variations that were detrimental may have been eliminated.

According to OMIM, the analysis of the genetic content of the human X chromosome to date implicates mutations in 271 protein coding genes as contributing to X-linked diseases. The identification of these mutations has revealed that some

8. During primate evolution, new genes were formed by duplications that were transposed to other regions of the genome. Most of the new genes on the Y were progressively recruited to enhance male germline function.

clinically distinct disorders are attributable to mutations in the same gene; for example, gout and Lesch Nyhan syndrome are classified as different disorders, but both are caused by different mutations in the *HPRT* gene (*Appendix A*). The difference in the disorders is attributable to the differences in the degree of enzyme deficiency caused by the mutations.

Perhaps surprising, the parts of genes that are encoded into proteins represent just 1.7% of the DNA sequence of the X, with highly reiterated sequences, noncoding introns, pseudogenes, and RNA genes making up the bulk of the chromosome. The interspersed repeats account for 56% of the X chromosome sequence. Prominent among them is the family of long interspersed elements (LINEs) that account for 29%. The significance of these sequences remains to be seen and is discussed in chapter 7.

Comparisons of the human X sequence with those of other organisms reveal something about the linear order of genes on the mammalian X chromosome. Over the last 100 million years of mammalian evolution, the order has not changed in humans, cats, dogs, pigs, and horses. But segments of the X chromosome of mice and rats have become rearranged many times over the same period, which may reflect the fact that the animals sequenced were laboratory animals selected for ability to inbreed; they are not necessarily representative of their species as a whole. Keep this in mind because such observations help to explain the species differences in the details of X inactivation between mouse and man (see chapters 8–10).

It is the extensive loss of Y chromosomal genes that produced the single X in males, while maintaining the two X chromosomes in females. This necessitated the evolution of compensatory mechanisms to equalize the sex difference in numbers of X chromosomes. As you will see, such mechanisms not only silence one of the human X chromosomes to equalize the dose of X-linked genes, but also increase the transcription of genes on the X chromosome in both sexes in order to balance the single dose of expressed X-linked genes with the double dosage of autosomal genes (see section 11.1, "Coping with a Monosomy X"). What we still do not know is the time relationship between the loss of Y genes and the onset of silencing of X-linked genes in females, or upregulation of X-linked genes in both sexes and how it was accomplished. This is difficult to determine because it happened at least 150 mya. In section 7.3 you will see that the new blocks of genes, arriving on the human X chromosome at different times during its evolution, eventually come under the influence of the inactivating machinery. And, studies in plants, which are in process of losing Y-chromosome genes, tell us that X-linked allele expression in males increases as Y-linked allele expression decreases. This suggests that some steps in dosage compensation can quickly evolve *de novo* after the Y genes are lost, at least in plants [29].

2.7. SUMMARY AND SPECULATIONS

Our sex chromosomes arose *de novo* from a pair of ancestral autosomes and have evolved such that today the X chromosome is a vigorous gene-laden chromosome—whereas the Y chromosome is gene-poor except for those genes involved in male sexual functions. Therefore, other putative male-specific attributes are likely to be due to modifications not involving the DNA sequence, or to environmental and social factors, rather than to sex differences in the genetic blueprint.

It is the effective loss of an X chromosome during the remodeling of the Y that accounts for the sex difference in the number of X chromosomes. And it is this difference that necessitates X dosage compensation.

The dynamic changes to the proto-sex chromosomes in males involve not only subtractions and inactivation of chunks of the future Y chromosome, but also additions of blocks of DNA to the future X chromosome, and the remodeling will continue. The elimination of Y-homologous DNA is most complete in the region of the X chromosome essential for X inactivation. This region of the X needs to be prevented from recombining with the Y—as much as the *SRY* gene needs to be kept off the X. Clearly, what has been lost from the Y was expendable and what remains on the conserved portion of the X includes all that is essential for dosage compensation.

The fact that there are still functional genes that recombine in the pseudoautosomal pairing region has implications for individuals with abnormal numbers of X or Y chromosomes. As one might expect, if both alleles are functional, they are not subject to X inactivation. Therefore, it is likely that these pseudoautosomal genes, and other genes which are transcribed from all X and Y chromosomes—and therefore equally transcribed in chromosomally normal males and females—are the genes responsible for some of the somatic abnormalities in males and females with sex chromosome aneuploidies like Turner or Klinefelter syndromes.

3

X Chromosome Dosage Compensation

An Overview

This chapter provides an overview of how individuals whose sex is determined by XX and XY chromosomes equalize the expression of their X-linked genes. It considers why modulation of this kind is needed, and the different mechanisms used for this purpose. The modulation is referred to as *sex dosage compensation,* a term first used by the *Drosophila* geneticist and Nobel Prize winner Hermann Muller [31]. It is also called X dosage compensation because the adjustments always affect the X chromosome. Yet, most species that need X dosage compensation have their own unique version of the process. This is true not only for animals but also plants.[1] Although understanding mosaic females does not require knowing the details of dosage compensation in flies, worms, and birds, the survey of the various recognized mechanisms in this chapter not only illustrates the remarkable versatility of biology but also helps to put our own version of dosage compensation in proper perspective.

Here, we consider the variety of ways that have evolved, independently, so that males and females will have the same amount of X-linked gene products. Some organisms balance the sex dosage, while maintaining the functional output of the pair of sex chromosomes. However, X inactivation, our own method of dosage compensation, creates a monosomy X in both sexes—that is, only one working set of X-linked genes in females as well as males, in contrast to their two working sets of all the autosomal genes. As a consequence, X inactivation requires another layer of compensation—one that balances the output of autosomal and X-linked genes. Why we might need parity between outputs of sex chromosomes and autosomes, and how this is accomplished, is considered in Chapter 11.1, "Coping with a Monosomy X."

---

1. A recent study of the plant *S. latifolia* suggests a compensatory mechanism for the evolutionary loss of Y chromosomal genes. How this is achieved is not yet known [29].

3.1. X CHROMOSOME DOSAGE COMPENSATION

In many species with the XX/XY mechanism of sex determination, the Y chromosome is either nonexistent or genetically impoverished except for the few genes with a role in sex determination and spermatogenesis. Because most of the genes on the X chromosome have no partner on the Y chromosome, males have only one set of X-linked genes, while females have two sets. This results in a sex difference in the quantity of proteins encoded by the X-linked genes. Pregnancy outcomes in human females tell us that a dosage adjustment is essential for normal embryogenesis, because individuals who express both sets of X-linked genes die *in utero*—we never see them. The survival of females requires that the proteins encoded by their X-linked genes be present in the same amount as in males. Even individuals with a partial imbalance in the amounts of X-encoded proteins are seldom seen and are always quite abnormal (see "Ring X Chromosomes" in section 11.5). Why, you may ask, does the adjustment reduce the protein levels in females and not increase the levels in males? The answer is that adjusting the expression of the female X is the mammalian way of doing it, but the other possibility works just as well in other species (figure 3-1). And because the mechanisms of dosage compensation arose independently, there are a variety of ways to solve the 1X:2X problem.

Because the solution requires a means of equalizing the amount of protein encoded by X-linked genes, any compensatory mechanism needs to adjust the levels of protein expression so that it is the same in both sexes. Clearly, the adjustment can be made locus by locus—regulating one gene at a time—and in some cases this is the means used for the fine-tuning. However, it is more expedient to do this in one fell swoop, rather than individually. In fact, the major means to achieve dosage compensation in all organisms that need it is to modulate the expression of all the genes on the chromosome as a block, rather than individually.

Regulation at the Level of Transcription

Whenever X dosage compensation takes place, its *modus operandi* is to modulate the amounts of proteins that are made either by enhancing, reducing, or silencing the expression of groups of X-linked genes. Therefore, dosage compensation is a global process, affecting the amount of RNA transcripts that mediate protein synthesis. To compensate for sex difference in X chromosome dosage, we equalize the amounts of RNA transcripts that are produced by adjustments in the mechanisms that regulate the process of transcription. The nature of this transcriptional regulation has been best studied in three very different groups of organisms: (1) the fruit fly, in particular, *Drosophila melanogaster*; (2) the nematode *Caenorhabditis elegans*; and (3) mammals, including marsupials.

Mechanisms of X Dosage Compensation
Involve Transcritional Modulation

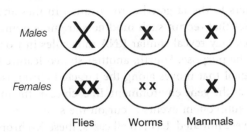

Figure 3-1. Overview of X dosage compensation in several organisms showing that mechanisms of X dosage compensation involve transcriptional modulation. The size of the X chromosome reflects its level of transcription, with increased transcription of the single X in male flies, reduced transcription of the two X chromosomes in female worms, and transcription of only one X chromosome in female mammals.

The diagram in figure 3-1 shows the three ways that such an adjustment can be made at the level of transcription: (1) increase the amount of transcripts from the single X in males to equal the output of the two X chromosomes in females, (2) reduce the level of transcription of each of the two X chromosomes in females so that they jointly equal that of the single male X, or (3) silence all but one X in cells of both sexes. In fact, all these mechanisms are used. In flies, both female X chromosomes are transcribed at normal levels because the single male X is over-transcribed approximately 2-fold [32, 33]. Female worms also use both X chromosomes, but they reduce the level of transcription on each of them by half [34]. And in mammals—and only mammals—females use only one of their X chromosomes; the other is silenced.

Therefore, several parallel strategies for dosage compensation have arisen during evolution. The modifications—although always targeted to an X chromosome—are targeted to different X chromosomes (sometimes the X in males, and other times one or more X chromosomes in females). And the mechanisms of dosage compensation in different species are mediated by different players and are adapted to the special needs of the organism.

Despite species differences in the chromosome that is targeted for regulation and in the details of dosage compensation, some features are similar for all species. First, the compensatory mechanisms are always closely associated with mechanisms of sex determination; that is, some of the molecular mechanisms are involved in both developmental processes. And if dosage compensation does not work for some reason, then the individual does not complete its development—as a female in the case of humans, or as a male in the case of flies. Second, all the compensatory adjustments are directed at the level of transcription, and in all cases they affect the transcriptional output of the targeted X chromosome—or chromosomes in the case of worms. Third, all strategies involve the remodeling of the architecture of the targeted X chromosome to achieve this transcriptional change. In all cases, these modifications affect the major part of the targeted chromosome(s), not just pieces of one—or the other. In all cases, the transcriptional modification is mediated by molecules that recruit the chromosome remodelers to the targeted chromosome. In flies and eutherian mammals, the molecules that recruit such modifiers are noncoding RNA transcripts, and further studies may reveal similar RNA molecules in worms, or other molecules that serve the purpose. Fourth, another shared feature is the existence of an inactivating signal that moves along the targeted chromosome, evoking further modification of the gene environment. In each case, the modifications occur *in cis*—that is, all subsequent events occur on the same chromosome where the original changes were initiated. Last, in all cases, these X-chromosome-wide regulatory mechanisms are superimposed upon the gene-specific mechanisms that locally control the function of individual X-linked genes. Such regulatory features target the promoters or untranslated regions of individual genes, determining when in development, and in which tissues, a gene is expressed. Therefore, dosage compensation is an extra layer of regulation and a more global regulation that is added on to those that regulate the gene-specific spatial and temporal expression of individual X-linked genes.

3.2. HETEROCHROMATIN AND CHROMOSOME SILENCING

Chromatin Remodeling Regulates Transcription

The expression of any gene is strongly influenced by its local environment. The genes of higher organisms consist of strands of DNA, which are packaged with proteins in a complex called *chromatin*. This chromatin is further organized into individual chromosomes to facilitate proper segregation of the genes to daughter cells during cell division (figure 3-2). This chromatin has another essential function: to block the expression of genes that should not be expressed—because the time or place (tissue) is not appropriate. To do this, the genes that need blocking are packaged so as to make them inaccessible to the transcriptional machinery of the cell. The packaging is mediated by *histone* proteins, which are the major proteins in chromatin; they make up the core for the DNA to wrap around, and therefore they provide the physical environment for the genes. The physical nature of the chromatin influences its ability to support transcriptional activity—determining not only whether or not a gene is transcribed but also when it is transcribed or how many transcripts are produced. Chromatin is said to be "active" or "repressed," depending upon modifications of the histone proteins (figure 3-2). This, in turn, determines the degree of compaction, or folding, of the chromatin. For any gene to be fully transcribed, it must be embedded in "active" chromatin; the chromatin must be loosely compacted, and accessible to the RNA polymerase enzymes and other protein factors that are essential for transcription. When the chromatin is "inactive," it is tightly compacted and repressed—and not "open" to the enzymes that carry out transcription. Therefore, the gene(s) embedded in "closed" chromatin cannot be transcribed.

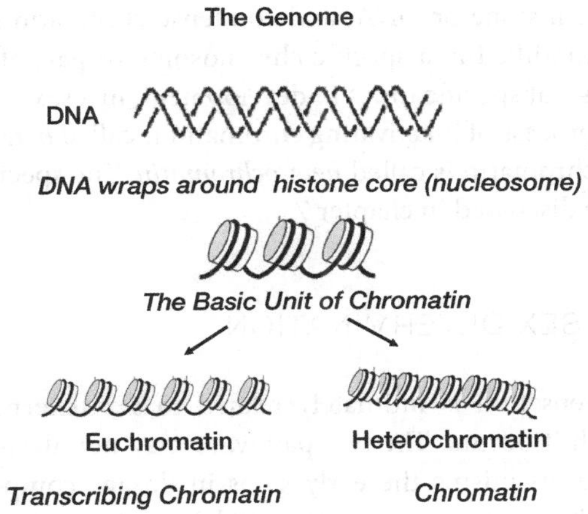

The Genome

DNA

DNA wraps around histone core (nucleosome)

The Basic Unit of Chromatin

Euchromatin   Heterochromatin

Transcribing Chromatin   *Chromatin*

Figure 3-2. Diagram depicting the genome, which consists of the genetic component (the DNA and genes) and the epigenetic component (chromatin). Chromatin is classified as either *euchromatin* or *heterochromatin*, depending on the *nucleosome* spacing and histone modifications.

Variations in Chromatin Organization Are Mediated by Complexes That Remodel Chromatin and Modify Histones

The configuration of chromatin of a particular chromosome is not static but varies during development and from one tissue to another, presumably driven by the developmental program of tissue-specific genes. Setting up a particular chromatin configuration requires many steps, and the complexes are formed by many proteins; some of these steps and proteins are known (see section 7.1, "Spreading Inactivation by Modifying Chromatin"). However, the factors that initiate the change from closed to open chromatin, and the reverse, are not yet well understood. We know that at least some of these initiation events require a unique kind of noncoding RNA molecule. Such RNA molecules differ from the messenger RNA molecules because they are not translated into protein. Instead, these molecules stay in the nucleus, bind to the chromosome itself, and start the process of chromatin modification. In the case of the human X chromosome, the binding of this RNA to the chromosome is referred to as *coating* or *painting* the chromosome. The spreading of these RNA molecules along the X chromosome enables the chromatin-modifying activities to spread long distances from specific initiation sites.

Although the initial steps that trigger the chromatin modulation are not the same for all organisms, the final steps in the cascade—those that actually create the architectural changes—are common ones; they are widely used throughout the genome to silence or activate chromatin wherever and whenever this is needed. This involves chemical modification of the histone proteins to compact or loosen the chromatin. The result of such localized activities that acetylate and deacetylate histone, methylate histone or DNA, and condense chromatin is that chromatin structure can be modified in a specific chromosome or part of it—in one tissue and not the others—at specific times in development, in a sex- and chromosome-specific way. The process of inactivating chromatin is called *heterochromatization*, and the silenced chromatin is called *heterochromatin*. The specific steps involved in this process are discussed in chapter 7.

3.3. ROLE IN SEX DETERMINATION

Sex dosage compensation is intimately related to sex determination in every organism in which it occurs. The two pathways may not always be interdependent, but in some organisms the early steps in dosage compensation and sex determination pathways are common ones [36]. In each case, one of the two sexes must undergo dosage compensation, or it cannot become a female or a male. Male flies cannot survive unless they jazz up the transcription of their single X chromosome to equal that of the two X chromosomes in females. The failure to dampen X-chromosome transcript levels causes sex-specific lethality in worms. Similarly, for a human female to survive, she must silence one of her two X chromosomes. Thus, mutations that disrupt X chromosome dosage compensation in any species cause male- or female-specific lethality.

3.4. MECHANISMS OF DOSAGE COMPENSATION IN OTHER ORGANISMS

The Nobel Prize winning biologist Francois Jacob suggested that evolution is not an engineer but a tinkerer [37]. And he added that, unlike engineers, different tinkerers who tackle the *same* problem most likely come up with *different* solutions. For me, there is no more compelling evidence of this than the various solutions to the 1X:2X problem. Despite the common themes of X dosage compensation, it should not be surprising that the ways to accomplish the transcriptional regulation differ among such diverse organisms.

Because the various means that have evolved to achieve dosage compensation provide extraordinary insights into the role of tinkering in the evolution of such mechanisms, and the species differences in X inactivation among mammals, it seems worthwhile to consider them in some detail. Therefore, below are brief descriptions of the process in flies and worms—not only to show how different the solutions to the same problem can be, but also to remind us that there is a great deal of serendipity involved in solving biological problems. I have also included birds because the evidence so far suggests that they may have yet another solution to the problem. A caveat is that all the details of the underlying mechanisms for all organisms are not yet known, but the general schemes are thought to be valid. For more detailed reviews of dosage compensation in these organisms, the reader is referred to Conrad and Akhtar [38], and Meyer [39].

Dosage Compensation in Fruit Flies

The Y chromosome of *Drosophila melanogaster* is smaller than the X and, like the human Y, consists mostly of heterochromatin. Unlike our Y, their Y chromosome arose *de novo*, and its genetic content differs from one fly species to another. The only Y-specific genes are those expressed only in the testes, but none is male determining, and sex is determined by the ratio of X chromosomes to autosomes. Dosage compensation is targeted at the single X in males and results in it being transcribed at about a 2-fold higher level than either X in the female. To my mind, this method of dosage compensation is the simplest, because it involves only one chromosome, the male X chromosome. And the amount of transcripts from the targeted chromosome is increased so that its output is equal to that of the two X chromosomes; therefore, two sets of X-linked genes are expressed in both sexes comparable to the two sets of genes expressed from all the other chromosomes. Hence, the output from genes on the X chromosomes and autosomes is balanced (Figure 10-1b).

The compensatory process requires the assessment of the number of X chromosomes in each cell and the translation of the information either to initiate dosage compensation on the single X in males, or to prevent it from happening in XX females. It begins early in the embryonic development of flies when an autosomal gene called *sex lethal* (*Sxl*) is turned on—in response to the presence of two X chromosomes in the female.[2] *Sxl* is one of several on and off switches that control whether or not dosage compensation takes place. In males, *Sxl* is always in the off position, and therefore its expression is female specific. When *Sxl* is transcribed, it blocks the synthesis of a protein that is essential for dosage compensation in males. This male-specific *MSL2* (*male sex lethal-2*) gene encodes the most important protein in a complex of at least five proteins, together called the male sex lethal (MSL) complex[3] or, alternatively, the dosage compensation complex (DCC). In female flies, the DCC does not form because of absence of MSL2. In males, the MSL complex binds to several dozen positions along the X chromosome (entry sites), then spreads to coat nearly the entire chromosome, and ultimately increases its level of transcription. You may wonder how binding of the protein complex to the chromosome increases its transcription. The answer is that a component of the MSL complex is an acetylase that can modify histone proteins. It seems that acetylation of the histones throughout the male X chromosome is the most essential step in *up*-regulating transcription because it "loosens" the chromatin structure, giving the transcriptional machinery greater access to the gene. The

2. The molecular mechanisms for sensing two X chromosomes seems to depend on greater expression of several X-linked genes in females, in an interplay between relative number of RNA or protein molecules encoded by the X and autosomes.

3. The four other MSL proteins are transcribed, albeit at low levels, in females, so MSL2 is the only male-specific protein in the complex. It is thought to provide X specificity to the MSL complex.

result is a near-doubling of DNA Polymerase II activity at the promoters of male X-linked genes. Also included in the complex are the two redundant noncoding RNAs, roX1 and roX2 (encoded by the X chromosome), which together associate with the genes (not between genes) throughout the length of the male X chromosome and lure the MSL complex to wherever they are[4]—no matter where they are. The MSL complex is virtually a chromatin-remodeling machine [33, 40]. What is not yet understood is how the fine-tuning is accomplished such that the level of up-regulation is precisely 2-fold.

Dosage Compensation in Roundworms

The small roundworm *Caenorhabditis elegans* has long been a favorite model organism for investigating embryonic development because its development takes place in only 16 hours in a petri dish and is visible because the skin of these developing worms is transparent. The sex of *C. elegans* is determined by the number of X chromosomes, but in this case the XX individual is not female but a *hermaphrodite* (having both ovaries and testes) that reproduces either by fertilizing itself or by cross-fertilization with the male. The male roundworm has an X0 karyotype; a homologue for the X was entirely lost during evolution. In these nematodes, X dosage compensation is carried out in the XX hermaphrodite by reducing the transcriptional level of each of her X chromosomes by half. Therefore, the combined output of the two X chromosomes in the hermaphrodite is equal to that in the X0 male. Because hermaphrodites modify both of their X chromosomes, there is no need to distinguish one X from the other.

Very early in development of the XX worm, the presence of two X chromosomes is sensed or "counted" by a subset of X-linked genes called X signal elements; the target of these signal molecules is the *xol-1* gene, which is the worm's master sex-determining gene—the one that initiates male development. The way that the *xol-1* protein initiates male development in normal males is by turning off the activities of genes that control the hermaphrodite program of development. In the case of the XX hermaphrodites, these X signal elements prevent male development by turning off the transcription of the male-determining *xol-1*. With *xol-1* repressed, the worm develops as a hermaphrodite. The developmental program for hermaphrodites includes the activation of dosage compensation—so repression of the *xol-1* gene activates the process of dosage compensation.[5] Therefore, *xol-1* is ultimately responsible not only for sex differentiation of the X0 male but

4. A unique aspect of dosage compensation in flies is the presence of multiple entry sites for the MSL complex along the male X chromosome that serve as initiation sites for spreading. Therefore, the spread of transcriptional silence is segmental rather than contiguous as it is on mammalian X chromosomes. Worms also have multiple recognition sites for spreading, which may preclude the need for a non-coding Xist-like RNA.

5. If *xol-1* is not turned on in X0 (male) embryos, X-linked genes are underexpressed, whereas inappropriate inactivation of *xol-1* in XX embryos causes lethality from overexpression of X-linked genes.

also for down-regulating the expression of X chromosome genes in the XX hermaphrodite [34].

As in flies, dosage compensation in worms is mediated by a specialized protein complex (here, it is also called the dosage compensation complex orDCC). Some components of this complex are also involved in condensation of chromosomes to aid their segregation during cell division). This complex assembles on both X chromosomes of hermaphrodites to repress their transcription by half. The mechanism by which the DCC down-regulates transcription remains unclear but it is mediated in part by inducing chromatin modifications[6] that compact the targeted chromosomes. The fact that proteins used for chromosome compaction during cell division have been recruited for the task of regulating X-chromosome-wide gene expression illustrates how evolution uses materials already on hand to accomplish novel functions. Experimental manipulation in worms has revealed multiple recognition elements along the X chromosomes that attract the DCC so that it can modify the chromatin of both X chromosomes. The multiple recognition sites direct the spreading of the inactivating signals all along each X chromosome *in cis*.

Dosage Compensation in Birds

There is relatively less information about dosage compensation in birds, but I have included them here because they are excellent examples of the extremes of variation in such basic processes as sex differentiation and dosage compensation. Birds are very different from mammals, flies, and worms. Their sex chromosomes are not called X and Y but Z and W. And it is the male who has two of the same sex chromosomes, a homologous pair of Z chromosomes, and therefore is the homogametic sex. Females are the ones with two nonhomologous sex chromosomes, Z and W, and they are the heterogametic sex. Studies of chromosome behavior in birds is also complicated by the fact that, in addition to their large chromosomes, they have many mini chromosomes, and their genomes are less understood than those of worms, flies, and mammals. Therefore, it is not surprising that the evidence for dosage compensation is limited and controversial. Large scale studies of gene expression in avian tissues suggest that a significant portion of genes on the short arm of the Z chromosome show robust dosage compensation not seen elsewhere on the chromosome; in such genes, the levels of expression are the same for males and females. Because males have two Z chromosomes and females only one, equal expression suggests that some Z-linked genes are compensated. How this is accomplished is not clear. Such partial dosage compensation could result from piecemeal up-regulation of Z-linked genes in females. In any case, because transcripts come from both Z chromosomes in males [41], it is unlikely that their dosage compensation involves chromosome inactivation. Rather, it may be a

6. For example, the DCC regulates the methylation state of lysine 20 of histone H4 leading to higher levels on both X chromosomes than on autosomes [35].

variation of the dosage compensation found in flies. Indirect evidence suggests that the Z chromosome in the female may be overexpressed like the X in male flies [42]. Or, birds may have another yet unknown variation on the theme of sex dosage compensation.

3.5. MECHANISMS OF DOSAGE COMPENSATION IN MAMMALS

The most primitive mammals, the monotremes, which live in Australia, have a curious mixture of features [43]. Although they resemble reptiles and birds in skeletal features and they lay eggs, they are clearly mammals: They have fur, mammary glands, and suckle their young. Recent DNA analysis indicates that monotremes diverged from therians about 166 mya, before the split into marsupials and eutherians. Based on the study of 10 X-linked genes in the duck-billed platypus, it seems that some but not all are expressed in equal amounts in males and females—in some cases only a single allele is expressed [44]—but how this is achieved is still unknown. Because the platypus has multiple Xs with gene content unrelated to that of the human X, and because the homologous X chromosomes do not differ epigenetically, if there is sex dosage compensation in monotremes, the process is likely to differ from the chromosome-wide inactivation in therians [45].

Susumu Ohno was right to assume that placental mammals would share their mechanism of X dosage compensation. Clearly, the evidence indicates that all of the placental mammals and also the pouched marsupials use X inactivation as their means of sex dosage compensation. In fact, as far as we know, X inactivation is unique to placental and pouched mammals.

X inactivation serves to equalize the output of X genes in males and females by ensuring that only a single X functions in both sexes. There is no need for compensation in XY male cells with their single X, but there is a need to silence the additional X in XX female cells. In the case of cells with more than two X chromosomes, all X chromosomes but one are silenced (figure 3-3 shows the three inactive X chromosomes in an individual with four X chromosomes). Thus, the targets of dosage compensation in both male and female mammals are all the X chromosomes in excess of one. Because females with more than one active X do not survive, X inactivation is an essential part of female sex differentiation. Although the details may differ, all placental mammals accomplish dosage compensation using the same basic molecular mechanisms. The method of silencing X chromosomes is to globally modify their chromatin so that genes on most of the chromosome become transcriptionally inert.

The inactive X chromosome in mammalian females is often referred to as the *heterochromatic X*; this term initially was used to reflect its unique staining properties in mitotic chromosomes that had been fixed on slides for microscopic examination. The unique staining was due to the condensation of the chromatin. Now, the word *heterochromatin* is used to describe any large block of repressed chromatin that remains condensed throughout most of the cell cycle. In contrast to

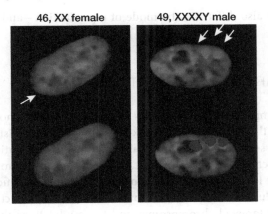

Figure 3-3. Barr bodies in interphase nuclei from a normal human female (left) and from a 4XY male (right) with one and three inactive X chromosomes, respectively. Top, DAPI stain; bottom, *XIST* RNA (red). Arrows show the position of the Barr body in DAPI-stained cells, which is difficult to visualize. Note that the Barr body is almost completely covered by *XIST* RNA, the silencing noncoding RNA in cells of eutherian mammals. [See color plate.]

the rest of the chromatin in the genome (called euchromatin, or true chromatin), heterochromatin is characterized by its ability to inhibit transcriptional activity in its vicinity. Not only does it block transcription, but it also maintains the silence of genes embedded within it, even those that accidentally (by translocation and rearrangement of chromosomal segments) come within its sphere of influence. Characteristically, the chromatin making up mammalian heterochromatin has few acetylated histones, and the regulatory regions of the genes therein are often methylated. The repressed chromatin of the inactive X is *underacetylated* in contrast to the *hyperacetylated* state of the up-regulated X chromosome in male flies.

The photomicrographs of the nuclei of human interphase cells in figure 3-3 show that heterochromatin of the inactive X can be visualized microscopically as a *Barr body*, or *sex chromatin body* during cell division because it is compacted, at a time when the euchromatin of all the other chromosomes is stretched out, in the process of being transcribed. In addition to the inactive X chromosome, the regions around the centromere of all chromosomes and other nontranscribed regions of a chromosome are made up of large blocks of heterochromatin. As in flies and roundworms, dosage compensation in eutherian mammals is also mediated by a protein complex that binds to the X chromosome to initiate its inactivation. As in flies, this protein complex includes a noncoding RNA (called *Xist*, for inactive X-specific transcript), which attracts the protein complex to the chromosome. The X chromosomes that remain functional in both sexes lack this RNA because its transcription was repressed very early in embryonic development.

The differences in dosage compensation among worms, flies, and mammals no doubt originate in the vast differences in their evolutionary biology as well as in their embryonic development. For example, these organisms differ in the way that sex is determined—the Y chromosome is the major sex determinant only in mammals. They also differ—in the mode of reproduction—and only mammals have placentas.

3.6. SUMMARY AND SPECULATIONS

The need to compensate for differences in dosage of X chromosomal genes in organisms with the XX/XY or XX/X sex-determining mechanism is a universal problem, but we see that the solution is far from universal. Evolution has come up with unique mechanisms to do the job. Although there are common features— regulation at the level of transcription, mediated through modifications of chromatin—each solution has its own innovative features that include differences in the nature of targeted chromosomes and the modulations that are induced. Because evolution has produced so much variation among diverse species of animals, we should not be surprised to see variations *within* related species even if they use the same basic mechanism. It is the study of many different species that tells us most about the essential elements and distinguishes the themes from the variations.

The Discovery of
X Chromosome Inactivation

In 1961 Mary Lyon, a geneticist working on the genetic hazards of radiation at the Medical Research Council Radiobiology Unit in Harwell, England (figure 4-1), proposed a truly innovative hypothesis to explain some unexpected results in her analysis of mutations affecting the coat color of female mice. In a one-page letter published in the journal *Nature*, she suggested that only one of the two X chromosomes of females functioned in each cell, and the other became inactive early in embryogenesis [46]. Although her paper came as a tremendous surprise to the scientific community, her hypothesis did not arise *de novo*. The time was ripe for such a proposal, as there had been several seminal observations made by other geneticists and cell biologists that should have led one to think of this possibility. In fact, Liane Russell, an American mouse geneticist, also suggested that only one X was active in a paper published in *Science* at about the same time [47]. Based on her own observations of mice with abnormal sex chromosomes, Russell had come to the same conclusion as Lyon. However, Russell's concept was largely buried in her nine-page paper reporting the functions and aberrant behavior of sex chromosomes.[1] Ernest Beutler, a colleague of Ohno, made a similar proposal to explain his observations of heterozygotes for *G6PD* deficiency consistent with mixtures of normal and *G6PD*-deficient red cells [48]. Clearly, it was Lyon's elegant and unambiguous statement of her hypothesis that made it so memorable and compelling.

According to Lyon's own account [49], "The first inkling that the X-chromosome might behave strangely came with the discovery of the first mouse X-linked gene in 1953." This mutation was discovered because it resulted in the death of males and an unusual pattern of white spotting in the coat of females carrying one copy of the mutant gene (*heterozygotes*). In most heterozygous mutations affecting pigment, the coat color would be diluted or the same as the normal pigmentation. Only when the heterozygous genes were on the X chromosome was there

---

1. Lyon made us understand what Russell meant by "Genic balance in mammals requires the action of one X in a manner which precludes realization of its heterochromatic potentialities; only any additional X's present assume the properties characteristic of heterochromatin" [47, p. 1798].

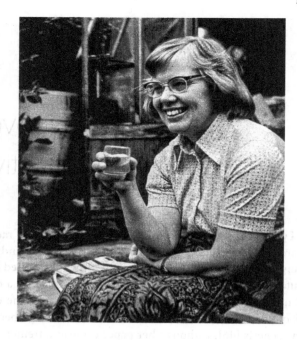

Figure 4-1. Dr. Mary Lyon. From [427], *Genetical Research*, p. 82, with permission.

a mixture of patches of both normal and abnormal pigment, resembling mosaic tiles. Such unusual variegation of skin pigment was confirmed in female mice carrying other X-linked genes affecting coat color. However, Lyon did not fully appreciate these observations until becoming aware of other relevant findings.

One influential finding was the serendipitous discovery of *sex chromatin*. Four years earlier, Murray Barr and Evart Bertram [50] noticed the presence in cat nerve cells of a dotlike structure, which they called a "nucleolar satellite" because it was always adjacent to the nucleus of the cell. This "body," which stained like chromatin, was seen in female cats but not in males. They went on to show that this "sex chromatin body," or "Barr body," as it was later called, was a general feature of female cells of many species, including humans (see figure 3-3). (I remember when Bertram, by then a teaching assistant in my medical school anatomy class, showed me the sex chromatin in a microscopic specimen). The availability of a marker that could distinguish males from females—even in tissue from the lining of the cheek (buccal smear)—was immediately applied to the study of individuals with abnormal sexual development. The ability to examine chromosomes directly would not be possible until 1956, so sex chromatin provided a screening test for sexual abnormalities not possible previously. By 1954, the test had shown that infertile females with the syndrome of gonadal agenesis and short stature described by Henry Turner (Turner syndrome) had no sex chromatin body (see Turner syndrome in *Appendix B* and figure 4-2). Also surprising, the infertile males with the syndrome described by Harry Klinefelter (Klinefelter syndrome) did have a sex chromatin body. When chromosome analysis became possible, the number of X chromosomes present in a cell corresponded exactly to one more than the number of Barr bodies in that cell. That is, individuals with two X chromosomes (normal females, and males with Klinefelter syndrome, 47,XXY) had a single Barr body, those with three X chromosomes had two Barr bodies, and males with one X chromosome had none.

Yet, the significance of the sex chromatin body was not appreciated until later, because many believed it was a structure formed by the crossing of the two X chromosomes in the cell. The true origin of the Barr body became apparent in 1959 when Susumu Ohno reported that it was derived from a single X chromosome [51]. He showed that there was a single condensed chromosome in the nucleus of liver cells from female rats (figure 4-3) and in a subsequent paper he extended his observations to mice [52]. Like sex chromatin, this intensely stained chromosome was not seen in male cells. Ohno suggested that it was an X chromosome.

What is surprising is that the single heterochromatic X was not interpreted as an inactive X chromosome until Lyon and Russell proposed it was.[2] According

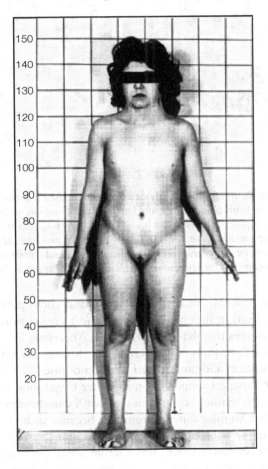

Figure 4-2. Girl with 45,X Turner syndrome.

2. Ohno once told me that he had indeed discussed the likelihood of a single active X in his paper reporting the single heterochromatic chromosome, but that he had to eliminate it from the discussion because a reviewer thought it not relevant enough.

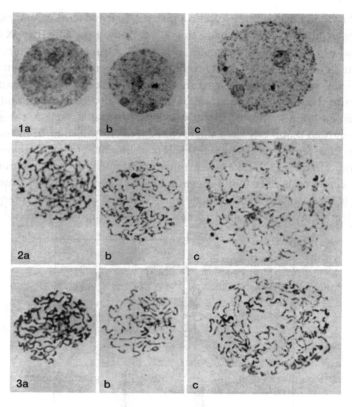

Figure 4-3. The sex chromatin (Barr body) is a single condensed X chromosome. Shown are interphase (1a–c), early prophase (2a–c), and late prophase (3a–c) in rat liver cells: male cells in column a, female diploid cells in column b, and female tetraploid cells in column c. Note that in interphase, sex chromatin is seen only in female nuclei. At prophase, all the chromosomes are threadlike, except for one condensed chromosome in diploid female cells (2b, c) and two condensed chromosomes in the tetraploid cells (3b, c). From Ohno et al. [51].

to Lyon, this was probably because, until then, ideas about genetics were dominated by observations in flies, where it is not the Y chromosome but the number of X chromosomes that determines sex [49]. Therefore, individuals are male even if they lack a Y chromosome (referred to as X0) but are female if they have two X chromosomes in addition to their Y chromosome (XXY) (see section 3.4, "Mechanisms of Dosage Compensation in Other Organisms"). The association between the sex chromatin body and an inactive X chromosome had to wait for the realization that X0 mice differed from flies because such mice were females, not males, and fertile females to boot. Welshons and Russell's 1959 paper [53] reporting that the X0 mouse (39,X) was a fertile female provided the final information necessary for formulating the X inactivation hypothesis; it meant that a single X chromosome might be enough—and that the other X chromosome in female cells could be inactive. Shortly thereafter, the human X0 female (45,X) was identified by *karyotyping* girls with Turner syndrome [54], and the XXY karyotype (47,XXY) was found in males with Klinefelter syndrome [55].

4.1. THE LYON HYPOTHESIS

In her original 1961 statement of the hypothesis in *Nature* [46], Mary Lyon proposed that female mice needed only one working X chromosome and that the inactive one would take on the appearance of a condensed chromosome, like the one observed by Ohno et al. [51] (figure 4-3). Further, she suggested that because either parental chromosome could be inactive, females would be mosaics—having two types of cells each with a different working X. In heterozygous female mice that have only one functional X-linked coat color gene because their other copy is defective, this would result in visible patches, some mutant and others with normal color (figure 4-4). Lyon next tried to explain why the patches that she observed were large instead of the salt-and-pepper kind of intermingling of mutant and normal cells one might have expected. She recognized that the patches could be clones of cells and that they reflect the fact that the silent state was heritable from one cell to another. She reasoned that if the inactivation event occurred early enough in development—perhaps at the *gastrula* stage when Barr bodies are first observed—and if the inactive state was clonally inherited, and if

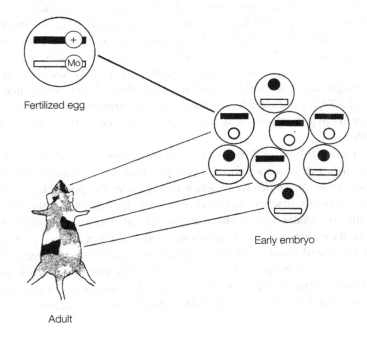

Figure 4-4. Lyon's own diagram of her hypothesis. This figure explains the origin of the pattern of white spotting in the coat of a mouse heterozygous for a mutation in the *mottled* gene. The inactive X is indicated by a circle, the active X by a rod. The mutant X is white, the wild-type X is black. White and black patches are due to clonal growth after random inactivation; in black patches the wild-type (+) allele is expressed, and in white patches the mutant (Mo) allele is expressed. Gray patches are contributed by autosomal coat color genes. Reprinted from *Genetical Research* [428], with permission.

cell mixing was restricted, then the mosaic patches would be large. In any case, the existence of patches implied that X inactivation was inherited; this meant that once inactivated, an X chromosome was committed to inactivity and that it would be maintained inactive in all the cells derived from the original one.

Although the possibility that X inactivation occurred in other mammals was mentioned in Lyon's 1961 *Nature* paper, the hypothesis was expanded to humans and other mammals in her second paper published the next year in the *American Journal of Human Genetics* [56]. In this remarkable paper, she discusses the various expectations predicated upon the hypothesis. Because of the mottled coat color patterns she had observed in heterozygous females carrying a mutant coat color gene, she predicted that all sex-linked color genes of the mouse should show the same kind of mottling effect—and this seems to be the case. Further, she predicted that because mottling requires mosaic expression from *two* X chromosomes, it should occur in XXY males but not in X0 females.[3] Because X-linked ocular albinism was the only human sex-linked pigment gene known at that time, she surveyed the literature for effects of known X-linked mutations in heterozygous females. In keeping with her predictions, she found that some females partially manifested these mutations. This was surprising because women heterozygous for recessive autosomal mutations usually do not manifest diseases.[4] Lyon also provided a valid explanation for the somatic abnormalities (i.e., short stature and webbing of the neck) in X0 Turner females; she predicted, "The X chromosome of man [the human X chromosome] has a short pairing segment, that is not normally inactivated, and that it is duplication or deficiency of this region which gives rise to the abnormal phenotypes observed" [56, p. 144] Also, she suggested that the single active X would explain some puzzling observations, such as the viability of XXXXY individuals with three extra X chromosomes.[5] She concluded that while her hypothesis stood up so far against these predictions, more evidence was needed.

The evidence in Lyons's 1962 paper convinced most of us that only a single X-linked allele was expressed in each cell. However, the variegated patterns and mosaicism were not sufficient evidence to eliminate the possibility that genes were independently inactive on one chromosome or the other. Therefore, while the hypothesis explained many observations, it needed to be experimentally confirmed. To show that an *entire* X chromosome was inactive, and not parts of both of them, Lyon bred female mice whose X chromosomes were both marked, each by a different coat color gene. In this way, she could determine if two genes on different copies of the X chromosome could ever be inactive in the same cell. The results indicated that only one of them in each cell could be inactive.

---

3. Calico cats are another example of mutants for X-linked skin pigment genes. Male calico cats are always XXY.

4. For autosomal recessive mutations, even if one allele is completely deficient, the activity contributed by the normal allele is usually sufficient for normal function.

5. Most individuals with more than two copies of a chromosome do not survive.

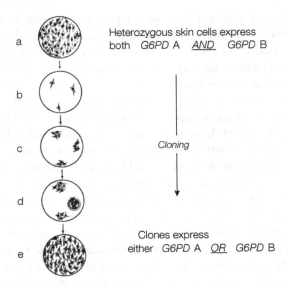

a. Heterozygous skin cells express
both G6PD A *AND* G6PD B

b.

Cloning

c.

d.

e. Clones express
either G6PD A *OR* G6PD B

Figure 4-5. Testing the Lyon hypothesis using clones derived from single cells: the Davidson, Nitowski, and Childs experiment [57]. *a.* Dish containing uncloned skin cells heterozygous for *G6PD*, expressing both A and B enzymes. *b.* Dish containing single cells, plated from dilute cell suspensions from the dish in *a.* *c.* Proliferating clones. *d.* When large enough, clones are removed with cloning cylinder and replated. *e.* Individual clonal culture— all cells therein derived from the one originally plated—ready for analysis. The clonal cultures express only one of the two enzymes. See section 5.3, and figure 5-6.

It was Ronald Davidson, Harold Nitowsky, and Barton Childs [57] who provided the most compelling test of the hypothesis using cells from human females carrying markers that distinguished one of their X chromosomes from the other (figure 4-5). These cells, derived from skin, were heterozygous for two different alleles of the X-linked gene encoding the enzyme glucose 6–phosphate dehydrogenase (*G6PD*). One X chromosome in each cell carried the *G6PD A* allele; the other X chromosome had the homologous *G6PD B* allele. Analysis of colonies originating from single cells showed that each *clone* (made up of at least 2,000 cells derived from the original one) expressed only one of the two alleles present in the parent cell. This showed beyond any doubt that only one X chromosome was functioning in each cell. It also showed that X inactivation, once it occurred, was irreversible in these skin cells and that the silence of the inactive X was clonally transmitted from one cell to all its daughter cells.

4.2. GENERAL SCHEME OF MAMMALIAN DOSAGE COMPENSATION

In the decades since Mary Lyon first proposed that mammalian females undergo X inactivation, we have learned a good deal about the characteristics of this

developmental event. Figure 4-6 shows the process of X inactivation schemati-
cally. Clearly, both X chromosomes function at least to some degree during the
early cleavage divisions of the zygote (discussed in chapter 6). However, one of
them subsequently differentiates in such a way that it no longer can be transcribed:
The chromosome becomes heterochromatic, which effectively silences most of its
genes. This event, which is called *cis* inactivation for reasons discussed further
below, is initiated in the mouse embryo at about the time of implantation—during the blastocyst stage of development and in human embryos by gastrulation.
Inactivation is associated with a switch in the time that the chromosome replicates
its DNA in anticipation of cell division, and the inactive X becomes the last chromosome to replicate itself. A late-replicating X chromosome is one of the earliest
signs that inactivation has occurred; relatively condensed during interphase, this
chromosome is visible cytologically as the Barr body or sex chromatin mass in the
nucleus of the cell (see figure 3-3). Inactivation does not require differences in the
parental origin of the chromosomes or in their gene content. In most mammals,
the choice of which X chromosome will be active (a step that precedes the silencing step) is random regarding parental origin of the chromosome (figure 4-6).
Therefore, the X chromosome inherited from the father has the same possibility
of being turned off as the X inherited from the mother. Silencing is mediated by
the synthesis of a special type of noncoding RNA molecule from a locus on the
X chromosome. These molecules spread along the chromosome, modifying the

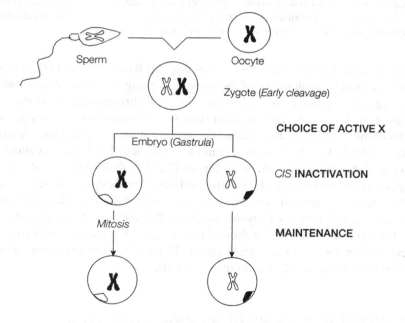

Figure 4-6. Simple scheme of X inactivation in female cells. The maternally inherited X
is black; the paternally inherited X is white. The inactive X is shown as a Barr body close
to the nuclear membrane. The first step is choice of active X, followed by *cis* inactivation of
the other. A cell transmits the same inactive X to all its progeny. Adapted from figure 1 of
Migeon [420].

underlying chromosome and thereby inducing transcriptional silence (see chapters 6 and 7). Once silenced, the inactive X usually remains mute in all progeny cells, and therefore the inactivation pattern is clonally inherited. X inactivation also occurs in cells that are destined to be ovarian germ cells. However, reactivation of the silent X is programmed to occur in oocytes during their maturation. These are the only cells in which there is a program to reverse X inactivation. In all the other cells (referred to as somatic cells), X inactivation is usually irreversible and faithfully transmitted (see chapters 6 and 7).

The program responsible for X inactivation occurs only during embryonic development. Adding X chromosomes (by hybridization and selection) past the stage when inactivation is initiated has no effect [58; B. R. Migeon, unpublished observations]. Removing the X-linked locus responsible for the silencing RNA after the critical time in development does not affect the immediate silence of the inactive X [59], but may have some long term effects (see section 6.4, "The Master Control Region: XIC and *Xist*").

The rules of inactivation are as follows: There is a single X in diploid cells of both sexes; all the others are inactivated—no matter the number of X chromosomes in the cell. Either X, the one inherited from mother or the one from father, can be functional or mute. There are some interesting exceptions: In marsupials and in some nonhuman placental tissues, the paternally inherited X is always nonoperative (discussed in chapter 9).

The X inactivation hypothesis was provocative and stimulated a large number of studies—at first to test its validity, and later to obtain insights into the molecular basis for silencing an entire chromosome. These studies have provided a wealth of observations about the process and about the genetic consequences of having a single active X. These findings not only validate Lyon's original conclusions and predictions but also stimulate new hypotheses about regulation of genes on the X chromosome and throughout our genome.

4.3. SUMMARY AND SPECULATIONS

The most remarkable thing about X inactivation is that the two homologous X chromosomes in women have different activity states, even though they have essentially the same DNA content and are contained within the same nucleus. Having independently carried out their individual differentiation, they differ remarkably from one another. The fact that an X chromosome can be inactive in one cell but active in another means that it is not the genes themselves but factors that regulate the genes—so-called *epigenetic* factors—that are responsible for the silent X. In fact, X inactivation studies have provided the first evidence of the major role played by epigenetic factors in gene regulation, and made us aware of their role throughout our genome, in cell differentiation, cancer, and genetic diseases (see chapter 12). Most likely, further exploration of X inactivation will continue to provide knowledge about the function and malfunction of our cells.

Experimental Models
for X Inactivation Studies

You may wonder how one learns about X inactivation, because it occurs very early in development when the embryo is implanting itself into its niche in the uterus. Direct observations of the embryo at this time are usually precluded simply because of inaccessibility. Even the mouse embryo is burrowed into the uterus—out of sight during the critical window of development when X inactivation occurs. The experimental models that have provided alternatives to direct observation include genetic mutations that interfere with dosage compensation, cultured cells and clones that carry these mutations, mouse–human cell hybrids, embryonic stem cells, and transgenic mice. What I have learned is that progress in scientific discovery depends to a large extent on developments in technology that enable us to ask the important questions.

5.1. SPONTANEOUS HUMAN MUTATIONS THAT INTERFERE WITH INACTIVATION

The best way to get around problems of inaccessibility is to find individuals who cannot carry out the process of interest because of mutations in essential genes. Mutations affecting all steps in the developmental pathway may spontaneously occur—or be induced—thereby providing insights into the functions perturbed by that alteration. Unfortunately, in the case of X inactivation, most mutations that interfere with this essential process are likely to be lethal and therefore not available for study. To our knowledge, there are no normal mammalian females with two working sets of X-linked genes in the same *somatic* cell[1]; presumably, having two active X chromosomes—referred to as *functional X disomy*—is incompatible with survival during gestation. In fact, spontaneous mutations that interfere with X inactivation have not been identified in any species except ours, probably because only humans bring their problems to the attention of physicians. Their need for medical attention has revealed the existence of a few females who survived gestation despite having mutations that interfered with

1. Both X chromosomes are expressed in oogonia.

X inactivation; they had severe clinical abnormalities, which include mental retardation and a constellation of other congenital malformations (discussed in in section 11.5). Such clinically abnormal females have more than one active X because one of their X chromosomes lacks essential DNA sequences needed for inactivation. The deleted segments removed not only the X inactivation center (XIC), the region of the X needed for inactivation (see section 6.4), but also a large amount of the rest of the X chromosome. Chromosomes that lack the XIC are usually very small. If less of the chromosome were deleted, then a greater number of genes would be expressed from both X chromosomes, hence increasing the functional disomy and decreasing the ability to survive in utero. In the case of tiny X chromosomes, the extensive deletions usually involve both the short arm and the long arm of the X chromosome, and this often leads to the formation of rings (figure 5-1; see also figure 11-1). Tiny ring X chromosomes like these have been used to identify the essential regions of the human X chromosome needed for inactivation, by determining which of them can carry out inactivation and which cannot. Even though the chromosomes that fail to inactivate are extremely small, they are responsible for very abnormal phenotypes—evidence that even a small number of genes with two working copies is extremely detrimental (figure 5-2). The induced mutations that interfere with inactivation in mice are discussed below (see section 5.5).

Other Chromosome Studies

Further insights into these essential elements come from other structural abnormalities of the X chromosome. Rearrangements—which physically disrupt the

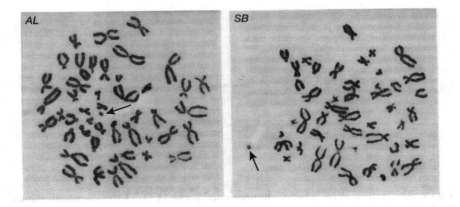

Figure 5-1. Tiny ring X chromosomes associated with severe phenotypes: metaphase spreads from two human females with mental retardation and congenital malformations due to their 46, X ring X karyotypes. Arrows point to the dotlike tiny ring X chromosomes that cannot inactivate. Adapted from figure 1 of Migeon et al. [120].

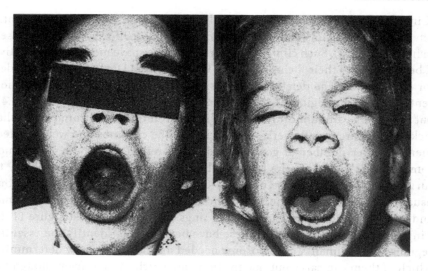

Figure 5-2. The severe Turner phenotype. Two unrelated girls with 46,X ring X chromosomes. Note the widely spaced eyes, prominent nostrils, large down-turned mouth, and low-set ears. From figure 1 of Kushnick et al. [422], with permission.

linear order of genes on a chromosome and attach part of the X to an autosomal chromosome—helped to identify the XIC region of the X chromosome critical for inactivation; the only part of the translocation chromosome that can be inactivated is the one with the DNA sequences needed for inactivation (figure 5-3; discussed in section 6.4, "The Master Control Region").

The replication status of an X chromosome can be visualized in *metaphase spreads* (cytological preparations of metaphase chromosome); the late-replicating

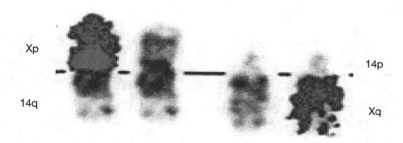

Figure 5-3. Translocation between chromosomes X and 14 (X/14 translocation), shown by "painting" the X chromosome. The break in both chromosomes occurred near the centromere. Shown are the two translocation chromosomes either banded with Giemsa or painted with X chromosome unique DNA (red). The positions of short (p) and long (q) arms of both X and 14 are indicated. Adapted from figure 1D of Morrison and Jeppesen [423], with permission. [See color plate.]

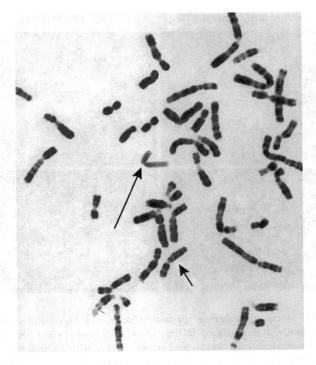

Figure 5-4. Late-replicating X chromosome. BrdU-induced R-banded metaphase from a human female. Inactive X chromosome (long arrow) replicates out of synchrony with the active X (short arrow) and the autosomes. Photomicrograph courtesy of Gail Stetten.

X chromosome is identified by using the thymidine analog BrdU to label the chromosome as it replicates, and the fluorescent dye acridine orange to detect the BrdU cytologically (figure 5-4).[2]

Fluorescent-labeled DNA probes that hybridize *in situ* with the DNA or RNA of the chromosome can be used to identify a chromosome in a metaphase spread by its DNA content and even its RNA expression (see figure 3-3). These procedures are referred to as FISH (fluorescence *in situ* hybridization). And by isolating specific individual chromosomes, one can prepare a hybridization probe consisting of DNA from all the unique genes on the chromosome and use it to identify the chromosome of interest by a method called "chromosome painting." Identifying the chromosome with a painting probe also permits us

2. Many recent studies of replication timing of individual genes are based on a simple FISH replication assay. The presence of double signals means the allele replicates early, whereas single signals indicate a late-replicating allele. Signals from the two chromosomes can be synchronous or asynchronous; that is, both alleles replicate early or late, or one replicates later than the other. However, the assay has been inconsistent with others, but only with regard to replication timing within the XIC. It has been suggested that the structure in this region may lead to lack of normal chromatid separation, so double signals would be missed [60].

Antibody to acetylated H4-K12   X & Y FISH Paints

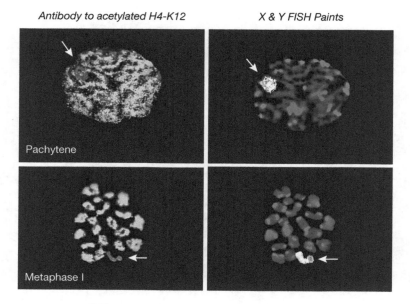

Figure 5-5. XY inactivation during spermatogenesis. The chromatin of the X and Y chromosomes (arrows) is repressed during spermatogenesis. Left: Chromosomes from mouse cells, at pachytene and metaphase I stages, labeled with an antibody to acetylated histone H4–K12 (green label indicates acetylation). Repressed chromosome regions are red (unlabeled). Right: Same cells labeled by X (pink) and Y (aqua) FISH chromosome paint to identify the sex chromosomes. Note: X and Y are underacetylated (red) from pachytene to round spermatid stage. Photomicrographs courtesy of Ahmad Khalil and Daniel Driscoll. [See color plate.]

to distinguish the component parts of translocation chromosomes, because the rearranged chromosome will be marked as a hybrid consisting of parts of two different chromosomes (figure 5-3). Finally, antibodies to the protein components of chromosomes can be fluorescently labeled and used as probes to study chromosome structure *in situ* (figure 5-5).

5.2. X-LINKED PROTEIN VARIANTS DISTINGUISH PARENTAL ORIGIN OF X CHROMOSOMES

In addition to the deleterious mutations that interfere with the ability to inactivate, other X-linked mutations serve as markers to distinguish active and inactive X chromosomes. Such mutations may encode defective proteins or merely variations of the normal ones. One such protein is the ubiquitous enzyme *G6PD* (see *Appendix A*, "Hemolytic Anemia [X-linked]"), an extraordinary probe for studies of X inactivation; the enzyme is dimeric with two subunits that associate as a pair of like or unlike subunits. Two relatively common (polymorphic) forms of this protein (*G6PD A* and *G6PD B*)[3] have normal activity but can be distinguished by their mobility on gels in an electric field. Heterozygosity for the *G6PD AB* variants provides the means to determine the number of active X chromosomes in a cell as well as the parental origin. Usually, heterozygous females express only one allele in each cell. However, if a cell has more than one functional X chromosome, then both *G6PD* alleles will be expressed. Biallelic expression can be detected from the presence of a heterodimer consisting of both A and B subunits of this dimeric enzyme. Such a heterodimer is seen in oocytes, which have two active X chromosomes (figure 5-6; see also figure 4-5). In contrast, the heterodimer is not seen in normal somatic cells; because of X inactivation the two subunits are synthesized in different cells, and so they never can form a hybrid dimer. Therefore, the absence of the heterodimer means that only one of the two alleles is being expressed in each cell. It is temping to speculate that if we had known about the dimeric structure of the *G6PD* enzyme before the Lyon hypothesis, then X inactivation might have been discovered much earlier because of the absence of the expected heterodimer. Even without knowledge that *G6PD* is a dimer, Davidson et al. [57] could deduce from cells heterozygous for the *G6PD AB* variants that only one variant or the other—and not both variants—was expressed.

5.3. CHARACTERIZING THE INACTIVE X IN HUMAN CELL CULTURES AND CLONES

Some features of the developmental program for X inactivation—such as maintenance of the inactive state and the cellular mosaicism—can be studied using fetal and adult cells in culture. In fact, most of our knowledge about the features of X inactivation in mammals has come from the studies of mammalian cells in culture. We can determine the effects of extra X chromosomes in both sexes by examining cells with varying numbers of X chromosomes (i.e., 47,XXY, 48,XXXX) and ploidy (triploids and tetraploids). Such studies have revealed that only one X is active in any diploid cell, irrespective of the number of X chromosomes present in that cell. Cultures of embryonic stem cells and mouse–human hybrid cells have been the major routes for exploring the molecular mechanisms responsible for dosage compensation (discussed below).

Cultivated skin cells were used to test the validity of the Lyon hypothesis because they can be cloned; that is, they can produce a sizable population of cells that are all progeny of the same cell. Until now, examination of the phenotype of individual cells has been difficult but can be done using cell clones consisting of many identical copies of the cell from which the clone was derived. Clones are obtained by isolating one cell from its neighbor; this is done by diluting suspensions of cultured cells and plating them at a low density (~10–20 cells per petri dish). When

3. *G6PD B* is the most common isozyme, with the *G6PD A* variant present in 12% of African American males. Another *G6PD A* variant common in African Americans leads to enzyme deficiency and causes hemolytic anemia.

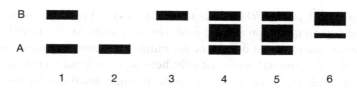

Figure 5-6. Diagram showing *G6PD* as a marker for the activity status of the X chromosome. Depicted is the expression of the enzyme in female cells heterozygous for the *G6PD A* and *B* enzymes in uncloned skin cells (1), cell clones expressing only *G6PD A* (2) or only *G6PD B* (3), oocytes expressing both variants as well as the *G6PD AB* heterodimer indicating that both alleles are being expressed in the same cell (4), triploid 69,XXY cell with two active X chromosomes (5), and a clone from human placenta with leaky X inactivation expressing a small amount of the AB heterodimer reflecting low level expression of the A enzyme encoded by the inactive X (6). Adapted from figure 1 of Migeon [424].

an individual cell has grown into a visible colony of approximately 10^6 cells, then the colony is enclosed within a cloning cylinder, detached by trypsin, and transferred to a small petri dish for further propagation (see figures 4-5 and 5-6).

Clonal cultures have been an especially useful experimental model, ever since Davidson et al. [57] first used them for this purpose. In this case the clones were derived from cells heterozygous for the *G6PD AB* alleles. Because all cells within a clone originate from a single cell—and because all clones expressed a single *G6PD* allele (and not the alleles from both X chromosomes)—Davidson and colleagues concluded that each clone has only a single active allele. This meant that each cell in the clone expressed the same allele, and therefore all cells in the clone had to have the same active X. This analysis of clones clearly showed that X inactivation occurs—and that once it occurs, it is faithfully transmitted. By showing that all the daughter cells inherit the same inactive X, they demonstrated the fidelity with which inactivation is maintained during mitosis in human cells.

The hypoxanthine phosphoribosyltransferase (HPRT) enzyme provides another sensitive probe for the study of X inactivation (*Appendix A*). In this case the variant protein is a mutant enzyme, associated with the syndrome first described by Lesch and Nyhan (*Appendix A*). Cultured cells with the normal enzyme or the deficient one can be distinguished at the cellular level, using an assay for uptake of radiolabeled (^{3}H) hypoxanthine, a substrate for the enzyme. Normal clones are labeled (figures 5-7 and 5-8a), whereas the mutant ones, which cannot incorporate the labeled substrate, are unlabeled. In addition, nutrient media are available that either favor or disfavor the growth of the HPRT-deficient cells (see figure 5-8b). Some mothers of Lesch Nyhan males are carriers and therefore heterozygous for the mutation; they have been shown to have cells of both types (figure 5-8a & b). The presence of mutant cells in females has been used as a test to identify carriers of the mutation [61].

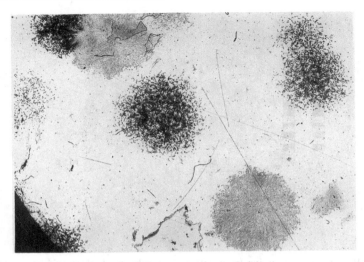

Figure 5-7. Lesch Nyhan heterozygote has both normal and mutant clones: Autoradiograph of skin fibroblast clones *in situ* from the mother of a Lesch Nyhan boy, showing the mutant (light) and normal (dark) clones. See figure 5-8a for explanation. From figure 1 of Migeon [329].

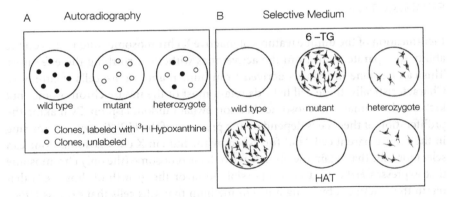

Figure 5-8. Diagrams showing identification of carriers of the Lesch Nyhan mutation, using autoradiography and selective media. *a.* Clones in petri dishes are labeled with ³H-hypoxanthine. After autoradiography, the clones consisting of normal cells, which incorporate the label, appear black (see figure 5-7), whereas the mutant clones are unlabeled (white). From figure 4 of Migeon [318]. *b.* Normal cells can grow in HAT medium [62] but not in medium containing 6-thioguanine (6-TG), an analog of hypoxanthine. Mutant cells cannot grow in HAT but grow well in 6-TG, because they do not incorporate this toxic analog. Both kinds of cells are present in the heterozygote. From figure 2 of Migeon [318].

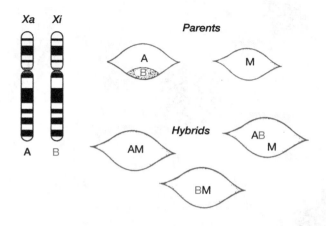

Figure 5-9. Separating inactive from active X in hybrids. A clone of human skin cells heterozygous for the AB variants of *G6PD* but expressing only the A enzyme (*G6PD B* on the inactive X) was fused with mouse cells, and hybrids were obtained. Because of the tendency to lose human chromosomes, hybrids contain only subsets of human chromosomes. All hybrids have the mouse active X chromosome (marked by the G6PD M enzyme). Some hybrids have *both* active (marked by the G6PDA enzyme) and inactive human X chromosomes (marked by the silent *G6PD B* allele). The rest have *either* active (AM) or inactive (BM) human X chromosomes. From figure 2 of Migeon et al. [220].

5.4. MOUSE–HUMAN HYBRIDS SEPARATE INACTIVE FROM ACTIVE X

Identification of the unique features of inactive X chromosomes often relies on the ability to separate them from the active ones without perturbing these features. This can be done in hybrids derived from human and mouse cells (figure 5-9). Characteristically, these cell hybrids retain most of the mouse chromosomes but kick out the human chromosomes in a somewhat random fashion. By making the proliferation of these cells depend on the presence of the *HPRT* enzyme—missing in the mouse parent cells[4] but furnished by the human X chromosome—one can select for cells that retain the human active X chromosome (the only chromosome that expresses *HPRT*).[5] It is also possible to favor the growth of those cells that retain the inactive X by using nutrient medium that kills cells that express *HPRT* (figure 5-8b).

4. One of the most useful technological advancements was the development of nutrient medium that could favor or disfavor mutations in somatic cells. Waclaw Szybalski was a pioneer in this technology. For example, he found that medium containing hypoxanthine (H) and thymidine (T) would allow cells to grow when the usual pathway to their synthesis was blocked by aminopterin (A), providing they had an intact *HPRT* gene, and so this HAT medium could be used to favor the growth of cells expressing *HPRT* [62].

5. The mouse cells used for hybridization have a mutation in their *HPRT* gene that makes it nonfunctional.

Hybrids having only the inactive X chromosome can be used to determine the activity status of genes on the inactive X. For example, they show that most genes on the X chromosome are subject to inactivation, but some of them seem to be partially expressed [63] (see section 7.3, "Escape from Inactivation"). Cell hybrids also have been used to identify the key gene in the inactivation process because it is expressed, paradoxically, only from the inactive X [64]. And hybrids provide the means to look for cells that can reverse the inactivation process [65]. Sometimes the foreign milieu of the mouse cell can destabilize the cellular mechanisms that maintain the silence of human X-linked genes, including DNA methylation and histone modification. Destabilization of this kind can reveal the means by which silence is locked in.

Hybrid cells are no longer needed, as they are other ways to look at expression from single chromosomes. RNA FISH provides an ideal means to look at expression of a few gene products in the cell, the number limited by the number of available fluorochromes (see figure 10-6).

One can now use large-scale expression assays using microarrays to quantitate the expression of many X-linked genes. In this way we can identify genes which escape X inactivation or are expressed at greater or lesser levels in males than females or from autosomes than X chromosomes. In addition, RNA transcripts obtained from tissues and sometimes even single cells can be quantified by sequencing them. A combination of such methods has been used to show an upregulation of X–linked genes so that they equal the output of a pair of autosomal genes. (See section 11.1, "Coping with a Monosomy X"). It is also now feasible to assay the gene products from single isolated cells.

5.5. MOUSE EMBRYONIC STEM CELLS FOR MANIPULATING THE EARLY STEPS IN X INACTIVATION

Recent studies show that the preimplantation human embryo has not yet undergone X inactivation up to the seven-day blastocyst [66]. Studies of the earliest postimplantation embryos obtainable from miscarriages show that X inactivation has already occurred [67] (figure 10-6). The inaccessibility of human embryonic specimens between gastrulation and 5–6 weeks postconception leave the window when X inactivation takes place out of view. In mice, however, it is possible to study that window into development using cultures of mouse embryonic stem cells. Gail Martin and her colleagues [68] showed that *totipotent* mouse cells (cells that give rise to all the cell types in the embryo) could be used as a model for X inactivation. They discovered a way to induce the process of X inactivation in embryonic carcinoma (EC) cells in petri dishes. While inducing these cells to differentiate into many cell types, these investigators noted that X inactivation occurred during the differentiation process. What they actually saw was that before differentiation females had greater amounts of X-linked proteins than males, but that the sex difference disappeared upon induction of differentiation. The availability of mouse embryonic stem (ES) cells that can recapitulate the events occurring during X inactivation has provided a similar experimental model but one that can be used to manipulate the process. Inactivation is induced by modifying the *in vitro*

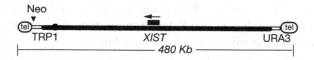

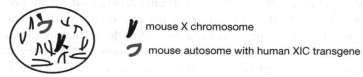

Figure 5-10. Diagram showing functional assay for human XIC activity. A yeast chromosome containing 480 kb of the XIC region on the human X chromosome is inserted as a transgene into an autosome in male mouse ES cells. If the transgene contains a DNA sequence that induces X inactivation, the sequence is considered to have XIC activity. The transgene shown is capable of inducing X inactivation in male mice [70].

culture conditions in which the cells are maintained.[6] Further, these ES cells can be manipulated—so as to interfere with function of the essential genes; usually, mutations are introduced into candidate genes.

Mouse ES cell technology has virtually revolutionized biology by providing the means to assess the function of many mammalian genes *in vivo*. ES cells carrying foreign genes (transfected genes or DNA from other organisms that integrate into the ES cell genome)—retain their totipotency; therefore, they have the potential to contribute to the development of mice that, in turn, will then carry the foreign genes. The altered ES cells can be transferred by micro-injection (monitored through a microscope) into the blastocyst cavity of a normal pregnant mouse to create chimeric mice containing both normal (host) and altered (ES) cells. These mice can be mated to obtain progeny that carry the foreign genes in all of their cells. Such techniques have been the best source of information about the early events in X inactivation in the mouse. And because ES cells can be used to make chimeric mice that carry the induced mutations (figure 5-10), the effect of the alterations on the development of mice can be assessed. Therefore, whereas it is difficult to study normal X inactivation in the mouse, the affect of perturbations can be determined in mice carrying induced mutations. One caveat is that some of the manipulations and induced mutations may perturb the chromatin of the region and influence more than just the gene or element under analysis. Another disadvantage in using this mouse model is that inbred mice are not heterozygous the way human females are. To solve the problem of lack of markers to distinguish one X from the other, mouse geneticists often create hybrid mice made up of two crossbreeding species whose alleles differ. This introduces another level of complexity into an already complex system, because it is not clear that X inactivation in the interspecies hybrid mice is comparable to that in wild-type mice.

6. Cells maintained on feeder layers in the presence of special differentiation inhibitor are removed from inhibiting conditions, and the blastocysts, which form in suspension culture, undergo differentiation. The process of X inactivation is induced during days 1–5 of this differentiation process that culminates in tissue specialization.

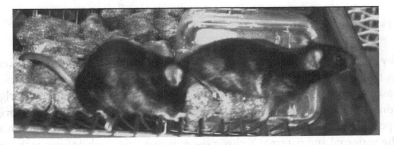

Figure 5-11. Chimeric mice derived from ES cells carrying the human XIC transgene, shown in figure 5-10. The ES cell contribution to the chimera is low and can be seen as the light (agouti) patches of color in fur, best seen on the underside of the mice. From figure 5 of Migeon et al. [111].

Recent developments in reproductive techniques have led to the development of nutrient medium that can support the short-term growth of fertilized eggs or zygotes created in petri dishes. These specimens are maintained in culture to the appropriate stages. This has enabled mouse scientists for the first time to examine X inactivation from early cleavage stages to blastocyst stage.

5.6. TRANSGENIC MICE AS A FUNCTIONAL ASSAY

As one means to analyze the function of a gene or region of the chromosome, relatively large segments of the genome can be transferred from one animal to another, either by injecting them into oocytes or using ES cell technology, as described in the previous section. In this way, abnormal human genes can be inserted into mice or human mutations can be introduced into the relevant mouse gene to determine how they affect the development of the embryo. This technology can also be used to determine how much of a transferred segment is needed for function. Transfecting a 450 kb region of the mouse X chromosome containing the region of the putative X inactivation center into mouse ES cells showed that it was capable of inducing X inactivation. It inserted itself into an autosome in male mice and was able to silence the chromosome from which it was expressed [69]. Comparable studies have been carried out using segments of the human X chromosome [70] (figures 5-10 and 5-11). In this way, studies of the events occurring during human embryogenesis, which are not accessible during human development, can be carried out using mice as the experimental model. Human ES cells have been derived from germ cells and blastocysts, but the limited number of specimens currently available do not proliferate in culture as well as the mouse ES cells. In addition, the earliest available material to date seems to have already completed X inactivation, so an inducible system like mouse ES cells is not yet available. The latest experimental models are stem cells obtained by reprogramming human adult somatic cells. However, the X inactivation status of these cells is highly variable and unstable because the epigenetic reprogramming is usually incomplete [71, 72]. Yet, it is likely that new techniques will be developed to get around even these limitations.

5.7. ASSAYS FOR X INACTIVATION PATTERNS IN HETEROZYGOTES

It is by examining the distribution of the two populations of cells in mosaic heterozygotes that we know about the effect of X inactivation on clinical manifestations of disease. Although the choice of active X is random regarding parental origin at the onset of dosage compensation in the fetus, the composition of these original cell populations often changes subsequently. Differences in the proteins encoded by the maternal and paternal X chromosomes may selectively influence the proliferation of the expressing cells. In this way, one cell population may overgrow the other (discussed in chapter 11). The proportion of each type of cell—at least in blood cells, which are the most accessible—can be determined using polymorphic differences that can distinguish the parental chromosomes. A good way of doing this would be to look at the proportion of cells expressing the maternal version of a protein compared to those expressing the paternal one. *G6PD* isozymes provide a good means to do this (figure 5-12). However, not all individuals have these useful variants, so that other means to carry out such an assay have evolved. One can use any difference in the RNA encoded by an expressed gene to distinguish the parental origin of chromosome that is active in the cell, and RT-PCR (reverse-transcriptase polymerase chain reaction) analysis has made this possible.

However, more often a DNA assay has been used for this purpose because preparing RNA for analysis is often troublesome and demanding. DNA polymorphisms can distinguish the parental X chromosomes from one another, but the problem is to distinguish between active and inactive X. In absence of gene expression, other characteristics of an inactive X can distinguish it from the active one. Such an assay has been developed using (1) the common polymorphic variation in the X-linked *androgen receptor* (*AR*) gene (*Appendix A*) to identify the parental origin of the X chromosomes, and (2) DNA methylation to distinguish active from inactive X. This analysis, referred to as the HUMARA assay (human AR assay), is described in more detail in chapter 12 and figure 12-8. These assays have revealed the selective advantage of the cells that express the normal alleles in carriers of many X-linked diseases, and why some girls manifest diseases that are usually seen only in males.

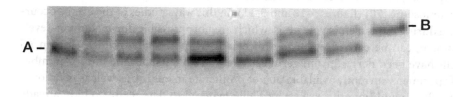

Figure 5-12. **Range of expression of *G6PD* enzymes in heterozygous women** (cellulose acetate electrophoresis): nine women showing differences in the ratio of A:B enzymes expressed in the their blood cells, ranging from lack of the cells expressing B in lane 1 to lack of the cells expressing A in lane 9.

5.8. SUMMARY AND SPECULATIONS

Because X inactivation occurs so early in embryonic development, the means to directly observe what is happening is difficult, if not impossible. However, using cell cultures—especially those with gene or protein variants—has provided insights into some of these events. The ability to separate the active human X from the inactive one in cell hybrids has helped identify the differences between them. Also, studies of mice during embryonic development and the induction of X inactivation in mouse embryonic stem cells provide the means to manipulate the process so as to learn which of the induced perturbations might adversely affect it. However, it is necessary to keep in mind that insights from perturbations in stem cells of one organism may not necessarily reflect what is happening during normal development, or the essential components of the inactivation process in other organisms. The best way to identify the underlying molecular mechanisms and distinguish the theme from its variations is to study the process in several mammals.

PART TWO

Themes and Variations of X Inactivation

6

Theme 1

The Initial Steps—Creating the Active and Inactive X

This chapter and the next deal with the features of X inactivation that are shared among mammals, the ones that reflect the basic themes responsible for the single active X in diploid cells. What all mammals have in common is that (1) the XX female—like the XY male—has only a single working X chromosome in each of her somatic cells, and (2) individuals of either sex with more than one X chromosome are cellular mosaics. Up to now, I have referred to the mammalian version of X dosage compensation as *X inactivation*, which is what it is most often called. However, the term is probably misleading because it implies that silencing an X chromosome is the primary thrust of our method of dosage compensation. Clearly, inactivation of X chromosomes is the means to eliminate the extra set of X transcripts in females, but it is not the defining step in the process; in fact, silencing X chromosomes is more of a default pathway. The *primary event* in mammalian X dosage compensation is *choosing* the future active X chromosome. Any chromosome that is not so designated will be silenced by the action of an extraordinary gene that is present on the X chromosomes of eutherian mammals. The inactive X transcript gene, *Xist*, is discussed in great detail later in this chapter, but for the moment, it is important to know that *Xist* has the power to initiate the transcriptional inactivation of any chromosome from which it is adequately transcribed. If the *Xist* locus were fully transcribed from all the X chromosomes in a cell, none of them would be functional. If all the X chromosomes in a cell were silenced, the embryo could not survive.[1] Therefore, to have an active X in each cell, it is necessary to repress the *Xist* locus on one X chromosome in that cell. Silencing X chromosomes is the default pathway, whereas ensuring that each cell has a single active X is the real thrust of our method of X dosage compensation.

6.1. CHARACTERISTICS OF THE INACTIVE X CHROMOSOME

Although the single active X is the hallmark of mammalian X dosage compensation, the inactive X is the chromosome that is targeted for chromatin modification.

---

1. Mouse embryos without an X (39,Y) do not survive beyond the two-cell stage.

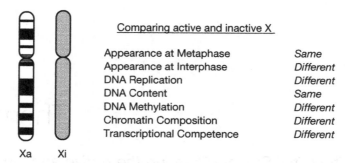

Figure 6-1. Comparing the human X chromosomes: active (Xa) versus inactive (Xi).

Historically, the inactive X has been the chromosome of major interest to most mammalian geneticists, and for good reason. Its physical and genetic character-istics are truly unique (figure 6-1), so it is easily distinguished from the active X and all the autosomes. The ability to compare the active and inactive X within the same cell has taught us a lot about how both expressed and repressed states are programmed and maintained—not only on the X chromosome but also on autosomes. Discernible differences in the two chromosomes are very subtle during mitosis when cells are actively dividing, but they are readily detectable during the interphase stage of the cell cycle, when transcription and chromosome replication occur. And the inactive X differs not only from its homologue but also from all the other chromosomes with respect to transcriptional activity, patterns of DNA meth-ylation, time of DNA replication, and the chemical composition of its chromatin.

The Inactive X Looks the Same as Its Homologue at Metaphase

In the mitotic-metaphase spreads used for chromosome analysis, the two chro-mosomes look almost the same. Both of the human X chromosomes are the sev-enth largest chromosome in size[2] and are submetacentric—the shorter arm (Xp) is separated from the longer one (Xq) by the centromere (see figure 2-2). Only the cognoscenti could distinguish the inactive X at this stage, by its being slightly more condensed than the active one. Often in metaphase cells it resembles the let-ter C with a bend placing the ends of the two arms (telomeres) closer to each other (figure 5-4 shows the curve in the late-replicating X). These features most likely represent residual effects of the more distinctive behavior of these chromosomes during interphase.

The Inactive X Is Condensed during Interphase

During the time when it replicates and carries out its transcriptional activities, the active X resembles all the autosomes—stretched out into threadlike molecules. In

2. Based on length in megabases.

striking contrast, the inactive X is relatively condensed and is seen as the sex chromatin mass or Barr body, close to the nuclear membrane (see figure 3-3). At least in some cells, the Barr body seems to have a nonlinear form with the telomeres of the short arm and long arm approaching each other [73], which may explain the curving of the inactive X chromosome that is seen in some metaphase cells. It has been suggested that in interphase cells the inactive X is folded according to the arrangement of its heterochromatin [74].

The Inactive X Is Late Replicating

Another difference between the two X chromosomes is the time when they begin to replicate themselves in anticipation of cell division. Although the male X chromosome and the active X in female cells initiate their replication later than most autosomes, the inactive X chromosome is the very last chromosome to begin its replication. This was determined by labeling human chromosomes with a tagged version of the DNA precursor thymidine during the DNA synthetic period [75, 76].[3] These studies showed that inactive X chromosomes—no matter how many in the cell—are late-replicating chromosomes; that is, they are the only chromosomes that incorporate thymidine at the very end of the period of DNA synthesis. Late replication is often used as a marker for an inactive X chromosome (see figure 5-4) [77].

The Inactive X Has Chromatin That Is Transcriptionally Inactive

As might be expected from its name, another difference between inactive and active X chromosomes is that the active X is extensively transcribed, whereas the inactive one has only limited transcriptional activity—most of it confined to the pseudoautosomal regions.[4] The differential transcriptional activity results from differences in the nature of the chromatin of the two chromosomes. The chromatin of the expressed regions of the active X is euchromatin—"open" and accessible to the transcriptional machinery, whereas the chromatin—of the corresponding regions of the inactive X, which are not expressed is heterochromatin—"closed" and inaccessible (see figure 3-2). The dissimilar chromatin can be visualized by labeling the chromosomes with antibodies to the acetylated forms of the core histone proteins, notably histones H3 and H4. In this case, the inactive X, unlike its homologue and all the autosomes, fails to label because its histones are characteristically underacetylated. The extensive underacetylation of histone H4 is also used as a cytological marker to identify an inactive X chromosome (figure 6-2).

3. The presence of the label is detected when the chromosome preparations are covered with a photographic emulsion because silver grains deposit at the site of the label. BrdU incorporation along with acridine orange is another method to visualize chromosome replication.

4. Other transcription from the inactive X is discussed in chapter 7.

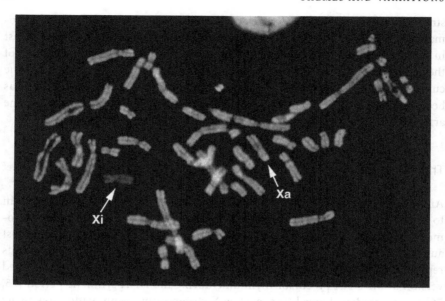

Figure 6-2. The inactive X has unacetylated histone H4: metaphase spread from a human female, labeled by an antibody to acetylated histone H4 (green), showing that the active X (Xa) is labeled (green) whereas the inactive X (Xi) is unlabeled (red because it lacks sufficient acetylated H4). Photomicrograph courtesy of Peter Jeppesen. [See color plate.]

The Inactive X Has Methylated CpG Islands

The two chromosomes also differ in DNA methylation: the clustered CpG di-nucleotides (CpG islands) in the 5′ regions of many X-linked genes are unmethylated on the transcriptionally active X and methylated on the silent one (discussed in section 7.2, "Maintaining Inactivation by DNA Methylation of CpG Islands").

The Inactive X Transcribes *Xist*

The last major difference between the two X chromosomes is that the *Xist* gene[5] is extensively transcribed only from the inactive X. *Xist* is a gene whose essential product is not a protein but a regulatory RNA. Located within the X inactivation center (XIC), *Xist* is the essential gene in the process of *cis*-limited inactivation (*cis inactivation*). In this case, the term *cis* refers to mechanisms that affect the locus itself or the chromatin in the immediate vicinity of the gene—that is, *on the same*

---

5. This gene is named *XIST* in humans and *Xist* in other mammals. For convenience, I will refer to it generically as *Xist*, except when referring specifically to the human gene.

chromosome as the gene of interest. Gene promoters and enhancers are considered *cis* regulators of transcription, as are mutations that affect the DNA sequence of the relevant gene. Almost everything else is considered a *trans* mechanism because the relevant gene products are encoded by one chromosome, but their site of action is on other chromosomes. Transcription factors are good examples of factors that act *in trans*. Encoded by one gene, these proteins are synthesized in the cytoplasm and reenter the nucleus to regulate other genes. *Trans*-acting factors often bind to DNA or chromatin, acting as effector molecules. However, these two mechanisms are not mutually exclusive. For instance, the events that lead to the inactivation of an X chromosome start at one site in the chromosome (the XIC) and progress along the same chromosome *in cis*, inducing further modifications that affect only this chromosome and its chromatin. Yet, the chromatin changes that are induced *in cis* are dependent on a series of *trans* factors—that is, the enzymes needed to modify the chromatin.

6.2. TIME OF INITIATION IN THE EMBRYO

The process of X dosage compensation in mammals has two major components. The first is choosing the active X chromosome, which is primarily a *trans* mechanism. The second, silencing all the rest of the X chromosomes in the cell, is primarily a *cis* mechanism. Inaccessibility and lack of sensitive assays have made it difficult to determine exactly when the active X is chosen or when the inactive X is silenced. However, the availability of cytological markers for histone modifications and chromosome replication has provided some insights. Although the time when the choice is made is still not known, determining the sequence of events involved in X silencing is now feasible using such markers of inactive chromatin and inactive alleles. The presence of a Barr body in interphase cells or a late replicating X has long been used as evidence that inactivation of the chromosome has already taken place.

Huynh and Lee [78] proposed that mouse embryos inherit a preinactivated paternal X chromosome, and therefore X inactivation begins earlier than originally thought. They suggested that transcriptional silence is initiated during spermatogenesis inactivating the paternal X. The inactive state is relaxed during the early stages of embryonic development, leading to random inactivation in the embryo proper. However, the evidence is more consistent with the notion that the *cis* inactivation process is initiated in the embryo rather than in parental gametes. First, asynchronous DNA replication (a marker for an inactive X chromosome) is notably absent in female embryos from the first cleavage (two-cell stage) to the mid-blastocyst stage, and the late-replicating X and Barr body are seen for the first time in the future placental tissues (referred to as *trophectoderm*) when they start to differentiate [79] (Table 6-1). Second, both X chromosomes are expressed during the early cleavage divisions based on the greater quantity of X-encoded proteins in female mice than in male mice; subsequently, the level in females decreases to equal that in males [80–83]. The most compelling evidence that both X chromosomes are expressed in the early embryo comes from studies using differences in X-linked alleles to determine which X chromosome is being expressed [84]. Even better, it has been shown that both parental alleles are being expressed simultaneously based on the presence of hybrid molecules (heterodimers) not seen under other conditions [85–87]. Some of the most elegant evidence that X inactivation begins in the blastocyst comes from Huynh and Lee [88] and Mak et al. [89], who studied several X-linked loci with distinctive parental alleles. Taken together, the two studies show that both parental alleles are expressed at the stage 2.5 days postconception (p.c.) but that the genes closest to the region of the XIC express less of one allele than the other (figure 6-3). However, with time, more of the paternal allele is expressed (day 3.5 p.c. and later stages; figure 6-4). Mak et al. [89] have interpreted their findings as emergence of the paternal X chromosome from a transient repressed state acquired by the inactivation of both sex chromosomes (X and Y) during spermatogenesis—an interpretation close to my own. In fact, all of the observations are completely consistent with the derepression of paternal alleles that were *temporarily* inactivated during spermatogenesis. Khahil et al. [90] show the paternal X and Y chromosomes are indeed inactivated during spermatogenesis at a time when they form a *sex chromosome body* or XY body (see figure 5-5). The active chromatin state of the XY body observed prior to inactivation is restored before fertilization occurs (XY body inactivation or meiotic sex chromosome inactivation [MSCI]). All of these studies present indisputable evidence that an imprint acquired during spermatogenesis persists during the early cleavage stages, especially in the region of the XIC, and is released before the onset of X inactivation in the mouse embryo proper. XY inactivation during male meiosis (MSCI) has its own unique characteristics, which are discussed further in section 10.2, "Paternal X Inactivation." In any case, by day 6 p.c., at the time when X inactivation is initiated in the female mouse embryo (in the inner cell mass of the blastocyst), two alleles are functional at loci where only the maternal allele had functioned previously.

Such differences in interpretation of data remind me of the important role that *semantics* plays in how we interpret scientific evidence. With regard to when it occurs, like most developmental processes, X inactivation has a beginning and an end. It seems fitting to define the time when a chromosome becomes inactive as the time when heterochromatization, condensation, and late replication have occurred. What is clear is that the process of dosage compensation that begins with the selection of the future active X occurs long before the process of *cis* inactivation is complete. Based on when an inactive X chromosome is first observed in embryonic tissues, *cis* inactivation is complete at various times during the early development of mammals (Table 6-1). Recent studies reporting the variable times of onset of the process in human and rabbit embryos are discussed in section 10.6, "Effect of Inactivation Timing."

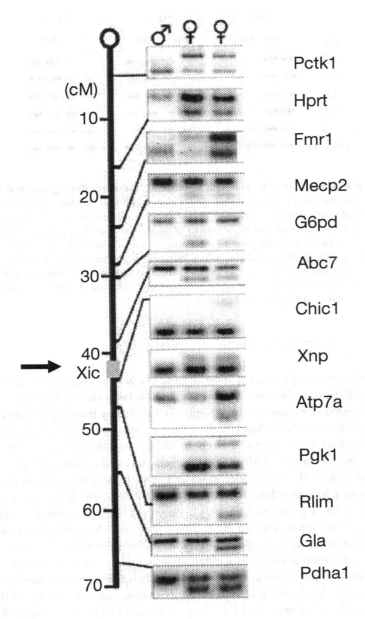

Figure 6-3. Partial repression of genes on the paternal mouse X: Allele-specific analysis of the RNA transcript from polymorphic X-linked genes of F1 embryos from an interspecies cross (*Castaneous* female × *Mus musculus* male); shown are one male and two females at the 16-cell stage; the male expresses his only allele (the maternal one), whereas females express both to some extent. However, many paternal alleles (not all) are expressed less (note less intense bands). Arrow points to the XIC. Adapted from figure 2b of Huynh and Lee [88], with permission of Macmillan Publishers, Ltd.

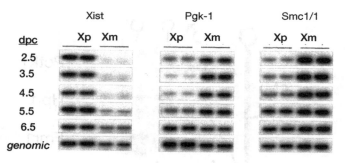

Figure 6-4. Release of the paternal X imprint acquired during spermatogenesis.
Quantitative expression of the parental *Xist*, *Pgk-1*, and *Smc1/1* alleles in mice from 2.5 to
6.5 days postconception (p.c.). The bottom row shows the pattern in the adult mouse control.
As expected, the maternal *Xist* allele is not well expressed until the onset of X inactivation
at day 5.5 p.c. In contrast, the paternal *Pgk1* and *Smc1* alleles are expressed at low levels (or
not in many cells) until day 5.5 p.c., when they are up-regulated at the time that random
X inactivation begins in the mouse embryo. The conclusion of this study is that loci on
the paternal X are gradually released from the imprint acquired during XY inactivation in
meiosis. Adapted from figure 4 of Mak et al. [89].

6.3. *CIS* INACTIVATION

The developmental program that turns an active X chromosome into an inactive
one is called *cis* inactivation because the process takes place within the confines
of the targeted chromosome. Inactivation is initiated by transcripts from the *Xist*
gene, and all events that follow take place on the same chromosome, *in cis*. Table 6-1
shows that the time during embryogenesis when *cis* inactivation occurs varies from
one mammal to another, earliest in marsupials, during the early cleavage stages; in
eutherian mammals, it coincides more or less with the time of implantation. In
some species, it occurs closer to the time of gastrulation, which has been called the
most important time of one's life [91] because it is the time when the embryonic
cells lose their totipotency and the embryo commits to becoming individualized.
Inactivation seems to be coupled with tissue differentiation [79, 92, 93], occurring
earliest in placental tissues, which differentiate before tissues of the embryo proper.
The factors that contribute to inactivation act only within a small temporal window
of embryonic development (48 hours in mouse embryonic stem [ES] cells). Wutz
and Jaenisch [94] showed that for a very short time inactivation is reversible, but
then it becomes irreversible, at least in these cells.[6] After this critical time, the window of opportunity has closed, and it is no longer possible to induce X inactivation;
adding or subtracting X chromosomes or other essential factors after this has no
effect.

6. Inactivation is reversible in germ cells and can be induced to reverse in human placental
cells.

Table 6-1. Time of X Inactivation in Mammalian Embryos

Subjects	Gestation Length (days)	Time of Implantation (days)	First Sightings of Inactive X[a] (days)	Location
Bovine	280	>20	7–9	Preimplantation Blastocyst[b]
			14–15	Embryo proper
Cat	63	12–14	6–14	Trophoblast
			19	Embryo neural tube
Horse	340	7–14	7.5–10.5	Trophoblast
			11.5–12.5	Embryonic disc
Human	270	6–7	10–12	Placenta
			12–14	Syncytioblast
			18–20	Embryo proper
Macaque	169		10–12	Placenta
			19	Embryo proper
Marsupial	32–34		Unilaminar blastocyst	Totipotent cells[b]
Mouse	19–21	4.5–6	3.5	Trophectoderm[b]
			4.5	Primitive endoderm
			5.5–6.5	Inner cell mass
Rabbit	30–32	>6	5	Embryo proper
Rat	21–23	5–7	6	Trophoblast[b]
			7	Inner cell mass
			12–16	Spinal ganglion

[a] Determined by Barr body or late-replicating X.
[b] Imprinted (paternal) X inactivation.

It has been customary to think of the *cis* inactivation program for silencing X chromosomes as having three major steps. The first step occurs during the early stages of embryogenesis, targeting the X inactivation center, a localized (<1 kb) region of the X chromosome (see figure 6-5). The second step is the propagation of this inactivation signal to the rest of the chromosome by inducing modifications in the chromatin, rendering it transcriptionally inert. The third step is the acquisition of further, more enduring modifications that maintain the transcriptional silence of the inactive X during all subsequent cell divisions. Such chromatin and DNA changes are considered *epigenetic*, because they do not alter the DNA code for proteins; instead, they modify the DNA either by adding molecules to it, or by altering its surroundings. These epigenetic modifications not only alter gene expression, but also they are transmitted from one somatic cell to its progeny; with some exceptions, they are not usually passed on through the germ line to the next generation.

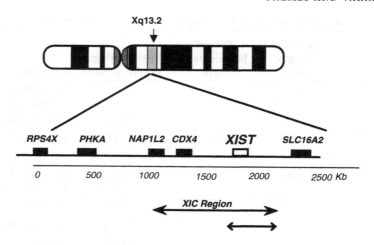

Figure 6-5. Zooming in on the human XIC and the *XIST* locus in Xq13.2. The longer arrow indicates the location of the XIC region as defined by patient studies. The shorter arrow shows the XIC region as narrowed by transfection studies.

6.4. THE MASTER CONTROL REGION: XIC AND *XIST*

It is the master control region, a complex X-linked locus called the X inactivation center (XIC), that distinguishes the mammalian X from all other chromosomes. Figure 6-5 shows this region (Xq13.2) of the human X chromosome. The concept of a localized region from which inactivation is initiated and spread bidirectionally along the chromosome was suggested by Liane Russell [95] and was supported by the behavior of *X-autosome translocations* in mice [96] (see section 11.6). When, by chance, breaks occur simultaneously in an X chromosome and a nearby autosome, parts of the X may be exchanged with the autosome; as a result, chromatin from the X chromosome is placed next to that of the autosome. If the exchange is reciprocal, it is said to be balanced. Because empiric observations of balanced translocations have shown that only one part of the bisected X chromosome is subject to inactivation, such translocations identified the region of the mouse X chromosome that was essential for inactivation (the *D region*). Its counterpart on the human X chromosome was identified by Eva Therman and her colleagues [97, 98], who noted that any translocation chromosome capable of being inactivated included the region of the long arm of the X chromosome closest to the centromere. She postulated that this segment of the X—which she named the *X inactivation center*—was essential for inactivation. The XIC region on the human X turned out to be homologous to the D region of the mouse X. And it happened that the D region included a putative gene that Bruce Cattanach and his colleagues called *Xce* (X controlling element) because it seemed to affect the randomness of X inactivation [99]. Subsequent studies show that this region of the X chromosome in both species is the one that responds to an initial signal and starts the cascade of events, which transmits inactivity throughout the chromosome. Not only does the XIC control the initiation of X inactivation, and its propagation along the future inactive chromosome, but also it must have an important role in protecting the future active X from being silenced.

Location of the XIC

The XIC region was first mapped to band Xq13 on the human X and to the D region on the mouse X, based on studies of rearranged chromosomes. Although the conserved region in both species includes several megabases, (MB) the XIC segment was narrowed to less than 1 MB by studies of X chromosomes carrying deletions that do not interfere with inactivation [100]. The region has been further delimited in both species by experiments that transfer parts of the putative XIC region into mouse ES cells to determine if they could function, based on their ability to induce inactivation [69, 70, 101, 102] (see section 5.6, "Transgenic Mice as a Functional Assay").

The Genetic Content of the XIC

The XIC region is relatively poor in protein-coding genes and enriched in repetitive DNA sequences and non-coding RNAs [30, 103]. Within the XIC is the unique *Xist* gene, which is the gene that initiates *cis* inactivation; it can silence only the chromosome on which it resides (figure 6-5; see also figure 8-1 for a close-up of the XIC). This gene was named the *X inactive specific transcript* (*Xist*) because it is expressed only from an inactive X chromosome, and its only product is a regulatory RNA transcript [104]. As sometimes happens, it was identified serendipitously during the search for an unrelated gene.[7] *Xist* has unique characteristics (table 6-2). Its large (>17 kb) transcripts are abundant.[8] Like most messenger RNAs the *Xist* transcripts are polyadenylated and the majority of them are spliced, but unlike most messenger RNA's *Xist* transcripts do not code for a protein. This noncoding RNA remains within the nucleus close to the chromosome from which it was synthesized (figure 6-6). *Xist* has been identified in many mammals: humans [104], mice [105], cows [103], rabbits, horses [106], several species of vole [107], cat, mole [77], rat, shrew, dog, pig, guinea pig, armadillo and

---

7. It was first identified by Andrea Ballabio with an antibody for steroid sulfatase, which is surprising and to this day unexplained, because steroid sulfatase is located very far away from *XIST* near the short-arm telomere of the X. Ballabio, seeing that it mapped to the long arm of the X, sent the *XIST* clone to Huntington Willard, knowing of his interest in genes that might escape X inactivation. On finding that it was expressed only from the inactive X, Willard and his student Carolyn Brown went on to clone the whole gene and discovered that it was a noncoding RNA [64, 104].

8. The human *XIST* locus spans 32,063 base pairs in Xq13. The major *XIST* transcript is an RNA of 17,225 base pairs, which includes the largest exon on the X (exon1: 11,333 base pairs). There may be longer transcripts generated by alternative splicing [104].

Table 6-2. CHARACTERISTICS OF HUMAN XIST

1.	A large noncoding RNA
2.	Encoded by a gene in the XIC in Xq13.2
3.	Transcribed only from the inactive X, and from every inactive X; repressed on the active X
4.	Transcripts remain in the nucleus near the site of synthesis
5.	The RNA accumulates and surrounds the inactive X
6.	Essential and sufficient for *cis* inactivation
7.	Functions only during a critical window of embryonic development; may have a role in maintaining silence.
8.	If adequately transcribed, acts as a silencer, even when ectopically inserted into an autosome
9.	Silences by inducing modifications to render chromatin transcriptionally incompetent
10.	DNA sequence is not well conserved through evolution, but promoter elements are
11.	The human gene is functional in mice

elephant [108]. *Xist* seems to be unique to eutherian mammals as careful analysis of marsupials and monotremes has failed to find such an RNA [109]. However, there is a candidate for an *Xist* substitute in marsupials (see section 8–3, "The Effect of Map Changes on X Inactivation in Mouse and Man").

Clearly, all eutherian mammals have their own version of *Xist*—or an analogous X-linked gene—capable of inducing *cis* inactivation. Yet there is not strict sequence homology among *Xist* genes (overall identity <50%). Shared features of the gene include its genomic organization, promoter region, transcription start sites, tandem repeats, and many intron–exon boundaries [110]. The number of exons is variable because of variable alternate spicing due to many splice site mutations. *Xist* exon 4 has homology with an exon of a protein coding gene, Lnx3, on chick chromosome 4, consistent with it having evolved from that gene [77, 109]. Characteristics of the conserved tandem repeats in the *Xist* promoter are discussed in "The *Xist* Promoter Region" below.

Despite low overall DNA sequence homology between human and mouse *Xist*, human *XIST* transcripts coming from a transgene are recognized by mouse ES cells [70, 102, 111] Moreover, this human transgene can induce X inactivation in *male* mice [70]. Although the sequences are not very similar, the A repeats in the promoter region are conserved, all species having seven to nine repeats. Conservation of this repeat structure implies that features of the gene other than linear DNA sequence are important in inducing inactivation. *Xist* RNA has the intrinsic ability to bind to the region from which it is synthesized and will do so even when the *Xist* gene is translocated to an autosome. Therefore, the noncoding *Xist* RNA transcripts are similar in some ways to the non-coding roX RNAs involved in dosage compensation in flies (see chapter 3). Just as *Xist* transgenes

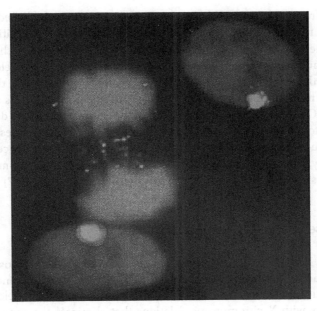

Figure 6-6. *XIST RNA* **coats the human inactive X chromosome in adult fibroblasts, except in mitosis.** Shown is the FISH analysis of human fibroblasts labeled with an *XIST* DNA probe that hybridized to *XIST* RNA. The RNA that coats the Barr body in interphase disappears from the chromosome when the cell divides, and then reforms by new transcription. This may not occur in mouse cells [118]. Photomicrograph from figure 9E of Clemson et al. [425], with permission. [See color plate.]

can exert effects on adjacent autosomal chromatin in mammals, roX transgenes inserted on autosomes in flies can cause site-specific histone acetylation of distantly linked genes that are not normally targets of dosage compensation.[9]

Xist is expressed at a low level in mouse embryos as early as the two- to four-cell stage, long before the onset of inactivation [112, 113]. Human embryos at the 5- to 10-cell stage express *XIST* irrespective of their sex, indicating that the maternal X in males also transcribes *XIST* [114]. However, at that time very little *XIST* RNA is made—certainly not enough to inactivate the chromosome. Then *Xist* is up-regulated on one or more X chromosomes prior to when allelic inactivation is observed, after which *Xist* expression becomes limited to a single X per cell [66]. In mice, *Xist* is up-regulated concomitantly with inactivation of the expressing chromosome [66]. However, in the inner cell mass of rabbit, human, and monkey cells, *Xist* is upregulated on both X chromosomes quite early—far in advance of silencing, dissociating the upregulation of *Xist* from the inactivation process, and suggesting that choice of active X occurs after the initial *Xist* up-regulation [66]; this is also true for the horse [115]. *Xist* continues to be fully

9. However, in contrast to *Xist*, there are two roX RNAs in flies, encoded by separate X-linked genes, with overlapping roles in *increasing* the transcription of the male X chromosome, rather than silencing female X chromosomes.

expressed from an inactive X long after X inactivation is established, and there is evidence that Xist RNA may be processed differently after the critical stage in embryogenesis [116]. Because its transcripts remain close to the chromosome, *Xist* could and may play a role in *maintaining* X inactivation. Yet deletion of the locus from the inactive X in human somatic cells does not reactivate the chromosome [59], no doubt because there are other means to maintain its silence (see chapter 7). On the other hand, recent studies show that when *Xist* is deleted from their hematopoietic cells, *in utero,* female mice develop highly aggressive myeloproliferative neoplasms at 2–5 months of age. That the blood cancer cells had significantly higher expression levels of X-linked genes than autosomes suggests that *Xist* has a role in the maintenance process, at least in mice [117].

Xist Is Essential for *Cis* Inactivation

The role of *Xist* in dosage compensation is to silence all X chromosomes from which it is adequately transcribed. Persuasive evidence that *Xist* is indispensable for *cis* inactivation comes from studies of mice with induced *Xist* deletions [119] and humans with X chromosome deletions that eliminate the gene [120–122]. In each case, when *Xist* is not present or not functional, its chromosome cannot inactivate. Further evidence from XIC transgenes [69, 70, 123, 431] makes it clear that, when adequately transcribed, *Xist* is capable of inducing inactivation wherever it resides—even when inserted into an autosome [124, 431].

6.5. SILENCING THE INACTIVE X CHROMOSOME

Another feature of mammalian X dosage compensation is that the silencing mechanisms act at the level of the chromosome, not individual genes. They provide an economical means to silence a big block of chromatin and many genes all at once, obviating the need for the piecemeal process of silencing one gene at a time. Therefore, *cis* X inactivation is a process that affects the chromosome as a whole entity, and not merely bits and pieces of it. Studies of how our X chromosome has evolved suggest that, over time, most of the autosomal genes that translocate to the X chromosome are not fully transcribed from the inactive X. Yet inactivation of these alleles does not seem to occur locus by locus in a piecemeal fashion. Instead, these new arrivals come under the sphere of influence of *Xist* and the inactivating wave and are eventually incorporated into the single silencing process (see figure 7-3).

Role of *Xist* in *Cis* Inactivation

The *Xist* locus seems to be expressed at three levels: off, low, and fully transcribed. Sensitive assays show that prior to inactivation there are low-level *Xist* transcripts from every X chromosome in mouse and human embryos of both sexes [114, 125]. In the mouse, these transcripts are seen at the earliest cleavage stages and persist until transcription is up-regulated on the future *inactive* X chromosomes. Such low-level transcription is not enough to silence chromatin, and its purpose remains to be seen; it may, or may not, be essential for the inactivation program. The silencing function of *Xist* seems to require its full transcription. And even when fully transcribed, *Xist* may not be able to silence the chromosome unless other components of the silencing process—like the chromatin modifiers or other competence factors—are available in sufficient concentrations in the cell.

How *Xist* expression is up-regulated is not yet completely understood. From observations of mouse ES cells, up-regulation seems to involve the stabilization of *Xist* RNA and its subsequent accumulation, because no difference in the rate of *Xist* transcription was found in low-level–expressing ES cells and high-level–expressing somatic cells [126]. There is also evidence supporting a role for the pathway involved in degradation of nonsense RNA in *Xist* upregulation, in a manner not yet elucidated [127].[10] Because the onset of inactivation is coupled with tissue differentiation, the up-regulation of *Xist* requires the down-regulation of pluripotency factors such as Nanog, Oct4/Pou5F1, and Sox2, which repress *Xist* expression in pluripotent cells [128]. The pluripotency factors no doubt do this indirectly as the binding site for them in the first intron of *Xist* can be excised without effect [129]. In addition, at least in the mouse, it seems that the up-regulation and activation of *Xist* requires some X-linked competency factors considered further in Chapter 10. In any case, tissue-specific enhancers, acting on any *Xist* locus that has not been specifically repressed, could mediate its activation and up-regulation.

At some time before *Xist* is fully expressed from the future inactive X chromosomes, it needs to be turned off on the future active X chromosome in cells of both sexes. *Xist* is not fully expressed from any active X chromosome. The only time it is expressed in a normal male is during spermatogenesis when the male X chromosome is inactive or recovering from transcriptional repression.[11] *Xist* expression at that time is considerable but, based on limited evidence, is not essential for inactivation of the XY body during male meiosis; a partially deleted *Xist* gene—one that interrupts X inactivation in females—does not interfere with either MSCI or normal spermatogenesis in mice [130].

Cis inactivation requires that *Xist* transcripts accumulate around the chromosome from which they are transcribed during the appropriate window of

10. The demonstrated role of the nonsense–mRNA decay pathway is to survey newly synthesized RNA and eliminate transcripts that are incomplete, thus preventing the cell from being clogged up with senseless transcripts. There is no evidence that this pathway can directly up-regulate nuclear transcripts, but up-regulation of *Xist* could be mediated indirectly by degrading some interacting molecule.

11. *XIST* is expressed in the somatic cells of Klinefelter males because, like women, they have two X chromosomes.

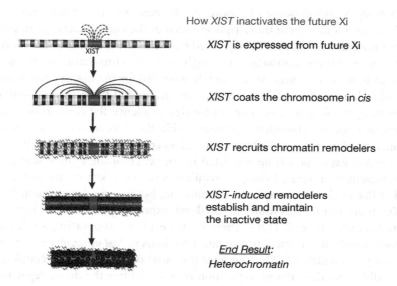

How *XIST* inactivates the future Xi

XIST is expressed from future Xi

XIST coats the chromosome in *cis*

XIST recruits chromatin remodelers

XIST-induced remodelers establish and maintain the inactive state

End Result:

Heterochromatin

Figure 6-7. Diagram showing how Xist RNA inactivates the future inactive X (Xi). Adapted from figure 5 of Avner and Heard [167], reproduced with permission from *Nature Reviews Genetics*, 2001, Macmillan Magazines Ltd. [See color plate.]

development (figure 6-6). This accumulation of *Xist* RNA is referred to as *coating* the chromosome, and in the mouse, it rapidly (within one or two cell cycles) induces inactivation of the chromosome (figure 6-7). Studies in mouse ES cells tell us that *Xist* transcripts are ineffective after this time and in fact are no longer needed. The intimate association of *Xist* molecules with its chromosome seems to be mediated by functionally redundant sequences within the gene. The fact that up-regulation of *Xist* on the future *inactive* X is associated with turning off the low-level expression on the future *active* X raises the possibility of cross-talk from inactive to active X chromosomes. In fact, there is some evidence of a transient association between the two chromosomes at the onset of inactivation in mouse ES cells [131, 132]. All the details are not yet known, but clearly the *Xist* transcripts recruit and interact with *trans* factors to modify the underlying chromatin, causing it to become transcriptionally inert in the manner characteristic of heterochromatin throughout the genome (see section 7.1, "Spreading Inactivation by Modifying Chromatin.")

The *Xist* Promoter Region

The conserved portion of *Xist* resides in the 5′ region of the gene, the so-called *A repeats* that in the human gene are 7.5 copies of a conserved 26-mer sequence, some of them in tandem. At least 5 of them are required for silencing [119]. Recently, these repeats have been shown to mediate duplex formation *in vitro* whose integrity is required for silencing; mutations abrogate the silencing function of these repeats *in* vivo [133]. In addition, a 14-mer hairpin in this region has been shown to adopt a novel AUCG tetraloop fold, whose integrity is also required for silencing [134]. It is thought that the complete A repeat region, stabilized by inter-repeat duplex formation, provides the means for the AUCG tetraloops to attract relevant *trans*-acting factors. RepA, a short transcript emanating from *Xist* intron 1, which encompasses the A-repeats, is thought to participate in this process. There is abundant evidence that mutations in the *Xist* gene can influence the randomness of X inactivation. If the *Xist* locus on one X is defective, then that chromosome cannot be inactivated, and in surviving cells it will always be an active X. Minor modifications in nucleotides of the *Xist* promoter may cause more subtle effects, such as increasing or decreasing the probability that the chromosome will be an inactive X. Two rare mutations have been described in the human *XIST* promoter, both occurring at nucleotide-43C [135, 136]. One of them makes the chromosome more likely to be inactive, whereas the other decreases the chance that it will be an inactive X. Pugacheva et al. [137] showed that these mutations alter the only binding site within the *XIST* promoter for a protein that interacts with DNA to influence transcription in a variety of ways, as yet not well understood.[12] Both mutations influence binding affinity, albeit in opposite directions. Yet, the influence of these mutations by themselves seems relatively subtle because in both cases the same mutations were also present in family members in whom X inactivation was random, not unbalanced [135, 136]

Other Genes within the XIC

Thus far, the evidence suggests that *Xist* is the most essential of the genes required to initiate *cis* inactivation. A human 480 kb XIC transgene that includes *XIST* can induce random X inactivation in male chimeric mice [70] (see figures 5-10 and 5–11). An *XIST* transgene containing only a few kilobases of flanking sequences can induce heterochromatin formation in human sarcoma cells [139], a mouse transgene containing effectively only the *Xist* locus induced silencing in mouse ES cells [123]. And a 16 kb *XIST* cDNA can silence the extra chromosome 21 in trisomy 21 human stem cells [431]. The essential sequences in the mouse XIC have been narrowed to approximately 80 kb [101], but this exclusion is complicated by the fact that, in mice, the *Tsix* locus, which overlaps *Xist*, must be included because it is needed for normal placental function in that species [140] (see "The *Tsix* Antisense Transcript Locus," below). In addition, there have been many evolutionary changes in the content of the XIC, quite close to *Xist* (see figure 8-1). Conceivably, *Xist* and adjacent elements are all that are essential for human XIC function.

12. CTCF is the name of the multifunctional protein (CTC binding factor) that binds to CCCTC in DNA and facilitates the formation of boundary elements that block enhancer activity and otherwise influence the chromatin environment of a gene. It has been implicated as a transcriptional repressor in the silencing of some imprinted autosomal genes and is thought to be critical for long range silencing. Encoded by human chromosome 16, CTCF is postulated to have a regulatory role in *Tsix-Xist* interactions in the mouse [138].

The *Xce* and *Xite* Loci

Before the discovery of *Xist*, the most likely candidate for its role was the X chromosome controlling element (*Xce*) locus within the mouse XIC [140], because it seems to affect the randomness of the choice of the active X chromosome. However, this locus maps outside the *Xist* locus, and it is now thought to play a more supportive role. Simmler and colleagues [142] suggest that *Xce* acts at some distance to regulate *Xist* expression. The nature of the *Xce* locus is not known because it still has not been identified definitively. Recent studies suggest that the number and diversity of loci that define *Xce* may be more complex than originally envisioned [143]. Ogawa and Lee [144] suggest it may be one and the same as a transcribed DNA element downstream of *Xist*, which they believe regulates *Xist* indirectly; they call this element *Xite* (*X inactivation intergenic transcription elements*). One might expect to find an analogous locus (*XCE* or *XITE*) on the human X chromosome. However, the *Xite* locus maps to a region of the mouse XIC that has been disrupted on the human X chromosome during mammalian evolution (figure 8-1) and it is not present in the DNA sequence of the human X chromosome. In addition, as *Xite* sequences are found in mouse and rat, but not vole, Shevchenko et al. [145] suggest that may have emerged and evolved only in those species.

The *Tsix* Antisense Transcript Locus

Within the XIC of both humans and mice is another noncoding RNA transcript, just downstream from *Xist* (figure 8-1). This one is called *Tsix* (which is *Xist* spelled backward) because it transcribes from the opposite DNA strand as *Xist*, overlaps the *Xist* locus, and is *antisense* to it (see figures 8-1 and 10-5). In the mouse, *Tsix* transcripts overlap the entire *Xist* locus, and they inhibit expression of the maternal *Xist* allele in placental cells [142] and on the future active X in ES cells [146, 147]. By repressing the accumulation of *Xist* transcripts, mouse *Tsix* blocks the cascade of events that lead to transcriptional repression of the chromosome. Based solely on observations in mice, *Tsix* has been proposed to have a critical role in protecting the future active X from inactivation—not only when the X is always maternal but also when randomly chosen [148, 149]. The prevailing thought is that the *Tsix* RNA interacts directly with the *Xist* transcripts to repress *Xist* function in the mouse [150, 151]. On the other hand, it has also been proposed that *Tsix* transcripts induce chromatin modification over the entire *Xist–Tsix* region but do not directly repress *Xist* transcripts [152]. This would mean that *Tsix* acts as a chromatin modifier and not as a transcriptional repressor.

In any case, the human version of the gene does not perform either function [67, 153]. Human *TSIX* is antisense to *XIST* but carries a deletion in its promoter region, the same one experimentally induced by Lee and her colleagues and shown by them to interrupt the function of mouse *Tsix* [147, 149] (see figure 10-5). Most important, human *TSIX* transcripts are ineffectual, because they do not repress

XIST in cis and, in fact, are coexpressed with *XIST* from the *inactive* X throughout female embryonic development [67] (see figure 10-6). *TSIX* is not transcribed in male human embryos, and its expression in female cells gradually ceases after birth. Despite being homozygous for the *TSIX* deletion, human females undergo random X inactivation. Therefore, *TSIX* repression of *XIST* cannot be essential in our species. Because its structure and function differ significantly in mouse and man, *Tsix* is discussed in more detail along with other species variations in chapter 10.

Other Noncoding Transcripts in the XIC

Along with a few protein encoding genes, there are other noncoding genes contiguous with *Xist* [103] (table 8-1, figure 8-1). None of the protein coding genes within the human XIC has been shown to have a role in X inactivation. On the other hand, studies in mice implicate three other noncoding RNAs within the mouse XIC, *Xite*, *JpX*, and *Ftx*, as regulators of *Xist*. Except for *Xist*, none has yet been shown to play a role in inactivating human X chromosomes, or in maintaining the single active X. Another gene within the mouse XIC is an E3 ubiquitin ligase, *Rnf12a*, which is thought to be an *Xist* activator [129]. However, it does not map within the human XIC [154].

Shevchenko et al. [145] found that not all functional elements flanking *Xist* in mice were well conserved even within rodents. They observed that non-coding RNA transcripts in the region surrounding *Xist* can appear, disappear, change their promoters, exon-intron structure and borders. Because no common conserved elements located 3′ to *Xist* have been identified in eutherians, they suggest that the XIC functional elements may be at least partially species-specific. One suspects that some DNA elements in the vicinity of *Xist*—perhaps species specific—may function as enhancers or receptors for the *trans*-acting molecules involved in the steps that precede *cis* inactivation having to do with designating the *active* X chromosome. The mouse *Xist* regulators within the XIC are considered further in section 8.3.

6.6. SINGLE ACTIVE X VERSUS X INACTIVATION

The use of the term *X inactivation* to describe the mammalian method of dosage compensation has certainly influenced the way we think about the process, as well as the studies we carry out. I would have preferred that Lyon's hypothesis be referred to as *the single active X hypothesis* as it seems more appropriate in light of the evidence on hand. The difference between the *single active X hypothesis* and the *X inactivation hypothesis* has to do with whether underlying mechanisms count X chromosomes to determine how many should be inactive—that is, *choose the inactive X(s)*, or they maintain the activity of a single X chromosome per cell— that is, *choose the active X*.

In the case of the *X inactivation hypothesis*, the argument is that *Xist* is up-regulated *only* on future inactive X chromosomes that previously were marked for inactivation by some chromosome-counting gene. The active X remains active because in the default pathway unmarked *Xist* loci are not up-regulated. In the case of the *single active X hypothesis*, there is no need to count X chromosomes; the *Xist* locus needs to be repressed on only one chromosome per diploid cell, no matter the number of X chromosomes. Because *Xist* is a chromatin silencer, the *Xist* allele on the future active X must be repressed before the critical time in embryogenesis when it is expressed in sufficient quantities to initiate the cascade of events that silence the chromosome. Any other X chromosomes in the cell will be inactivated by upregulation of their *Xist* allele according to the developmental program for chromosomes with an active *Xist* gene.

Given the evidence from diploid cells, it is not readily apparent which choice pathway is operative; both are plausible. However, as you will see, it is the study of human 69,XXX and 69,XXY triploid cells that provides compelling evidence that it is the active X, rather than the inactive X, which is chosen (figures 6-8 & 6-9; see also triploidy below and in section 11.7).

No Need to Count X Chromosomes

The major dogma about mammalian X inactivation insists that the counting of X chromosomes is the essential first step in X dosage compensation (e.g., see references [58, 113, 151, 165–167]). No doubt this reflects the influence of other mechanisms of dosage compensation on our thinking about our own species: The notion of counting X chromosomes relative to sets of autosomes is a holdover from the X:autosome ratio that underlies dosage compensation in flies. However, the mammalian method of dosage compensation arose independently and is not directly derived from that in flies. There is no compelling evidence that the number of X chromosomes to be inactivated is counted in some way. Observations of mouse ES cells suggest that the activity state of the two X homologues is *sensed* prior to the up-regulation of *Xist* by a physical association of the two inactivation centers [131, 132]. Yet, how this relates to counting, and whether it occurs in mouse embryos or in other species, remains to be seen.

I suggest that counting the future inactive X chromosomes is not required for the following reasons. All the observations of individuals with multiple X chromosomes tell us that inherent in the ontogeny of an X chromosome is the program for transcriptional inactivation. By default, *all* of the X chromosomes in a cell might be inactivated unless some event occurs to turn off the *Xist* locus on one of them. The evidence also indicates that, regardless of the number present, only one X chromosome is chosen in each diploid cell; the designated chromosome, whose X inactivation center receives a "mark," would remain active, and all the others (having an unblocked inactivation center) would be subsequently inactivated (see figure 6-8). Therefore, in light of what is known about dosage compensation in mammals, it seems to me that X inactivation is not about counting inactive X chromosomes, and there is no need to count the active one; in viable diploid cells, only a single X chromosome is active—no matter how many X chromosomes are present—and all the rest (the total number of X chromosomes minus one) are silenced.

To those who assume that *Xist* is programmed to be silent, and its expression is induced only on the future inactive X chromosomes, I would argue that *Xist* has all the hallmarks of a housekeeping gene (ubiquitous expression and regulatory CpG island with SP-1 binding site), and this class of genes is programmed to be expressed without induction. *XIST* is expressed, from all X chromosomes in human zygotes of either sex, albeit at low levels, until the time in embryogenesis when the locus on the future active X is turned off, and methylated in both males and females. Then, I would point out that silencing X chromosomes individually is a far more complex program than the one to silence all *Xist*-expressing chromosomes. One would need a flexible mechanism that could accommodate the zero to four or five X chromosomes that might need to be silenced in male or female cells with more than one X chromosome. Although biology is often more complex than it need be, it would be much simpler to maintain the activity of just one X chromosome per diploid cell, as one X remains active in males with four X chromosomes just as it does in females with two of them (see figure 3-3). I believe that all the evidence is most consistent with the notion that a single active X is explicit in the silencing program for diploid cells because of the limited number of molecules of *Xist* repressor that is available. The number of active X chromosomes in a cell is limited by the number of repressor molecules coming from an autosomal gene, and in diploid cells there is enough to keep one X chromosome and only one X chromosome active. It seems logical to me that the first step in X dosage compensation in both sexes is the designation of the future active X by *Xist* repression. Up-regulation of the *Xist* locus on any and all remaining X chromosomes is the default pathway [155]. Because the single active X hypothesis has much to support it, at least in human cells, the next section considers how an active X might be chosen.

6.7. CHOOSING THE ACTIVE X CHROMOSOME

Although the active X is not "counted" in female cells, it is "chosen" from among the other X chromosomes in the cell. The evidence to date indicates that the choice of active X chromosome requires the activity of a gene that is not on the X chromosome. By virtue of being the sole recipient of *Xist*-repressing molecules, the targeted chromosome is "chosen" to be the *active* X. Consistent with this is evidence that deleting *Xist* does not interfere with the "choice" of active X [166]. X chromosomes with either normal or mutated *Xist* can become the active X. Although *Xist* mutations do not influence the selection of the active X, they do influence the ability to inactivate. If the mutant allele cannot induce inactivation, at least some cells—those with wild-type X chromosome designated as the active X—will have two active X chromosomes and do not survive [155, 168] (see figure 10-1).

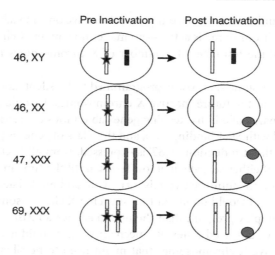

Figure 6-8. The blocking factor model for random X inactivation: The blocking factor (black star) protects one X chromosome from inactivation in diploid 46,XX, 46,XY, and 47,XXX cells, thus choosing the active X (white). Acquiring the factor precludes *XIST* transcription on that chromosome. The nonblocked chromosomes (gray) are inactivated by *XIST* transcription and become by default inactive Xs. In triploid cells (69,XXX), more than one X can be active, presumably because of the extra amount of *Xist* repressor, contributed by the extra autosomal set of chromosomes.

The Dual Function of the XIC

Clearly, the XIC has a major role in the cascade of events that silence inactive X chromosomes, because it is the region of the X chromosome that initiates *cis* inactivation. Although *XIST* may be sufficient to initiate *cis* inactivation, other genes or elements within the XIC are needed to protect the *active* X from inactivation in diploid cells of both sexes. Even though the process of repressing one *XIST* locus may involve other chromosomes or other regions of the X chromosome, some of the repressor molecules must make their way to enhancers of *XIST*. Therefore, the human XIC has a second important function: it must receive a signal(s) that represses the *XIST* gene on the future active X.

Trans-Acting Factors Inhibit *Xist* Expression on the Future Active X

The concept of a blocking factor that protects the active X from inactivation was suggested by Mary Lyon [156] and Sohaila Rastan [157] long before the *Xist* locus was discovered. Figure 6-8 shows how such a blocking factor might work. Although *cis*-acting elements probably participate in the process of repressing *Xist*, it is unlikely that repression of only one *Xist* gene and not the other(s) could be carried out entirely by an X-linked gene. It is difficult to imagine how an X-linked locus could randomly choose one *Xist* locus over the other. The repression of only one *Xist* gene—especially if chosen in a random fashion—seems to require a *trans*-acting factor, if not to silence *Xist* directly, then to choose the *cis* element

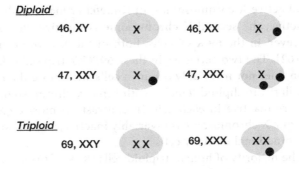

Rule: Diploid cells have a single active X
Triploid cells may have two active Xs

Figure 6-9. X inactivation differs in diploid and triploid cells, even when the sex chromosomes are the same. Black dots represent Barr bodies. Note: Only one X is active in diploid cells, whereas two may be active in triploid cells.

that will silence *Xist*. Such a *trans*-acting factor most likely comes from a nonsex chromosome. Autosomal genes with a role in X dosage compensation have been identified in other organisms. Dosage compensation in flies involves a number of X-linked and autosomal genes that act to "sense" the X-to-autosome ratio. These autosomal signal elements influence the early choice of sexual fate and antagonize X signal elements (see section 3.4, "Mechanisms of Dosage Compensation in Other Organisms").

Therefore, I would wager that one or more *trans*-acting factor(s) originating from an autosome is required for some step in blocking *Xist* transcription on the future active X. After all, *trans*-acting pluripotent factors are thought to block the upregulation of *Xist* very early in mouse development [118]. Other *trans*-acting molecules at later stages could be targeted to repress only one *Xist* allele in diploid cells of both sexes. Although little is known about the nature of these factors, clearly all of the mammalian species with a single active X must have some version of them.

Triploid Cells Have Two Active X Chromosomes

Evidence supporting the existence of an autosomal *trans*-acting factor comes from observations of triploid human embryos with 69,XXX or 69,XXY karyotypes (also see "Triploidy" in section 11.7 and *Appendix B*). Such fetuses have been identified among the products of conception that did not survive gestation. Studies of these triploid human fetuses show that the rules of X inactivation differ in cells with 69 rather than 46 chromosomes (figures 6-8 and 6-9). In addition to three sets of autosomes, triploid cells have three sex chromosomes rather than two, and they can be XXY, XXX, or XYY. Despite the same set of sex chromosomes, triploid males with 69,XXY chromosomes differ from diploid males with Klinefelter syndrome (47,XXY) in the number of active X chromosomes. In Klinefelter males, only one X chromosome is active; the second X chromosome is inactive, just as in normal females. However, in the 69,XXY cells, both of the X chromosomes may be active [158–162]. The two active Xs in these 69,XXY triploid cells tell us that X inactivation does not invariably occur in cells with more than one X chromosome. Similarly, in diploid females with three X chromosomes (47,XXX), two of them are inactive in each cell. In contrast, in most 69,XXX triploid females, only one X chromosome is invariably inactive, and two of the X chromosomes are functional in many cells.

In fact, in the majority of human triploid cells (87% of the 47 triploids studied), there are two active X chromosomes [162]. This suggests that the extra set of autosomes in triploid cells, although not sufficient in every cell, provides the means to keep more than one X chromosome active in many cells. The evidence from human triploid embryos suggests that if enough of this repressor is available, none of the X chromosome needs to be inactive (reviewed by Jacobs and Migeon [161] and by Migeon et al. [162]). The likely explanation for two active X chromosomes in triploid cells is (1) the active X is chosen by repression of its *XIST* locus, (2) the repressor is encoded by an autosome and is dosage sensitive, and (3) the extra dose of this key repressor enables the expression of more than one X in many triploid cells. The *modus operandi* of the putative *trans*-acting repressor is predicated on there being only a limited number of repressor molecules. Although in diploid cells the amount of autosomal *trans*-acting factor is enough to repress one *Xist* locus, the extra set of autosomes in triploid cells can mediate the repression of two of them. It is difficult to envision the features that make such molecules so exquisitely dosage sensitive. Most likely, only a small number of these signaling molecules are needed and their function is subject to cooperativity. That autosomes come in pairs means that at least two repressor molecules are targeting a single X chromosome in each diploid cell. For male cells there is no problem, because there is only a single X in the cell. But it is a bit tricky for females, because only one of the two X chromosomes can be designated the active X. Conceivably, this autosomal gene is imprinted such that only one parental allele is expressed, hence only one functional copy of the relevant gene per diploid cell. Or the products of the two alleles could dimerize and act together as a repressor unit. Alternatively, once the targeted X chromosome receives the first molecule, then all the other molecules are directed there subsequently. In that scenario, once one X chromosome receives the signal, the other cannot. One way of doing this would be an actual physical association between the relevant autosome and the future active X, such as the associations between nonhomologous chromosomes that have been implicated in other regulatory pathways [163, 164]. Not only can those genes whose proteins work together move to the same transcription site, but enhancers on one chromosome can meet up with genes that they regulate even if the genes are on other chromosomes.

In any case, the chance occurrence of cells in which both X chromosomes receive signals would lead to death of the cell because of the two active X chromosomes.

This might explain the large number of otherwise normal females that seem to be lost during preimplantation development (see section 1.1) The receptor for such molecules has not been identified but must reside within the XIC. While the promoter of *Xist* is a likely target, other binding sites close to the gene could also serve as the signal receptor.

Because triploids have enough *trans* factor to maintain the activity of two X chromosomes, my colleague Patricia Jacobs and I thought that we might be able to identify the relevant autosome by examining X inactivation in 47,XX females with trisomies for the various autosomes. In each case, our specimens came from miscarried products of conception. Several years ago we reported that the extra chromosome in 18 of the 22 autosomal trisomies did not affect the inactivation of the X [161]. Since then, we have examined trisomies of chromosomes 11 and 5, which can be added to the list of autosomes with no signs of involvement [162]. Conceivably, several genes, each on a different autosome, act in concert to maintain the activity of two X chromosomes in triploid cells. Or the presence of an additional set of chromosomes somehow limits the number of *Xist* up-regulators, or otherwise interferes with activation of *Xist*. On the other hand, the lack of trisomies for chromosome 1 and paucity of trisomies for chromosome 19—two chromosomes that could not be studied directly—suggest possible candidates for the triploidy effect. We have narrowed the candidate regions for these chromosomes by eliminating regions present in liveborn females, with partial trisomies who had a normal inactive X [162].

Genes That Could Affect the Choice of Active X

The choice of active X is usually random with respect to parental origin, because the *Xist* allele on either maternal or paternal X chromosome can be repressed. The program designating the active X is initiated much earlier than *cis* inactivation, probably during the early cleavage stages of embryogenesis. Most likely, one X chromosome is designated to be the future active X when its *Xist* locus is repressed. Of course, this chromosome must be able to respond to such a *trans*-acting signal so that the locus can be silenced.

When X inactivation is *imprinted*—as it is in the mouse placenta—the maternal *Xist* allele is always the target of repression. Either the paternal allele cannot be an active X, because of some modification acquired during spermatogenesis, or alternatively, the maternal X in imprinted tissues is a better target for these transacting molecules—or perhaps it is a combination of the two (discussed in section 10.4). If choice resides in the ability of the XIC to receive *trans*-acting molecules, the limiting *trans* factor might have a greater affinity for one parental X chromosome than the other because of differences in the ability to respond to these signals. Therefore, among the genes or genetic elements that can affect choice of active X are those in the XIC, which respond to these molecules.

The Role of Cell Selection in the Choice Process

Chapter 12 deals in great detail with the role of cell selection on the composition of mosaic populations created by X inactivation. However, here I introduce the concept of cell selection—that is, a selective advantage of one cell over another or others—to consider its role in the initial choice process. Cell selection is a dynamic process, with the potential to be an important determinant of development at every developmental stage. We are all familiar with the role of cell selection in malignant processes such as leukemia, where unfortunately the cancer cells—having acquired mutations leading to a growth advantage—proliferate faster than the normal cells and eventually replace them. Fortunately, mutations expressed during normal embryonic development most often have a neutral or detrimental effect on viability so that if there is any proliferative advantage, the normal cells usually have it. Selection during embryogenesis usually favors the proliferation of the more viable cell. If the mutation is severe enough, it will drastically interfere with the proliferation of the cells in which it is expressed, such that such cells are completely eliminated and are not detectable in the newborn. For selection to influence the choice of active X, there must be a difference in the rate of growth of some cell(s) within the mosaic cell populations. Therefore, cell selection has no role in choice of active X until *after* the choice is made and the individual becomes mosaic. If the X chromosome chosen as active X is inadequate, or if there is more than one active X chromosome per cell because of failure of the second X to inactivate, then the inadequate cells most often will be eliminated because they do not proliferate as well (see figure 10-1). It may be helpful to know that the early embryo has an excess of cells—more than the number needed for a viable human being. Therefore, loss of quite a few cells is well tolerated, especially during the earliest stages of embryogenesis when the active X is chosen (see chapter 12).

Choosing the active X—at least for females—is a rather demanding process, with the possibility of errors. In some cases, embryos may die, but often errors in the process may only lead to a loss of embryonic cells. The developmental biologist Scott Gilbert has reminded us that there are elements of chance and randomness during morphogenesis [169]. Many of these have to do with timing of these events, chance exposures to environmental inducers, and other haphazard factors. Because *stochastic* variation is the rule for many developmental events, even monozygotic twins will differ in their antibody repertoire, neural connections, and vascularization. The following chapters discuss how chance events that affect the composition of the cells in mosaic females influence their phenotypes. However, even at the initiation of the dosage compensation process, there seems to be a remarkable degree of randomness in choice of active X. Fortunately, most of the individuals or cells that cannot successfully complete the process do not survive.

6.8. SUMMARY AND SPECULATIONS

Because X inactivation was such an important component of the Lyon hypothesis, one might think that the major thrust and basic theme of dosage compensation in mammals are the inactivation of X chromosomes. And because the X:autosome ratio is important in dosage compensation in flies, one might expect that the earliest steps in inactivation would be to count the number of X chromosomes to determine how many need to be inactivated, and to mark them for inactivation. In fact, the first step in mammalian X dosage compensation is not likely to inactivate X chromosomes but to *maintain* a single active X in all cells, irrespective of the sex of the individual. Any X chromosome in addition to one in males as well as females is subject to inactivation because it was not designated to be the future active X chromosome.

You may ask why it is necessary to maintain the activity of one X chromosome. The answer is that (1) every cell needs an X chromosome to carry out essential cell functions; (2) every X chromosome carries one powerful gene—*Xist*—that is programmed to turn off the transcriptional activity of the chromosome from which it is transcribed; and consequently, (3) in each cell one X chromosome must be protected from inactivation. Therefore, I suggest that the earliest step in X inactivation is repressing the *Xist* locus on the future active X in cells of both males and females. It is likely that such a *Xist* repressor is an autosomal *trans*-acting factor.

So much for creating the active X chromosome. Now, what do we know about the initial steps in creating inactive X chromosomes? What we have learned from studies of mouse ES cells is that *Xist* cannot be adequately expressed in the presence of pluripotent factors, and so the silencing process must await the onset of tissue differentiation. In these cells *Xist* upregulation is abetted by a series of X-linked noncoding RNAs and the ubiquitin ligase *RNP12A*. Whether similar mechanisms are operative in nonrodent species, including us, must await the development of new experimental models that permit observation of very early embryogenesis, or relaxation of current limits for reproductive research.

Although single allele expression is characteristic of most genes on the X chromosome, it is not an exclusive property of X-linked genes. Some autosomal genes are subject to allelic selection. The immunoglobulin genes have their own unique way of choosing the expressed allele. It is not clear how the first allele is chosen to undergo the programmed rearrangement that is needed for it to function. In this case, the rearrangement of the gene is a chancy process, often not successful on the first try. However, once the proper rearrangement occurs, there is a feedback inhibition that prevents the other allele from undergoing recombination. And the manner in which only a single odorant receptor allele is chosen to be expressed in each olfactory sensory neuron has not yet been fully elucidated, but seems to involve physical contact between the chosen allele on one chromosome and an enhancer element on a nonhomologous chromosome [164]. At first glance it seems unlikely that the means of choosing single alleles is the same as those that choose an entire chromosome. However, it only takes repression of a single *Xist* allele to choose the active X—and to maintain the activity of an entire X chromosome. Therefore, there may be some common features.

7

Theme 2

Subsequent Steps—Spreading and Maintaining Inactivation

Chapter 6 considered the earliest steps in the process leading to a single active X chromosome in cells of both sexes. It introduced the *Xist* locus in the X inactivation center (XIC)—extraordinary because it functions not to encode proteins but to silence genes. Due to its unique features, under the appropriate conditions *Xist* can induce the inactivation of any X chromosome from which it is expressed. Because each cell needs an active X chromosome, one *Xist* locus per diploid cell must be silenced so that one X chromosome will escape inactivation. Therefore, the process of X dosage compensation in mammals starts with choosing the future active X by repressing its *Xist* locus. In subsequent steps, any X chromosome—except the one designated to be active—is inevitably silenced. This chromosome silencing process, called *cis* inactivation, begins with timely and sufficient *Xist* transcription from all X chromosomes whose *Xist* gene was not repressed; these are the future *inactive* X chromosomes. In mouse ES cells, up-regulation of *Xist* seems to require the expression of several noncoding elements within its XIC (see table 8-1). *Xist* up-regulation leads to synthesis of stable RNA transcripts that accumulate in the vicinity of their site of synthesis and surround the chromosome from which they were transcribed, thus initiating the inactivation process.

In this chapter, we move on to the next steps in the process of *cis* inactivation: the ones that spread the silencing signal from the *Xist* locus to the rest of the chromosome. In addition to silencing blocks of our X-linked genes, this cascade of events provides memory of the epigenetic modifications so that they can be faithfully transmitted to the cell's descendents. Therefore, we must consider some of the most enigmatic developmental mechanisms in human biology. The programs that regulate X chromosome activity are in many ways similar to those that determine how a pluripotent cell in the fetus, which is capable of giving rise to many tissues, differentiates into a specific liver cell and then produces more liver cells exactly like itself. Needless to say, the mechanisms underlying cell differentiation, cell memory, and long-term repression of blocks of genes are at the forefront of biomedical research. In fact, X inactivation provides a powerful research tool to explore such issues because both active and inactive forms of the X chromosomes coexist in the same cell. As chromatin modifications are such a hot topic of research and as X inactivation is such a good experimental model, more details of these events are known than earlier steps in the process. I have included many of them here to give some idea of the complexity and redundancy of the epigenetic modifications that convert an active chromosome to an inactive one.

7.1. SPREADING INACTIVATION BY MODIFYING CHROMATIN

The Role of *Xist*

The initial events in X inactivation are directed toward a limited region of the X chromosome—perhaps even a single locus. However, subsequent steps are targeted to the chromosome as a whole. The inactivating signal that emanates from the *Xist* locus needs to spread throughout the chromosome. This is accomplished when the *Xist* RNA molecules fan out from their site of synthesis in both directions and ostensibly cover the entire X chromosome. It seems that the target of *Xist* RNA may not be the genes themselves, as they have been observed to lie outside of the *Xist* RNA [170]; rather, the target may be repeat sequences in the core of the chromosome that lead directly to chromatin condensation, and ultimately to silencing the genes. Yet, it is important to distinguish the spreading of *Xist* RNA along the chromosome from the silencing of the underlying chromatin, as these are separate functions. *Xist* RNA molecules continue to coat the X chromosome long after X inactivation occurs, but they can initiate the silencing cascade only during the critical window of development at the onset of inactivation. The *Xist* RNA will spread, but not silence the underlying chromatin—if the RNA molecules fail to bind to the chromosome. Studies of DNA deletions that interfere with silencing [119] or molecules impeding the function of mouse *Xist* [171] show that not only must the RNA associate with the X chromosome, but it must also specifically bind to it.

The ability to bind chromatin depends upon conserved tandem repeat sequences within exon 1 of *Xist*. Perhaps these sequences are needed because they can form stem loop structures, recognizable by binding factors. In any case, they can even function when moved to an ectopic location within the gene. Jeon et al. [172] have reported studies of experimentally manipulated mouse ES cells, which suggest that the ubiquitously transcribed YY1 transcription factor is needed to keep *Xist* tethered to the X inactivation center, or it would otherwise diffuse. Yet, this does not explain why the inactivation process is induced only during a critical window of development. It has been suggested that differences in the processing of *Xist* RNA may be important in this regard [116]. And most likely, initiation of inactivation requires other competence factors that are available only at the critical time.

Transmitting Transcriptional Silence

All mammals use the same method to transmit transcriptional silence along the X chromosome. Silencing is mediated by changing the chromatin of the X from transcriptionally active to transcriptionally inert. The *Xist* RNA molecules interact with other cell components to modify the chromatin that they overlie, and these modifications are responsible for the transcriptional inhibition. Most likely, *Xist* itself is capable of recruiting all the factors needed to start the cascade that silences chromatin and this is its major role in the *cis* inactivation process.

In fact, none of the known chromatin modifiers are exclusive to the X inactivation process [148, 173]. Our genomes contain a lot of silent chromatin that surrounds the relatively small islands of expressed genes. In most cases, silencing of chromatin is the end result of a series of chromatin modifications (discussed later in the "Sequence of Events Involved in Silencing X Chromosomes" section). The features of inactive chromatin from the silent X seem to be generally the same as that of inactive chromatin elsewhere in the mammalian genome. But, they are not identical, as chromatin modifications (epigenetic marks) do vary somewhat between species and cell types ([118], table 1),

Heterochromatin and the Heterochromatinization of the Silent X

As described in the preliminary discussion of heterochromatin in chapter 3, chromatin is the complex of the DNA and proteins (mainly histone proteins) that provides the structure for the chromosomes and the milieu for the genes. The fundamental repeating subunit of chromatin is the *nucleosome*, which consists of an octamer of histone proteins (two molecules each of histones H2A, H2B, H3, and H4) wrapped with two loops (146 base pairs each) of DNA (the genes and the regulatory DNA; see figure 3-2). There are two kinds of chromatin, differing in structure and function. Chromatin that is transcriptionally active, or has the potential to be active under the right conditions, is called *euchromatin* or true chromatin. Although not all the genes in euchromatin are actively transcribing, they have the ability to be transcribed. In contrast, the chromatin that is transcriptionally inert, containing genes that are unable to be transcribed, is called *heterochromatin* to distinguish it from euchromatin. The process by which a large block of chromatin is silenced permanently is called *heterochromatization* (figure 3-2).

Heterochromatin differs from euchromatin regarding the specific modifications of the histone proteins in chromatin (*histone modifications*); among the possible modifications are acetylation, methylation, ubiquitination, phosphorylation, and sumoylation. Most modifications responsible for long-term silencing occur in the exposed tails of the histone proteins, at points where histones make contact with the DNA, and many are specific to the amino acid *lysine* (symbolized by K in the protein code). These covalent marks (often referred to as histone marks or histone code) can be added or removed by a variety of site-specific enzymes such as histone acetyltransferases (HAC) or deacetylases (HDAC) and histone methyltransferases

(HMT). The end result of these modifications is to make the chromatin environment of the gene either *permissive* or *nonpermissive* for transcription.

The modifications of lysines in the histones of actively transcribed euchromatin usually differ from those of heterochromatin[1]; the permissive modifications *open* the chromatin structure to permit the entry of molecules involved in transcription. In contrast, *heterochromatin* is typically a *closed* chromatin structure consisting of histones that are underacetylated and differentially methylated; closed chromatin is inaccessible to the transcription machinery and appears as more darkly staining regions in cytological preparations. With a few exceptions, the silencing modifications of histones of the inactive X are similar to those in heterochromatin wherever it occurs. The early models of X inactivation reviewed by Gartler and Riggs [174] did not consider the role of histone modification in the process. Although it was recognized that heterochromatization was part of X inactivation, the nature of heterochromatin was not understood. We now understand that histone modifications serve as a code to mark a region of a chromosome or locus for future transcriptional or silencing events. At the same time, the changes they induce, either alone or cooperatively, alter the environment of the gene so as to facilitate or inhibit its transcription.

Sequence of Events Involved in Silencing X Chromosomes

Several investigators have tried to sort out the various changes in chromatin of the silent X that are mediated by the *Xist* transcripts, and to determine the sequence in which they occur. Because it is not usually feasible to examine the early events when they occur in the embryo, mouse ES cells have been the major subject of such studies. In fact, ES cells in petri dishes provide a relatively simple model for this complicated developmental program. However, one caveat is that the observations of ES cells that have been experimentally induced to undergo X inactivation, may not accurately reflect what goes on in the embryo. Such studies are still in process, and we do not yet know the exact sequence of events in any mammal.

Having said that, we do know from studies of mouse ES cells that *Xist* accumulation—occurring shortly after induction—is the earliest sign that the process is underway [178, 179]. The earliest change in chromatin structure—occurring just after *Xist* RNA coating—is the loss of the histone modifications that mark active chromatin. The ability to compare the histone changes occurring on the future inactive X as it is silenced with the chromatin of the active X within the same cell is providing insights into the nature of the histone code.

Then, as *Xist* spreads along the chromosome, histones H3 and H4 undergo further lysine modifications characteristic of inactive chromatin mediated by the transient enrichment of the non-histone polycomb-group (PcG) protein complex on the future inactive X (discussed later in this section). Subsequently, the histone macro H2A variant, which has accumulated on the chromosome, becomes

1. Generally, acetylation of histones is associated with transcriptional activity, but the methylation modification is sometimes a permissive or active mark (i.e., H3K4) and other times a nonpermissive or repressive mark (i.e., H3K9me3, and H3K27me3).

ubiquitinated [180]. All the modifications that occur remodel the chromatin of the inactive X such that it is no longer competent for transcription.

An early step in the process is the formation of a transcriptionally inert compartment within the *Xist* RNA domain. Studies of mouse ES cells [181] suggest that the *Xist*-RNA-coated chromosome rapidly loses the basic transcriptional machinery such as RNA POL II, and transcription factor IID. At the same time the Cot1 repetitive RNA become depleted and the euchromatic histone modifications disappear. Enigmatically, the X-chromosome sequences lying within the *Xist* domain initially—the ones that are silenced first—seem to consist of repetitive DNAs. And then, the X-linked single copy genes, which were initially outside or at the edge of this Xist RNA coat, move into it as they are silenced [63].

For the chromatin aficionados, the following paragraphs present even more details about the sequence of silencing events:

Xist RNA coating induces dramatic changes in the chromatin of the inactive X. Based on studies of mouse ES cells, such alterations seem to occur in a stepwise fashion, within a couple of cell cycles (reviewed in [118]) The first step is the removal of the histone modifications generally associated with gene activity, such as di- and trimethylation of lysine 4 of histone H3 (H3K4me2/3), methylation of lysine 36 of histone H3 (H3K36me) and acetylation of histones H3 and H4. Figure 6-2 shows the striking under-acetylation of the inactive X chromosome in human cells.

Shortly after the loss of these *active* marks comes an enrichment of *repressive* marks mediated in part by the recruitment of *polycomb complexes*. These include trimethylation of lysine 27 of histone H3 (H3K2me3), dimethylation of lysine 9 of histone H3 (H3K9me2), and methylation of lysine 20 of histone H4 (H4K20me1). It has been proposed that H3K9 methylation provides the mark that promotes higher order heterochromatin formation on the inactive X [175]. It does this by attracting a protein complex, including the *heterochromatin protein HP1* that mediates the spread of silent chromatin to neighboring sequences.[2] The exact constitution of such chromatin marks differs to some extent among mammals. In any case, the imposition of these repressive marks is the means of spreading the inactivation throughout the chromosome.

During this time genes begin to be silenced, shifting from outside to inside the *Xist* RNA compartment. This is followed by a shift in the time when the inactive X replicates its DNA, which further impedes the establishment of transcription complexes.

Among proteins that associate with the inactive X chromosome at this time are the polycomb-group (PcG) proteins,[3] Eed and Ezh2, that mediate transcriptional

2. Another lysine modification affecting mainly histone H2B is ubiquitination. Apparently histone H2B must be ubiquinated in order for H3 to become methylated, and so on.

3. PcG proteins function as long-term repressors for genes expressed early in development of the embryo, after these early transcripts are no longer needed. PcG proteins do this during the development of many organisms, including flies, worms, and mammals. Among the several proteins in a complex is the histone methyltransferase (HMTase) Ezh2 that methylates H3K27. H3K27 can be mono-, di-, or trimethylated (1mH3K27, 2mH3K27, and 3mH3K27, respectively) and its methylation status mediates the repression.

silencing by both generating and recognizing histone modifications. However, this association is not specific to the X chromosome because it also occurs in the imprinting of human autosomal genes and in gene silencing in other organisms.[4] Recent studies implicate the Eed/Ezh2 PcG proteins in the early events leading to histone methylation. This protein complex has the enzymatic activity needed to methylate H3K9 and H3K27, making them repressive histones.

The enrichment of PcG proteins at the time of X chromosome silencing suggests that the complex was recruited by *Xist* for this purpose. In fact, mutant mice deficient in Eed (PcG) protein have a problem with methylating H3K27; yet, contrary to expectations, methylation of H3K27 is not essential for the *cis* inactivation process, because the deficiency of Eed causes only limited reactivation of X-linked genes [177]. Therefore, although Eed PcG complex is required for H3K27 methylation, it is not essential for inactivation, probably because other factors can carry out this function. This should give you some idea of the complexity involved in the early steps of the silencing process.

The early steps that induce inactivation of the chromosome are followed in short order by others, which serve to reinforce the silencing process. Among the later steps is the recruitment of the variants of histone H2 (macro H2A1 and A2). Another late acting factor is *Brca1*, the tumor suppressor gene that is mutated in some familial cases of breast cancer. BRAC1 protein localizes around the inactive X relatively late in the inactivation process, and is thought to contribute to the final steps in the heterochromatin process. Having ubiquitin ligase activity, BRAC1 may have some role in the ubiquitization of histone H2B on the inactive X. During inactivation of the sex body during spermatogenesis, BRAC1 recruits a phosphorylase that is needed to trigger chromatin condensation and transcriptional repression. It may play a similar role in the condensation and repression of the inactive X in somatic cells.

The last event to occur, at least in ES cells, is the methylation of the clustered CG dinucleotides (CpG islands), which locks in the inactive state [179] (see "Maintaining Inactivation by DNA Methylation of CpG Islands" below and figures 7-1 and 7-2). Thus, it seems that most of the histone modifications in the cascade of chromatin changes induced by *Xist* RNA are acquired early. They occur much earlier than DNA methylation, which is seen only *after* gene silencing is well underway. No doubt, these later changes are responsible and sufficient for the maintenance of the silent state of the inactive X in somatic cells. In any case, the many layers of modifications lead to establishing the inactive state and locking it in.

It should be apparent by now that the process of silencing the inactive X chromosome is quite complex and full of redundancy. Many of the specific details are still being worked out. The ability to examine the X chromosome in two different activity states within the same cell facilitates identification of all the players, those

4. From studies of an imprinted domain on mouse chromosome 7, we know that the PcG proteins mediate the acquisition of trimethylation at H3K27 there just as they do on the inactive X [176], showing that inactive chromatin is similar whether due to parental imprinting or X inactivation.

involved not just in X inactivation but also in heterochromatin assembly wherever it occurs. In fact, it is not clear if any of the observed chromatin modifications are unique for the inactive X chromosome. What is unique about the heterochromatization of the inactive X is the spread of the *Xist* RNA along the chromosome, which then induces the rest of the changes.

Way Stations for Spreading the Inactivation Signal

Evidence suggesting that the inactivating signal spreads better through X chromosomes than autosomes [182] has raised the possibility that X chromosomes are enriched for "way stations" [183] that enhance spreading—presumably by interacting with *Xist* RNA. If there are way stations to facilitate the spreading process, then their paucity in some areas of the X could play a role in the "escape" from inactivation (see section 7.3 Escape from Inactivation). Mary Lyon [184] has suggested that L1 elements (highly repetitive DNA sequences) serve this function, and there is some support for this. The mouse autosome containing the human *XIST* transgene did not spread the silencing signal very far when the autosome was depleted in L1 elements [70], and the human X has twice the number of recently evolved L1 elements as autosomes [185]. The density of L1s on the X is greatest in the evolutionarily oldest regions; their accumulation there may have resulted from the reduced recombination with the Y, because recombination tends to protect against invasion by repeat elements. However, the lack of L1 elements does not interfere with XCI in some mammalian species [186], and there is no evidence yet that *Xist* binds to them. And the putative species differences in way stations were no barrier to inactivating a chicken transgene on the mouse inactive X [187] (see section 8.3, "Stability of X Inactivation"). Whether, in fact, the *Xist* inactivating signal requires special genomic sequences in addition to the chromatin remodeling factors for efficient spreading remains to be seen.

In this regard, we must consider the spreading of X inactivation into the autosomal segments of translocation chromosomes (discussed further in section 10.5, "X-Autosome Translocations and Spreading of Inactivation"). Chromosomes like these contain a piece of an X chromosome attached to a piece of an autosome. When the X portion of the chromosome is inactivated, the silencing seems to spread from the X chromosomal segment near the translocation break point into neighboring autosomal segments. Based on clinical effects and chromosome replication analysis, it seems that the extent of spreading is limited and varies considerably depending on the chromatin of the attached autosomal segment. The striking effects of position on gene silencing were first recognized in flies when it was noticed that genes could be silenced by placing them next to heterochromatin. When a chromosome with an X-autosome translocation is the inactive X, the autosomal genes near the break point are often inactivated, but most of the distal autosomal genes are not. This limited autosomal spread has raised the possibility that the *Xist* transcripts travel less well in autosomal chromatin. Some have suggested that the spreading of the *Xist* signal is facilitated by other repeat sequences along the X chromosome (e.g., L1 sequences) that are less dense along autosomes. Others suggest specific DNA sequences may impede the spread of silencing molecules [188]. However, in some cases where the *Xist* locus was inserted into an autosome as a transgene, the *Xist* transcripts from the transgene coat a good portion of the autosome from which it is synthesized [69, 431]—at least initially.[5] Conceivably, the limited spread of inactivation into autosomal segments of X/ autosome translocations may not reflect the extent of spreading when X inactivation was initiated, but rather instability of the inactivation, subsequently, or poor survival of cells in which the silencing was more extensive.

Studies of X inactivation in such chromosomes using allele-specific RT-PCR (reverse-transcriptase polymerase chain reaction) is a more direct way to show how X inactivation spreads *in cis* through autosomal DNA. Sharp and colleagues [189] observed long-range silencing of autosomal genes located up to 45 MB from the translocation break point, and the extent of spreading could be visualized cytogenetically because the inactivated autosomal segment had the histone modifications characteristic of the inactive X. And the silenced autosomal genes are maintained by methylation of CpG islands just like the genes on the inactive X (see below). Spreading of gene silencing occurs in either a continuous or discontinuous fashion in different cases, suggesting that some autosomal DNA domains may not maintain the inactive state as well as others. Alternatively, spreading may be facilitated when the breakpoints occur in heterochromatic regions of autosomes.

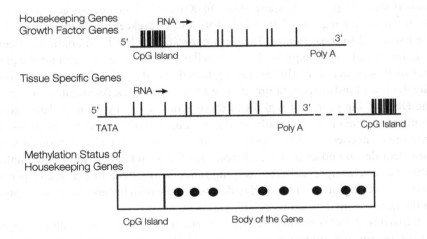

Figure 7-1. **Diagram showing distribution of CpG dinucleotides in the mammalian genome.** Top and center: CpGs are depicted by vertical bars; some are clustered (CpG islands). The CpG islands are in the promoter region of housekeeping genes and randomly distributed in tissue-specific genes. Bottom: The methylation pattern of a typical expressed housekeeping gene anywhere in the genome. The black dots denote methylated CpGs, which are seen here only in the body of the gene. See footnote 6.

5. There is evidence that in successive cell generations, the coating of the transfected autosome by the Xist transgene becomes less extensive.

7.2. MAINTAINING INACTIVATION BY DNA METHYLATION OF CPG ISLANDS

As you will see in chapter 8, not all mammals strictly maintain the transcriptional silence of genes on the inactive X from one cell to its progeny. However, those that do maintain inactivation use methylation of the DNA for this purpose. DNA methylation is known to be associated with heterochromatin and repressed genes. In mammals, the site of DNA methylation is the CpG dinucleotide. About 20% of the CpG dinucleotides occur in clusters, whereas the majority of them are scattered throughout the genome (~80%; see figure 7-1). In most of the nonclustered CpG dinucleotides, the cytosine that is 5′ to the guanine is methylated. The pattern of methylation often varies between cell types and during development. The methylation pattern serves as an epigenetic mark, providing a means to regulate gene expression throughout the genome. Methylation patterns are epigenetic marks because the methylation status of CpGs is faithfully transmitted from one cell to all its progeny; unmethylated CpGs remain unmethylated in all progeny of a cell, whereas the methylated CpGs are also faithfully reproduced because of the nature of the methylating enzymes (see later in this section). The prevailing view is that CpG methylation patterns stabilize chromatin structure in one of its alternative forms, thereby regulating access to the transcriptional machinery.

The CpG dinucleotides that are clustered into so-called islands are normally *unmethylated* (figure 7-1). Many of the 30,000 CpG islands in our genome occur in the promoter regions of growth factors and housekeeping genes—genes that are expressed in most tissues. The term *housekeeping* has been applied to genes that are constitutively expressed in each cell because they are needed for the general metabolic activities (housekeeping functions) that all cells must carry out. Genes of this kind are programmed to be active at all times. As might be expected, the DNA of the promoter regions of these genes is usually unmethylated, so as to maintain the open chromatin configuration, accessible to the transcriptional machinery needed for active genes. Figure 7-1 shows the distribution of CpG dinucleotides in housekeeping and tissue-specific genes; it also shows the methylation pattern in expressed housekeeping genes. Most often, the clustered CpGs in the promoter region are unmethylated, whereas the nonclustered ones in the body of the gene are methylated more or less.[6]

Experimental observations tell us that whenever the clustered CpGs in regulatory regions like promoters are methylated, the relevant gene is not expressed. How does the methylation of clustered CpG dinucleotides lead to transcriptional repression of the relevant gene? Methylation itself can preclude binding of those transcription factors that interact only with unmethylated sequences. Also,

---

6. Genome wide methylation studies distinguish the methylation patterns just outside the CpG island, within 2 kb of the gene promoter, called CpG island *shore* methylation [190]. These patterns may have some significance for the analysis of cancer genes and imprinted genes but as yet have no apparent relevance for X inactivation.

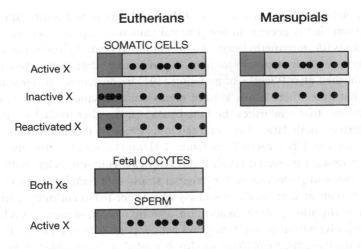

Figure 7-2. Diagram showing DNA methylation (denoted by black dots) **of X-linked housekeeping genes in cells of eutherian and marsupial mammals,** Shown is the active and inactive gene and the reactivated gene in somatic cells. Also shown is the methylation of the same genes in fetal oocytes (< 24 wks gestation) and sperm. The gene is depicted as a rectangle, with the darker square on the left representing the CpG island in the promoter region. Note: The CpG island is methylated only on the inactive X in somatic cells of eutherians. In contrast, the methylation in the body of the repressed gene is paradoxically less than that of the active X (see text in this section). Also note that when reactivated by 5-azacytidine the inactive X loses methylation in the CpG island, but the body methylation remains the same [214, 217].

methylated CpGs are recognized by methyl-binding proteins that in turn recruit the chromatin-modifying proteins to lock in transcriptional silence of inactive genes throughout the genome. (More details about this later in this section).

The CpG islands on the inactive X chromosome have been pressed into service for the job of maintaining X inactivation. In contrast to the active X and autosomes, the CpG islands on the inactive X are extensively methylated (figure 7-2). Parenthetically, studies of the CpG islands in inactive X chromosome genes were the first to show that CpG islands were regulatory elements of human housekeeping genes [191], further evidence that X inactivation is a lovely model system for gene regulation. Certainly, methylation of CpG islands is the major mechanism responsible for the faithful and enduring transmission of the inactive state through mitosis in most mammals. Studies of genes on the inactive X that are induced to reactivate by demethylating agents tells us that the only functional methylation is in the CpG islands [217] (see figure 7-2, reactivated X). Also striking is the relatively sparse methylation in the bodies of inactive X-linked genes. One possible explanation is that the relatively greater condensation of the inactive X could interfere with remethylation of newly replicated DNA. In any case it is consistent with observations from genome-wide studies that methylation in gene bodies is more characteristic of highly transcribed genes [192, 193].

DNA methylation patterns are established in the fetus by a combination of the methylation that is present in the parental gametes (eggs and sperm) and any adjustments (*de novo* methylation and programmed demethylation) made during the early embryonic stages. In humans, we know that adult methylation patterns are established after 9 weeks of gestation [194] because other patterns are seen before that time. There is one kind of methylating enzyme—capable of *de novo* methylation—that establishes the initial patterns. Another methylase maintains the pattern of methylation from one cell to its progeny; this maintenance-methylating enzyme, DNA methyltransferase 1 (Dnmt1), was the first mammalian DNA methylase discovered [195]. It does not efficiently methylate both strands of the DNA and prefers using the original strand as a template for methylating the newly replicated molecule—precisely what is needed to faithfully maintain an existent methylation pattern. In addition, a group of *de novo* methylases has been identified. Methyltransferase 3 enzymes act cooperatively to establish the initial methylation patterns. All of them are closely related and seem able to carry out the same function, but some are more tissue specific than others. Studies of a genetic disorder called the ICF syndrome (see *Appendix A*), resulting from a deficiency of one of these *de novo* methylases, Dnmt3b, provides evidence of both this redundancy and site specificity. This condition is not lethal because the other *de novo* methylases compensate in vital tissues. However, a unique function of Dnmt3b is the methylation of DNA sequences in the centromeric regions of chromosomes 1, 9, and 16, such that its deficiency leads to an abnormal degree of unraveling of blocks of heterochromatin in these regions, which leads to chromosome fragility. The reasons for the immunodeficiency and abnormal facial features are less clear; these tissues are either special sites for Dnmt3b methylating activity or sites in which the need for methylating capacity is greater than what can be provided by the other methylases alone. Dnmt3b probably has fewer functions than the other Dnmt3 methylases, at least in mice, because mice that are deficient in the others show more lethal effects. Of interest, another finding in ICF patients is that some of the genes on their inactive X chromosomes are not stably inactivated [196], suggesting a role for Dnmt3b in methylating CpG islands on the human inactive X.

It is the cooperative methylation of many CpG dinucleotides clustered in the island that maintains the silent state of the inactive X. In addition, this extensive methylation of CpG islands is responsible for faithful transmission of the same inactive X from one cell to its progeny. In an analogous way, the unmethylated state of the homologous CpG islands on the active X is also transmitted to the replicated X in daughter cells because Dnmt1, the maintenance methylase, effectively methylates only DNA that is already methylated on one strand (hemimethylated DNA).

Therefore, whether the CpG island is methylated or not, this methylation pattern is accurately replicated through mitosis, allowing faithful transmission of the inactive (or active) state and providing the mechanism for cell memory. Unlike the initial inactivating process that affects a large contiguous region of the chromosome, the process that maintains inactivation works in a *piecemeal* fashion. The reason for this is that the methylation status of CpG islands influences *only* the chromatin domain in its immediate vicinity. Because of the high fidelity with which DNA methylation is maintained, the silence of most genes on the inactive X is highly stable. Yet, methylated cytosines are "hot spots" of mutation because they can be changed to thymines by deamination,[7] giving rise to the commonest kind of mutations in coding sequences. Such CpG mutations are responsible for many inborn errors of metabolism, polymorphic variations, and somatic mutations leading to cancer. However, the accumulative effect of many methylated CpGs within the island means that single random deaminations have little consequence. For this reason, the locus rarely reactivates spontaneously, and reactivation usually requires manipulation such as cell hybridization, demethylating agents, or the milieu of a cancer cell. This is discussed further below in the "Induced X Reactivation in Placental Cells" section.

We are acquiring knowledge of the process by which CpG islands become methylated on the inactive X, yet remain unmethylated on the active X. Conceivably the islands on the transcriptionally active chromosome are protected from methylation by the presence of the protein complexes involved in transcription. As for the islands on the inactive X, clearly they are methylated only after the chromatin becomes transcriptionally inactive, and there is some evidence that trimethylation of histone H3 (H3K9) may be required for DNA methylation to occur [197]. On the inactive X, the methylation of CpG islands is sufficient, by itself, to *maintain* inactive chromatin, because it inhibits the binding of transcription complexes. It does this by means of at least three methylation binding proteins that selectively bind methylated CpG dinucleotides. These proteins mediate transcriptional repression through interaction with their corepressors, a complex of histone deacetylases that are key players in assembling transcriptional-silencing complexes. One of the methylation-binding proteins is encoded by the *MECP2* gene on the X chromosome. Mutations in this protein cause the syndrome described by Rett (see Rett syndrome, *Appendix A*). Because a deficiency of MeCP2 protein produces a limited range of abnormalities—primarily neurological—it seems that it is needed only to regulate a subset of methylated genes. There must be a good deal of redundancy in this function, so perhaps it is not surprising that *MECP2* mutations do not affect the inactivation status of most genes on the inactive X chromosome.

Although DNA methylation could maintain the silence of the inactive X by itself, it has help in the maintenance process. Some of the components of inactive chromatin serve to reinforce this repression, including the macro H2A1 variant of histone H2A. Enriched in the chromatin of the inactive X, it forms a macro-chromatin body in the nucleus after *Xist* accumulates around the future inactive X. This macro-body is formed even if the *Xist* that accumulates is mutant and incapable of silencing, and it disappears if the *Xist* locus is deleted after inactivation has occurred. *Xist* itself may also have a role in maintaining silence of the inactive

7. The product of deamination of methylated cytosine is thymine, leading to a transition mutation in the next round of replication.

X, as deleting *Xist* in blood cells of mice, although without immediate effect, leads after several months to hematologic malignancies, presumably because of reactivation of X-linked genes [117].

7.3. ESCAPE FROM INACTIVATION

To complicate matters, while inactivation seems to affect the chromosome as a whole, and most genes are silenced, some loci are transcribed from the inactive X. These "escapees" include not only genes in the pseudoautosomal region near the short-arm *telomeres*, but also some genes on the short arm and a few on the proximal long arm of the chromosome [198]. Carrel and Willard [63] published a profile of expression patterns based on an estimated 95% of assayable genes in fibroblast-based test systems.[8] In total, about 15% of X-linked genes escape inactivation to some degree, and the numbers of them in each regions of the X chromosome reflect the evolutionary history of the region. Figure 7-3 shows that they occur predominantly in the pseudoautosomal region of X and Y chromosomes (PAR1), which are transcribed from both sex chromosomes (i.e., *SHOX*; see tables 2-1 and 2-2). Other transcribed genes have homologues elsewhere on the Y chromosome (*ZFX, RPS4X*) or have Y pseudogenes (*STS*), and still others have no homologue in the male (*UBE1*)[9] Some of these genes are recent additions to the mammalian X chromosome, because they are not present on the marsupial X [22]. It has been suggested that the escapees, or genes expressed from the inactive X, are potential contributors to sexually dimorphic traits, to phenotypic variability among females heterozygous for X-linked conditions, and to clinical abnormalities in patients with abnormal X chromosomes. To me, what is even more impressive than the genes that are not fully inactive is the large number of genes that are completely silent. What is also apparent in figure 7-3 is that inactivation is not limited to the X conserved region (XCR). Most genes in the X added region (XAR) are subject to inactivation—often very stable inactivation, evidence that the *XIST* inactivation signal is spread effectively throughout most of the chromosome. As new blocks of genes are added to the X at different times during evolution, they come under the influence of the inactivating machinery.

The first gene shown to be expressed from the inactive X was the *STS* gene [199, 200]. In this case, the allele expressed from the inactive X contributed only about 30–50% of the activity of the normal allele. Less than full expression is not surprising because genes expressed from these regions of the chromosome are often embedded in inactive chromatin. In fact, most genes that escape inactivation are only minimally expressed. Figure 7-4 shows that, with the exception of the pseudoautosomal region (PAR1), most of the genes expressed from the inactive X have *less* than 15% activity. The fact that these alleles on the inactive X are

---

8. Nine hybrid cells with an inactive human X were assayed using RT-PCR. Figure 7–3 shows that, except for genes in PAR1, expression is variable among the various hybrids tested.

9. *UBE1* was lost from the Y chromosome during evolution of the primate lineage.

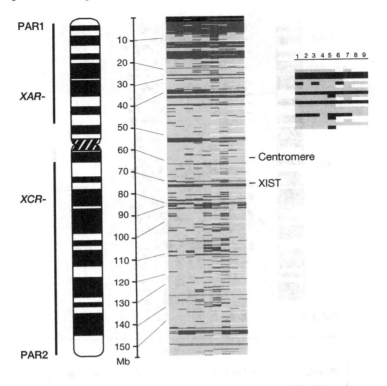

Figure 7-3. Genes that "escape" X inactivation: X inactivation profile of the human X chromosome (624 genes were examined). Pseudoautosomal (PAR1, PAR2), conserved (XCR), and added regions (XAR) of the X chromosome are indicated. Expression based on RNA analysis is shown for nine hybrid cell lines containing a normal inactive X chromosome, and no active X (each hybrid represented by a vertical row). Silent genes are yellow, PAR1 genes are purple, and genes with >5% activity are blue. Untested genes are white. Inset on the right shows the variability in expression among the nine hybrid clones. Adapted from figure 3 of Carrel and Willard [63], with permission of Macmillan Magazines Ltd. [See color plate.]

expressed at all means that many genes are not as dosage sensitive as others and do not need the rigorous control imposed by complete repression. Clearly, the genes that need rigorous control will not be found among those that escape inactivation, having acquired additional means to reinforce the silence process. Tighter controls for such genes would likely be favored by evolution. We must conclude that any leaky expression from the inactive X observed in normal females is not a big problem for them—which is precisely why we see it. And the variation in the expression in these genes may not differ from the extent of variation in the expression of autosomal genes. On the other hand, any extra expression contributed by alleles on the inactive X no doubt explains some of the clinical manifestations of sex chromosome aneuploidies (see chapter 11) and could influence the expression of some common diseases.

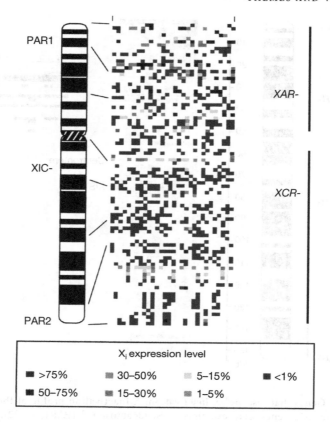

Figure 7-4. **Expression levels of genes that "escape" X inactivation:** expression based on RNA analysis of the inactive X in human fibroblasts, which express the same X in every cell (each sample is represented by a vertical row). Regions of the X are indicated as in figure 7-3. Note: The highest expression levels are seen in genes in PAR1 and the distal XAR. Adapted from figure 2 of Carrel and Willard [63], with permission of Macmillan Magazines Ltd. [See color plate.]

Although a good number of genes seem to be expressed to some extent from the inactive X, the time when these genes escape X inactivation has not been established for any of them. Some expressed genes may be new arrivals on the nonconserved part of the X, and not yet subject to the silencing process. Yet, it has been suggested that escape genes are passed over by the wave of inactivation that silences the chromosome. However, there is little compelling evidence that the inactivating signal skips over any segment of the conserved region of the X chromosome. X inactivation is a means to silence the chromosome as a whole, not in a piecemeal fashion. Even foreign transgenes on the X chromosome are subject to inactivation [187, 251]. Conceivably, there are DNA sequences or structural barriers to DNA or chromatin modifications. Such DNA sequences may have to do with maintenance rather than the spreading of the initial wave of inactivation. Recall that maintenance of the silent state is influenced by the activity status of chromatin domains. Not all genes on the *active* X are programmed to function in all tissues, and silent and functional genes could be separated from one another by boundary elements that separate active from inactive chromatin domains [201]. Escape from inactivation in some cases might be related to a disturbance in the position of such boundary elements caused by the evolutionary inversions in the chromosome. Aberrantly located boundary elements could prevent the propagation of DNA methylation and associated chromatin modifications within the *escape* domains, resulting in failure to maintain stable silencing.

I suggest that many of the genes considered to be escapees were initially inactivated but their inactive state was not well maintained. There is evidence supporting the concept of faulty maintenance; some genes, transcriptionally silent in the embryo, are expressed in the adult [202]. And escape from inactivation, in the few cases studied, is associated with failure to lock in the repressed state (lack of a CpG island in the vicinity of the gene, or hypomethylation of the relevant island; further discussed in chapter 9.2, "Genes That Escape Inactivation").

7.4. TRANSIENT X INACTIVATION IN GERM CELLS

A Developmental Program for X Reactivation Only in Oocytes

Although X inactivation cannot be reversed in somatic cells, it is reversible in germ cells. Studies of mouse oocytes indicate that one of the X chromosomes is inactive in oocyte progenitors before meiosis, but both X chromosomes are active in oocytes during the later stages of oogenesis. I have always wondered how oocytes tolerate having two active X chromosomes, whereas somatic cells cannot. Perhaps oocytes that are nurtured by their neighbors, the follicular cells, express a relatively reduced subset of genes. In any case, the X chromosome that was silenced in migrating primordial germ cells is reactivated in the progeny of these germ cells, close to the time when they initiate meiosis [86, 203]—no doubt to facilitate the pairing of the X chromosomes during meiosis. We know that that both X chromosomes are active in human fetal oocytes because they express the AB heterodimer of *G6PD* [204, 205] (see figure 5-6). Up to now, we know little about the sequence of events responsible for the programmed reversal of X inactivation in female germ cells during their ontogeny. Inactivation in these cells in both mouse and human females is accompanied by low-level *Xist* transcription [114, 125], but not by DNA methylation [210, 207]. It is likely that reactivation in these cells is facilitated because the inactive state is not locked in by DNA methylation [206, 207] or by the histone variants associated with stable X inactivation in somatic cells [203].

Inactivation of the X Chromosome in Male Germ Cells

X inactivation also occurs transiently during the ontogeny of the male gametes. At the pachytene stage of meiosis—which is the time that homologous chromosomes synapse in order to recombine—both X and Y chromosomes form a condensed chromatin domain, called the sex or XY body (see figure 5-5). There are dynamic chromatin changes during meiotic inactivation of the XY body. Studies of histone proteins indicate that inactivation of the XY body is indeed transient, with active chromatin restored to both chromosomes before the end of meiosis [90]. Inactivation of the X and Y chromosomes during spermatogenesis is commonly referred to as meiotic sex chromosome inactivation (MSCI). And *Xist* is expressed during this transient inactivation of the XY body in spermatogonial cells [208]. However, whereas partial disruption of the *Xist* gene on an X chromosome in female mice at the critical time interferes with inactivation, disruption of *Xist* on the X in male mice does not interfere with spermatogenesis [208]. Instead, the XY inactivation seems an adjustment to the lack of an extensive pairing region on the sex chromosome pair. The unpaired or unsynapsed regions of the X and Y are silenced in the same way as unpaired (unsynapsed) regions of meiotic chromosomes throughout the genome [209, 210]. The tumor suppressor protein BRCA1 is implicated in this silencing.[10] Inactivation of the male X chromosome during spermatogenesis may have been the impetus for the evolution of several testis-specific autosomal genes that carry out functions not carried out by the repressed X-linked genes. Phosphoglycerate kinase 2 (PGK2), an active processed retrogene on chromosome 19, expressed only during spermatogenesis, substitutes for PGK1 during its transient silencing during human male meiosis [211].

Epigenetic Reprogramming of the X Chromosome from Somatic Nuclei in Cloned Mice

Somatic cell nuclei can participate in embryogenesis if they are transplanted into the milieu of an oocyte. Procedures such as these have produced relatively small numbers of cloned animals. Cloning of this kind is an inefficient process because the reprogramming of the somatic nucleus does not always recapitulate what is needed for normal development. You may ask what is reprogramming, or, for that matter, what is programming. The developmental program for an individual consists of series of sequential events that are needed to carry out the differentiation of cells and tissues. It requires the coordinated expression of thousands of genes or more to carry out any of these programs. Gene expression depends not only on the transcriptional competency of genes but also on the milieu in which the genes function. Their chromatin is modified to permit the function of these genes at the appropriate times and to inhibit their function in other circumstances. Some of these epigenetic modifications, such as acetylation and ubiquitination, affect the histones of the chromatin, and others such as methylation modify both the histones and the DNA. The somatic cell has its own epigenetic program depending on what tissue it came from and what kind of function it fulfills. Lung cells have different epigenetic programming than skin cells; the two tissues have different DNA methylation patterns and they express different subsets of genes. When a

10. The nucleosomal core histone H2AX is phosphorylated within the XY chromatin domain just prior to MSCI, and this triggers the chromatin condensation and transcriptional repression. The enzyme that carries out this phosphorylation is recruited by BRCA1 at the onset of MSCI.

skin cell is transplanted into a totipotent oocyte, it undergoes epigenetic reprogramming that erases most of the epigenetic marks in its chromatin. It is the faulty epigenetic reprogramming that contributes to lethality of cloned embryos because some of their key developmental genes are inappropriately expressed.

How does the reprogramming of this somatic cell affect the inactivation status of the X chromosome? The chromatin of active and inactive X chromosomes has distinct epigenetic marks in somatic nuclei, and these marks influence their potential transcriptional status. The epigenetic program of the transplanted mouse X chromosomes is modified, but these modifications differ markedly from those that take place in normal embryos, because not all the epigenetic markers present on the chromosome when it was in a somatic cell are erased. Despite the disappearance of *Xist* RNA coating within 30 minutes of transplantation, the epigenetic memory of the inactive X persists in some cells of reprogrammed mouse embryos [212]. Subsequently, *Xist* is reexpressed from the original inactive X, and the silent *Xist* allele on the active X undergoes reactivation, resulting in unusual biallelic *Xist* RNA expression clouds. It seems that somatic-cell–derived embryos are unable to regulate X inactivation consistently, so that some of them have a mixture of cells with varying degrees of inactivation. While abnormal expression of X-linked genes occurs at all stages of clone development, it is clear that normal X inactivation occurs to some degree in these cloned embryos, but not all cells can do it successfully [213]. It is likely that the clones that survive are those that most closely recapitulate the normal program.

Recent attempts to obtain human stem cells by reprogramming human adult somatic cells suggest that the X inactivation status of such cells is also highly variable and unstable because the epigenetic reprogramming is usually incomplete [71, 72]. New techniques need to be developed to get around these limitations.

7.5. INDUCED X REACTIVATION IN PLACENTAL CELLS

X inactivation is extremely stable in human cells, and only fetal germ cells have a developmental program to reverse the process. The long-term silencing is mediated by the methylation of cytosine residues in clustered CpG dinucleotides on the inactive X. So it may not be surprising that a kind of leaky reactivation occurs in undermethylated tissues such as those of marsupials [214] and in placental tissues of humans [215] and mice [216]. In each case, the reactivated gene is not fully expressed. Reactivation of this kind is not associated with global changes in the chromosome; the hallmarks of an inactive X chromosome—late replication and chromosome condensation—are not affected. A similar piecemeal reactivation of one or several genes on the inactive X can be induced by agents that demethylate the relevant CpG islands (the islands within the reactivated genes, or nearby) in cultured somatic cells [217] and hybrid cells [218].

On the other hand, the experimental attempts to induce *global* reversal of X inactivation—of the kind that takes place in germ cells—have generally been unsuccessful. To date, the only human somatic tissue capable of global X reactivation is the placenta, specifically, cells from the chorionic villi (see figure 10-2). Unlike the inactive X in other somatic tissues, the inactive X in cells from term (newborn) placentas can be globally reactivated when the placental cells are hybridized with mouse cells [65]. The reactivated chromosomes are indeed active; they replicate synchronously with human autosomes and fully express genes that are usually silent on inactive X chromosomes: *G6PD*, *HPRT*, *PGK*, and *TIMP*. And this reactivation is associated with repression of the *XIST* gene on that chromosome [219].

The most likely explanation for why placental cells are competent to reverse the process is because they are undermethylated, and therefore the alleles on the poorly methylated inactive X are subject to leaky expression. However, hypomethylation is not enough because, even though placental cells at all stages have undermethylated DNA, not all of them can reverse inactivation. Placental cells from first-trimester *spontaneous* abortions also permit reactivation, but those from first-trimester *elective terminations* do not [220]. These differences in inducibility are not associated with obvious variations in histone H4 acetylation, DNA methylation, or *XIST* expression—hallmarks of the inactivation process—so other factors must have a role. One notable feature is that the reversal-competent cells, unlike the noncompetent ones, have ceased to proliferate *in vivo* and are either beginning or in the process of programmed cell death. Cessation of mitotic proliferation also characterizes oocytes at the stage they undergo X reactivation. Conceivably, along with undermethylation, the apoptotic changes accompanying cessation of cell proliferation contribute to the reversal of inactivation, not only in placental cells but also in oocytes entering meiosis.

7.6. ROLE OF DNA REPLICATION IN X INACTIVATION

The Role of DNA Replication

Until recently, the earliest visible sign that X inactivation had occurred was the asynchronous replication of one of the X chromosomes in female mouse cells [221]—that is, the inactive chromosome is seen first as out of synchrony with its active homologue, either earlier or later, but soon it is out of synchrony with all the other chromosomes, becoming the latest chromosome to begin its DNA synthesis. It replicates so late in the period of DNA synthesis (S phase) that it can be visualized in many cells as the only replicating chromosome in late S phase (see figure 5-4). The prevailing view is that asynchronous replication is a relatively late event in the inactivation process, occurring after the chromatin modifications (see above). However, there is evidence based on a FISH assay[11] (see below) that prior to inactivation in female ES cells, there are differences in the timing of replication of *Xist* and other X-linked alleles [225]. More likely, the initial events make the chromosome transcriptionally inactive, and this in turn alters the time at which

---

11. Recently, replication of X-linked genes has been studied using fluorescent in situ hybridization (FISH) at different stages in the cell cycle (see chapter 5). The use of this assay for the Xist locus has been controversial, because the results conflicted with observations based on other methodology. Because the locus is functional on the inactive X and silent on the active X, one expects that it would replicate earlier on the inactive X than on the active one. In fact, FISH

replication occurs. By virtue of its delayed replication, the inactive X chromosome loses its access to cell-cycle–specific transcription factors, and this modification provides another means to silence or maintain the silence of the chromosome. Replication timing is established locus by locus or chromatin domain by chromatin domain. Late replication is associated with a closed chromatin structure and therefore with repressed genes. When a locus on the inactive X chromosome is induced to reactivate, reactivation is associated with a switch to early (synchronous) replication of the locus [65, 220, 222]. Of interest, the only genes that escape inactivation are those that replicate like active X alleles, earlier in the S phase.

Evidence that delayed replication has a major role in the maintenance of X inactivation comes from studies of the ICF syndrome (see *Appendix A*), caused by a deficiency in one of the *de novo* DNA methyltransferases [196]. Mutations affecting *DNMT3B* are associated with hypomethylation—at times pronounced—of the CpG islands on the inactive X chromosome of affected individuals. Yet, despite the fact that demethylating agents induce reexpression of some silent alleles, many of the unmethylated genes in these individuals remain silent because the gene continues to be late replicating. This is consistent with the proposal that global long-term silencing, once established, can be maintained autonomously through late DNA replication [226]. Therefore, taken together, these observations suggest to me that replication timing is determined by the methylation status of the chromatin domain and not of the individual genes.

7.7. SUMMARY AND SPECULATIONS

Spreading of inactivation along the future inactive X chromosome requires a complex set of interactions between many gene products. The wave of inactivation emanates from the *Xist* locus in the XIC by means of the accumulating *Xist* RNA. These unique transcripts are capable of attracting the factors that actually modify the chromatin environment of the genes. The first changes that occur remove the marks of active chromatin, substituting those of inactive chromatin. These modifications—methylation, deacetylation, and ubiquitination—target lysines in the tails of the histone proteins. Once the critical modifications of histones are induced, they are reinforced by other epigenetic modifications of the DNA; that is, CpG methylation that provides the means for cell memory, and asynchronous DNA replication. And as if this were not enough, other variant proteins are recruited for the maintenance process. Chapter 13 presents further discussion of the phenotypic effect of epigenetic modifications. One can safely speculate that (1) mechanisms that interfere with inactivation will adversely affect embryonic development, and (2) any mutations that lock in this process will have a selective advantage during evolution.

---

assays show that this is true [222, 223]. However, other assays suggest the opposite is true [224]. It has been suggested that the FISH assay, which has been accurate for all other loci analyzed, cannot be used for XIST. The explanation is that the XIST region may have an unusual structure that invalidates the FISH assay.

8

Variations 1

The X Inactivation Center

In stating her hypothesis, Mary Lyon clearly implied that X inactivation was a general mechanism shared by most mammals. Yet, based on the abundant evidence of evolutionary tinkering, we should expect that the details of the inactivation process might differ among mammals. Nonetheless, because most of the recent experimental evidence comes from manipulating mouse embryos and embryonic stem cells, findings in the mouse have been considered to apply to all mammals. What has not been appreciated enough is that the process of X inactivation itself has been subject to its own evolution, resulting in many variations on the common themes. Because so few species of worms and flies have been studied, we do not know how much interspecies variation has occurred in their mechanisms of dosage compensation.

No doubt, the observed differences in the details of X inactivation among mammals are attributable to the considerable species differences in the staging of events during embryogenesis. By this, I mean the time of onset and the relationship to other developmental events occurring simultaneously—for example, the time between fertilization and the choice of active X. It is likely that innovations in the details of X dosage compensation were acquired during mammalian evolution to reinforce the basic themes. Such modifications were needed to accommodate the species differences in the timing of interacting developmental events (see chapter 10.6, "Effect of Inactivation Timing"). The important thing to remember is that any modifications observed today are those that survived because they did not interfere with our single active X. The problem is that modifications found in one species may not be recognized as variations, and may be interpreted more broadly than they deserve. Therefore, in this and the next chapter, I will try to distinguish the major players from the supporting ones as a means of identifying the essential molecular mechanisms, which I consider the basic themes.

8.1. VARIATIONS ON THE THEMES OF X INACTIVATION

Because X inactivation is the means of dosage compensation used only by mammals, and because much of the X chromosome has been conserved in eutherian mammals, it is almost certain that the mechanisms responsible for the single active X are the same for most of them. Yet, some features of the process differ among species—even among tissues of an individual. The major differences have to do with whether X inactivation is imprinted or random (discussed in chapter 10) and the stability of the inactive state (discussed in chapter 9) and even the role players (discussed in this chapter). Underlying such variations are differences in the physical map of the X inactivation center (XIC) region, temporal differences in the onset of developmental events, and of course, the role of tinkering in the evolution of biological processes [37, 155, 227] (see chapter 10.5, "Evolution and Tinkering"). Because X dosage compensation is an essential developmental program, such changes eliminate or add elements that modify, but do not meddle with, the indispensable components of the program. Instead, many of the species and tissue variations that we observe reinforce the essential program, adapting it to the special needs of the organism. Such variation adds complexity and nuance to the system, and it is also useful to experimentalists. Because the species lacking particular features can be considered mutants, species differences can be used to probe the molecular basis of the features that differ.

8.2. DIVERGENCE IN THE PHYSICAL MAP

Originally defined based on X autosome translocations, the XIC in both species was further delineated using transgenes to determine how much of the DNA in the region was needed to mediate inactivation of the autosome in which it inserted. The results indicate that approximately 80 kb is needed in mice [101] and no more than 480 kb in humans [70]. One needs to keep this in mind because more genes are now included in the region designated as the XIC than may be needed to inactivate a chromosome.

The XIC region, as currently defined in humans and mice (see figure 8-1 and table 8-1), is delimited by several X-linked protein coding genes (*NAP1L2*, *CDX4*, *CHIC1*, *CNBP2*, and *SLC16A2*) that have no apparent role in X dosage compensation. In fact, in most cases their function is not well defined and they are known only by their transcripts. More relevant is the group of noncoding RNAs, including *XIST* and its antisense homolog *TSIX* in both species (table 8-1).

According to Ohno [1], X-linked genes remained on the X chromosome, and were not distributed among several chromosomes during extensive mammalian speciation, in order not to perturb the mechanisms responsible for dosage compensation. Without knowledge of the DNA sequence and extensive comparative genomic studies that have been carried out recently, Ohno thought the conservation of the mammalian X chromosome was greater than it actually is. Now, we know that the content of the X chromosome and linear order of its genes differs considerably from one mammal to another, because innumerable translocations and inversions have occurred during their evolution. Nonetheless, Ohno was right about the need to maintain mechanisms of dosage compensation; clearly, any changes in DNA sequence that we observe today were permitted because they did not perturb dosage compensation. Such variations arise in part because of the random changes in the DNA blueprints, and they persist because they improve or at least do not interfere with essential processes. For example, duplication of gene function in one species permits them to eliminate genes that are still needed in other species.

Studies of loci on the X and Y chromosomes suggest that the heterochromatization of both chromosomes is an ongoing process—induced in response to a functional loss of homologous genes on the Y chromosome and new additions to the X. Therefore, perhaps it is not surprising that even the physical map of the XIC region differs among mammals [103, 107], reflecting the occurrence of microdeletions and inversions within this region. Such rearrangements change the orientation of some genes and eliminate others. In addition, there is evidence of invasion by dispersed repetitive DNA [107], and this has led to a major expansion of the human XIC region from that on the mouse X chromosome (figure 8-1). Also, the *SLC16A2* gene (also called *Xpct* in the mouse) that is within 800 kb of *Xist* has undergone an inversion so that its orientation differs on mouse and human X chromosomes (figure 8-1). In addition, other genes that neighbor *Xist* are functional in one species but are pseudogenes in another. These include the protein-coding *Ppnx* gene and the *Tsx* gene (within 100 kb of 3′ *Xist*), which are transcribed in the mouse and rat but are nonfunctional pseudogenes in humans [107, 153]. *TSX*, the human version of the mouse *Tsx* gene, has lost all but two exons, which are widely separated by interspersed DNA repeat sequences. In addition, extremely close to 5′ *Xist* in both species is a pseudogene of *Fxyd6*, a member of the large ion transport family (figure 8-1).

An important species difference in the physical map has to do with the *Tsix* locus, which is antisense to mouse *Xist* and inhibits expression of the maternal *Xist* allele in mouse placental tissue [131, 137, 138]. The human *TSIX* gene, starting <50 kb from *XIST*, is an expressed pseudogene, unable to repress *XIST* [153, 67] (considered further in chapter 10.4, "Does Antisense Transcription Have a Role?"). However, while the evolutionary change in *TSIX* interferes with its antisense function, it has not disrupted the function of *XIST*. In fact, none of the rearrangements in the region interferes with *cis* X inactivation or choice of active X.

Even the *Xist* locus itself has undergone evolutionary changes. What has been conserved is the overall organization of the gene, with some regions of considerable homology, including promoter region and the exon–intron boundaries. Both mouse and human genes have eight exons, but the intron–exon structure is not totally the same, nor is the DNA sequence itself. According to Chureau et al. [103], at the sequence level, *Xist* exons show an average identity of 66% (mouse vs. human) and 62% (mouse vs. bovine)—a figure close to the average conservation in *untranslated* (non-exon) regions of human and mouse analogous protein-coding genes. With the exception of a few blocks, *Xist* introns are weakly conserved. Although most protein-coding genes are generally rich in LINE (Long INterspersed Elements) repetitive sequences, the *Xist* gene in mouse, human, and bovine is relatively devoid of them, suggesting that insertion of LINE sequences

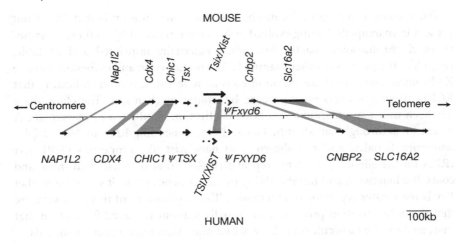

Figure 8-1. Diagram comparing the human and mouse XIC, showing known genes, and the expansion of the XIC in human relative to mouse. The human genes are in the region from 72–73.5 MB on the human X map, and the mouse genes reside in the region from 97.7 – 98.4 MB on the mouse X (http://genome.ucsc.edu). Note: The *Xist* and *Tsix* transcripts overlap each other in both species. Yet, they differ in initiation sites and extent of overlap (see figure 10-5). Also, *TSX*, the human counterpart of mouse *Tsx*, is disrupted [153], and the *Xite* element (*) has been identified only in the mouse [144]. Also note, the inversion in the *Slc16a2* gene. Incredibly close to *Xist* in both species is a pseudogene for *Fxyd6*. For clarity, ubiquitously expressed untranslated transcripts (*Jpx* and *Ftx*) [103] that map between *Xist and Cnbp2* in both species have been omitted, but actual map positions are shown in table 8-1. Courtesy of Iain McIntosh.

has been strongly counterselected. However, sequence divergence has not otherwise been constrained. The relatively low level of sequence homology among mammalian *Xist* genes suggests that its modus operandi must depend more on its secondary structure than on its DNA sequence. This idea is supported by the fact that despite poor conservation of the DNA sequence, a human *XIST* transgene can initiate X inactivation in male mice [70].

To add some perspective, comparing the degree of evolutionary tinkering among primates across the past 80 million years, the changes in the *Xist* gene are relatively small compared to those in the region around *Xist* [430].

Yet, a major variation in the mechanisms of X inactivation is that *Xist* is not present in marsupials, having evolved only in eutherians [109]. In these metatherians, X chromosome inactivation, albeit paternally imprinted and unstable, resembles the process in other mammals. The metatherian and eutherian inactive X chromosomes also share common epigenetic features, further indicating that XCI in these mammals must proceed by similar mechanisms. Therefore, there has been much speculation about how inactivation is initiated in marsupials. A recent breakthrough has identified a candidate noncoding RNA in *Monodelphis domestica* females, and has shown it to have *Xist* like properties [228]. *Rsx* (RNA-on-the-silent X) is a large repeat-rich RNA that is transcribed from, and coats, the inactive X and has the ability to silence genes *in cis*. It seems likely that *Rsx* is the master regulator in marsupials. The implications of this discovery are that the X inactivation process arose initially without the need for *Xist*. In that case, an *Xist*-like molecule must have arisen more than once among mammals.

8.3. THE EFFECT OF MAP CHANGES ON X INACTIVATION IN MOUSE AND HUMAN

Some of the physical changes within the XIC are likely to affect the way dosage compensation is carried out, and how the developmental process is initiated.

Table 8-1 compares the genetic elements within the X inactivation center of mouse and man. The differences between these elements reflect the species differences in the physical map of the XIC. Evolutionary changes that increased the size of the XIC in humans have at the same time eliminated two genes (*XITE* and *XCE*)[1] that have key functions in X inactivation in mice and made pseudogenes of two other genes (*TSX* & *TSIX*) [153].

In the mouse *Tsix* is the key repressor of *Xist* in ES cells and placental tissues. Expressed from the maternal X in placental tissue, it serves to repress *Xist* transcription from that chromosome. By repressing *Xist*, *Tsix* ensures that the maternal X-linked alleles will be expressed in every cell. Even though human *TSIX* is truncated, it is transcribed. In contrast to mouse *Tsix*, which is expressed from the *active* X *briefly* during the narrow window when inactivation occurs, the human *TSIX* transcripts emanate only from the *inactive* X, along with *XIST* transcripts, and are synthesized in the fetus, *throughout gestation* until shortly after birth. Not only do I wonder what these truncated transcripts could possibly contribute to the inactivation process, but also why they *cease* to be transcribed after birth. It may be that human *TSIX* is a run-off transcript, which is induced initially by some chromatin modification in the XIC, coincident with the up-regulation of *XIST* on the future inactive X and its transcription in the region helps increase the expression of *XIST*. In this case, one expects that some additional chromatin remodeling in the region turns off the *TSIX* transcripts after birth.

---

1. Ogawa and Lee [144] propose that *Xite* is the best candidate for the *Xce* locus, the classical modifier of the X chromosome inactivation ratios in several mouse species.

Table 8-1. GENETIC ELEMENTS WITHIN THE X INACTIVATION CENTER OF MAN AND MOUSE

Genes and Human Map Site[a] (Centromere–Telomere)	Description	XCI Function	Functional in Mouse	Functional in Man
NAPIL2 72432137–72434710[b]	Nucleosome assembler	None known	Yes	Transcript[b]
CDX4 72667090–72674421	Homeobox transcription factor	None known	Yes	Transcript
CHIC1 72782984–72906937	Cystein-rich hydrophobic domain	None known	Transcript	Transcript
TSX	Non coding RNA in testes & brain	None known	Yes	Pseudogene
XITE	Noncoding enhancer	Tsix regulator	Yes	Not found
XCE	Noncoding element	Skews XCI ratios	Yes	Not found
TSIX 73012040–73049066	Noncoding RNA	Xist repressor	Yes	Truncated transcript
XIST 73040495–73072588	Noncoding RNA	Chromatin silencer	Yes	Yes
JPX 73164159–73290217	Noncoding RNA	Xist regulatory switch	Yes	Transcript, untested
FTX 73247971–73513409	Noncoding RNA with micro-RNAs	Xist activator	Yes	Outside XIC, untested
CNBP2 (ZCCHC13) 73524025–73524869	Zinc finger protein	None known	Transcript, in testes	Transcript, in testes
XPCT (SLC16A2) 73744194–73753752	Solute transporter	None known	Yes	Yes
RNF12 (RLIM) 73802811–73834461	E3 ubiquitin ligase	Xist activator	Yes	Outside XIC, untested

[a] Map location of element on the human X in kilobases.
[b] Although the human protein coding genes are present by sequence data and homology, little is known of their function, if any, in human cells. Adapted from table 1 in Migeon [155].

Clearly, human *TSIX* is not the repressor of *XIST* in human cells. In fact, it is co-expressed with *XIST* from the *inactive* X in female fetal cells [67]. Chang and Brown studied the human XIC region in mouse embryonic stem cells and found that human *TSIX* lacks the regulatory elements found in mouse *Tsix*, lending further support to the argument that *TSIX* is not a regulator of human *XIST* [229]. They did identify some DNAse-hypersensitive sites upstream of *Xist*, implying other possible regulatory elements; these sites show conservation of human with other eutheria, but not with mice. All the evidence indicates that in human fetal cells *TSIX* does not repress *XIST* expression. We see that changes in the XIC that occurred during the evolution of mouse and man have influenced some details of the inactivation process. To my knowledge a functional *Tsix* gene has been identified only in rodents. I have previously proposed that *Tsix* repression of *Xist* is a unique feature of X inactivation in mice [230] but it seems that rats and voles also have a functional *Tsix* gene [145] so that it seems to be a special feature of X inactivation in rodents. We and other eutherians may use other X-linked genes to repress *XIST in cis* (see *XACT* later in this section). However we have not yet identified a *trans* gene(s) to repress *XIST* on the future active X.

Comparing the Gene Content of Human and Mouse X Inactivation Centers

Whereas *XIST* is the only gene thus far within the human XIC that is known to be essential to our mechanism of dosage compensation, several potential role players have been identified within the mouse XIC. We have already considered the roles of mouse *Xist* and *Tsix*. Table 8-1 shows that the master control region of human and mouse X chromosomes contain other noncoding elements. The content differs because the *Xite* and *Xce* noncoding elements have not been found in the human XIC or elsewhere in our genome. *Xite* and *Xce* may be one and the same [144]. In the mouse these elements regulate *Tsix* and skew XCI ratios, respectively.

There are two noncoding genes, namely *Jpx* and *Ftx*, that are present upstream of *Xist* on both mouse and human X chromosomes. Because they are upregulated on both X chromosomes at the time that ES cells differentiate, and partially escape X inactivation, both genes are thought to have a role in inactivating the mouse X chromosome. Some suggest that they activate *Xist in cis* by generating a transcriptionally active environment that spans *Xist* and flanking genes. Others like Tian et al. [231] propose that in the mouse *Jpx* is the switch that up-regulates *Xist* on the inactive X chromosome. The function of human *JPX*, which lies 90 kb upstream of *XIST*, remains to be seen. A noncoding RNA like *JPX* could play some role in the *XIST* up-regulation process, as part of the default pathway that silences future inactive X chromosomes.

The noncoding *Ftx* RNA is also thought to have a role in activating mouse *Xist* [232]. Less than a third of the exons of mouse *Ftx* are conserved in the human genome. Included within the gene in both genomes is a set of micro RNAs of unknown function, which differ somewhat in the two species. Of interest, human *FTX* lies outside of the limits of the human XIC [154].

The only protein-coding gene within the mouse XIC considered to have a role in X inactivation is *Rnf12*, an E3 ubiquitin ligase that regulates activities of different classes of transcription factors. In the mouse it seems to target the pluripotent factor *Rex1* for proteosomal degradation, which in turn up-regulates *Xist*. Residing 500 kb upstream of mouse *Xist*, *Rnf12* is the oft-mentioned candidate for the gene that counts the number of X chromosomes in the cell to determine how many to inactivate [129, 233]. When overexpressed in mouse ES cells, it induces ectopic initiation of *Xist* transcripts in male cells and *Xist* transcripts from both X chromosomes in female cells. Therefore, it can act in *trans* as well as *cis*. What is proposed is that the number of inactive Xs is determined by the number of expressing *Rnf12* loci. It is not yet known if the role of Rnf12 is limited to the imprinted X inactivation in early mouse embryos [234] As for the human *RNF12* gene, it resides 760 kb from *XIST*—outside the limits of the XIC, as defined by cytogenetic studies [154a]. Of course it could still play a role in X inactivation, but there is no means to test it's function in human cells at this time.

Whereas several genes within the mouse XIC seem to participate in the X inactivation process, *XIST* is the only gene known thus far within the human XIC to have a role in our mechanism of dosage compensation. The ban against the study of early human embryos, along with the fact that most of the human embryonic stem cells currently available have already finished their inactivation process, has made it difficult to test some of candidate genes within our XIC. However, based on differences already observed in the physical map of the XIC, we should not expect that regulators of *XIST* will be the same as in mice, nor that they need to lie within the human XIC.

XACT, a Long Noncoding Transcript Coating the Active X in Human Pluripotent Cells

We are increasingly aware of long (>200bp) non coding RNAs, the biggest class of RNAs that do not code for proteins. Xist was among the first to be discovered. Now, thousands of them have been annotated in the human transcriptome, The dozen or so that have been assigned a function seem to regulate transcription, either as activators or silencers. But, we know little of the vast majority of them. Recent studies suggest that some have evolved rapidly, and have been used as fodder for evolution. A novel development in the saga of our own mechanisms of X dosage compensation is the recent discovery of *XACT*, a very long noncoding RNA that is expressed from the human X chromosome, yet, surprisingly not from the XIC [235]. Synthesized from Xq23, between the protein coding genes, angiomotin (*AMOT*), and the hydrotryptamine receptor, *HTR2C*, this 251 kb unspliced transcript is transcribed from and coats the active X in female human embryonic stem (HES) cells that express *XIST*.

In female HES cells that do not express *XIST*, the *XACT* locus is bi-allelically transcribed, forming an *Xist*-like cloud over both X chromosomes. The same transcript coats the active X in male ES cells (C. Rougeulle. personal communication, July 2, 2013). Examination of several differentiated human tissues shows that *XACT* expression and its ability to coat the active X is restricted to pluripotent and early-differentiating cells [235].

Like *Tsix*, whose function seems to be limited to rodents, *XACT* has only recently evolved. Although the *Amot* and *Htr2c* genes are present in many mammals, the 5′LTR that corresponds to the promoter of *XACT* is present only in humans and chimpanzee, and not in macaques or more distally related species [235]. Therefore, *XACT* resembles mouse *Tsix* in being expressed from the active X chromosome for a short time during early differentiation, and it may contribute to protecting the active X from inactivation. Whether *XACT* coating of the active X is a cause or consequence of *XIST* repression remains to be seen. In any case, because like *Tsix* in rodents, it is an X-linked gene, and not present in most mammals, *XACT* may not be "the" *Xist* repressor that is involved in the initial choice of active X.

8.4 SUMMARY AND SPECULATIONS

Our accumulating knowledge of evolutionary mechanisms informs us to expect species differences in all developmental processes. Here we have considered variations on the theme of X inactivation, attributable to changes in the physical map of the inactivation center—some mediated by chance rearrangements and invasion of repetitive elements. Some of these changes eliminate genes in the human XIC that play a role in inactivating X chromosomes of mice. The loss of genes in one species that function in another suggests that some steps were no longer required, or were never needed, and therefore could be eliminated. In any case, they reflect species differences in the process. Surprisingly, we see that the noncoding RNA that serves as master regulator of the silencing process has evolved more than once during mammalian evolution. We also see that some rapidly evolving noncoding RNAs, like *Tsix* and perhaps *XACT,* can be pressed into service as species-specific reinforcers of developmental programs. Yet another remarkable example of evolutionary tinkering!

9

Variations 2

Stability of the Inactive X

Among the variable features of X inactivation is the stability of the inactive X. As discussed in chapter 7, the silence of genes on the inactive X is well maintained in the evolutionarily conserved region of human and mouse X chromosomes. Once inactivated, most of these genes remain silent through many cell divisions for the life of the individual, and they are not expressed in cultured cells established from these tissues. Although we know from markers of active chromatin (e.g., acetylated histone H4) that distinguish active from inactive X that most of the chromatin of the silent X is transcriptionally inactive, transcription studies of individual genes reveal some exceptions. The most prominent exception is the block of genes in the pseudoautosomal region PAR1 that remain active because these genes have active homologues on the Y chromosome. PAR1 genes are freely exchanged between X and Y chromosomes. Other exceptions are genes that are located mainly on the short arm of the X, and these expressed genes are referred to as genes that "escape" inactivation (see section 7.3, "Escape from Inactivation"). It is important to remember that the expression level of such genes is much reduced from that of their allele on the active X (figure 7-4), reflecting the fact that such genes are being expressed from heterochromatin. Of interest, most of the mouse counterparts of these escapees are completely silent on the mouse inactive X. Also, some genes that are stably inactivated in human adult tissues are inappropriately expressed in placental tissues [215]. And in striking contrast to human and mouse genes, most of the marsupial genes that have been analyzed are transcribed to some degree from the inactive X in some tissues [22]. In the case of these marsupial genes, this small amount of expression *in vivo* is dramatically up-regulated when cells are grown *in vitro*, and the silenced genes become fully active within a couple of subcultures [238]. Clearly, there are many species and tissue differences in the inactivation status of genes on the inactive X.

However, leaky X inactivation does not mean that these genes fail to be inactivated at onset. More likely, the expressed genes in the conserved portion of the inactive X were initially silenced but could not completely maintain their transcriptional repression. Evidence to support this hypothesis comes from studies of a few such escape genes. In fact, it is the study of loci that are usually subject to inactivation but are expressed in some tissues—or at some times but not always— that have helped define the role of DNA methylation in X inactivation.

9.1 STABILITY OF INACTIVATION AND DNA METHYLATION

Although DNA methylation was originally considered to be *the* mechanism for initiating the silence of the inactive X [174], it is now known to play its role only after gene repression has occurred [179, 214]. Therefore, DNA methylation is not the primary inactivator, but serves in most cells and at most loci as a cell memory device to lock in the silence of the locus once inactivated. Yet, inactive X chromosomes are not entirely silent and are not silent in all kinds of cells. All the available evidence tells us that this loss of memory is related either to lack of CpG islands within the gene's chromatin domain, or to undermethylation of the relevant CpG islands.

Early studies of X-linked housekeeping genes showed that the methylation of CpG islands occurs only after the onset of inactivation [239] and does not occur in inactivated marsupial genes [214], suggesting that DNA methylation was not needed to initiate inactivation but served to lock it in once it occurs [214, 240]. There is abundant evidence that DNA methylation of CpG islands is required for the stable maintenance of X inactivation. Demethylating agents such as 5-azacytidine are capable of reactivating genes on the inactive X [218]. Reactivation is piecemeal, reflecting the localized chromatin domain that is influenced by any specific demethylating event. Therefore, either a single gene or a group of neighboring genes within the chromatin domain may be derepressed [241]. There is little doubt that the leaky expression from alleles on the marsupial inactive X is due to the unmethylated status of CpG islands [214, 242]. This also explains why inactivation of marsupial genes is not well maintained in cell culture, as in this milieu, the levels of expression from the inactive X rapidly approach that of the active X [238]. In contrast, most genes on the human inactive X consistently maintain their silence during proliferation *in vitro* because it is locked in by DNA methylation. The extensive hypomethylation of CpG islands in human placental tissues [217, 243] also explains the extensive leaky expression in this tissue.

Dan Driscoll and I [206] showed that the CpG islands in human female germ cells have very little if any DNA methylation prior to the time when meiosis is initiated; the lack of such a lock-in device facilitates the complete reversal of X inactivation that is programmed to occur during the ontogeny of oocytes. In the same way, the undermethylated DNA of human male germ cells [206] facilitates the programmed reversibility of the inactive X during transient inactivation in spermatogenesis [244]. Unlike all other somatic cells, the chorionic villi of the human placenta can reverse X inactivation when hybridized with mouse cells. No doubt it is the extensive hypomethylation of CpG islands on the inactive X chromosome in these placental cells that makes them permissive for reversal of X inactivation [65] (see section 7.5, "Induced X Reactivation in Placental Cells").

9.2. GENES THAT ESCAPE INACTIVATION

As you now know, some X-linked genes are expressed from the inactive X (Figure 7-3). Characteristically, the level of expression of genes from the inactive X ranges from 5- >50% of normal activity depending on the permissiveness of their chromatin environment (Figure 7-4). A consistent feature of such escape genes in adult somatic cells is insufficient CpG island methylation. The CpG islands in the genes expressed from the PAR1 pseudoautosomal region are unmethylated [245, 246]. Also, not all X-linked genes have CpG islands in their promoter region or even in their neighborhood. One leaky human gene is *steroid sulfatase* [199], which has no CpG island, and its promoter is cytosine–guanine poor [247]. Compared to genes that are well inactivated, those that escape X inactivation have fewer CpG islands, particularly within the 2 kb upstream flanking sequence close to the promoter region. It seems that if the means to lock in inactivation is not available, then the locus may be reexpressed.

On the other hand genes on the inactive X, like the *F9* gene in liver cells, whose expression on the active X is limited to one tissue must have another means of repression, as there are no CpG islands anywhere in the vicinity of the gene [248].

The molecular mechanisms of escape are not well understood. It has been suggested that the distribution of LINE-1 repeat elements or DNA sequence motifs may be important factors. Some escape genes are depleted in long terminal repeats or adenine-thymine-rich repeats, or have insulator elements, like CTCF, that interfere with the transmission of the inactivating signal [249]. Yet, because X inactivation is a global event affecting the chromosome as a whole, it is unlikely that these genes were singled out to escape the wave of inactivation when it first occurred. There is no compelling evidence that the inactivating signal skips over any segment of the conserved region of the X chromosome. The fact that most genes in the XAR are stably silenced (see figure 7-3) shows that even newly added genes are not silenced one by one but come under the influence of the global silencing mechanism.

Evidence implicating poor maintenance of inactivation in "escape" genes comes from studies of the murine lysine-specific demethylase 5C gene (formerly called *Smcx* and *Jarid1C*). In this case the escape from inactivation is associated with initial inactivation but subsequent reactivation during embryonic development [202]. And the fact that a gene can escape inactivation in one tissue but remain fully silenced in another argues against the possibility of architectural deterrents to inactivation at onset.

Even transgenes on the X chromosome are subject to inactivation. Chong et al. [187] showed that during mouse embryogenesis a transgene containing active chromatin from a chicken (the entire chicken lysosome gene domain) is silenced when that chromosome is the inactive X, but not when on the active X. Similar studies were carried out with transgenes from the chicken beta globin locus containing a chromatin boundary element with a CTCF binding site. Insertion of CTCF binding sites into the mouse inactive X—in an attempt to insulate the transgene from inactivation—did not prevent silencing of the transgene. On the inactive X chromosome, both the insulator and transgene were almost completely methylated in contrast to the unmethylated status of the same transgene on the active X [251]. It is possible that some features of the DNA sequence in addition to the lack of CpG islands may characterize escape genes, but I expect that such features will influence maintenance of repression rather than confer resistance to the initial wave of *Xist*-induced inactivation.

Genes Expressed from the Inactive X Do Not Require Rigorous Dosage Control

If expressing two X chromosomes is so deleterious, why are some genes expressed from the inactive X chromosome in normal females? The answer is that not all genes need to be rigorously dosage compensated. Strict maintenance of the inactive state seems to be less important for marsupials than for eutherians, because the inactive paternal X is expressed to some extent in many of their tissues. And compensation is less essential in human placental tissues, which are discarded after birth, than in the embryo proper. Another important factor is the level of transcription of most of these escape genes. Alleles transcribed from the conserved region of the inactive X usually produce significantly fewer transcripts than do their homologous alleles on the active X [63, 200]. Most likely, genes are poorly expressed from the inactive X because they are being transcribed from a chromatin domain that is relatively repressed. With regard to the significance of this leakiness to cellular function, the extra expression in the cells is usually <15% greater than if the genes were completely repressed, and this is likely to be within the range of tolerable variation for such genes. I expect that the range of expression of alleles at autosomal loci—when it is adequately examined—will be just as variable. The fact that we observe a subset of genes that are expressed to some degree from the inactive X tells us that such expression is not detrimental and has little selective disadvantage; in fact, in some cases unmethylated CpG islands, or disruption of CpG islands in X-linked genes, may have been favored during evolution, as a means of increasing transcriptional activity of specific genes.

On the other hand, it is likely that even minimal expression of genes on the inactive X may have some undesired phenotypic effect. Such extra gene product may explain the detrimental effects of chromosomal aneuploidy in individuals with 45,X Turner syndrome, 47,XXY syndrome, and 47,XXX syndromes. Even if minimal, the transcripts from escape genes may contribute to excessive expression of the locus. Conceivably, even a small excess of gene expression might be responsible for some common disorders, especially those attributable to the collaborative effect of several variant genes.

In addition, escape genes also have the potential to ameliorate the deleterious phenotypic effects of some X-linked diseases in females. It is likely that human females heterozygous for mutations in the X-linked gene responsible for orofaciodigital syndrome type 1 (see chapter 12 and *Appendixes A* and *C*) are protected to some extent by the small amount of protein produced from the normal allele on their inactive X. As a consequence, these affected heterozygotes have much milder renal disease than their mouse counterparts, whose analogous gene on the inactive X is completely silent. Not having an escape gene, all the heterozygous mice are born with polycystic kidneys and survive only a short time after birth.

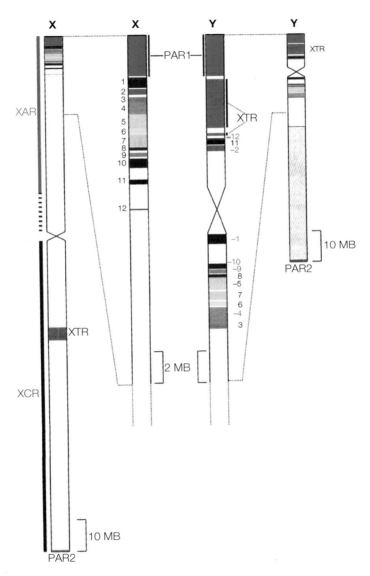

Figure 2-6. The human X and Y chromosomes, showing the location of homologous genes. The entire X and Y are shown using the same scale on the right and left sides of the figure, with expanded views in the center. The colored segments on X and Y show the position of homologous genes on the two sex chromosomes. The red numbers along the Y chromosome indicate that the segment is inverted with respect to the X. Adapted from Ross et al. [30], figure 6, with permission.

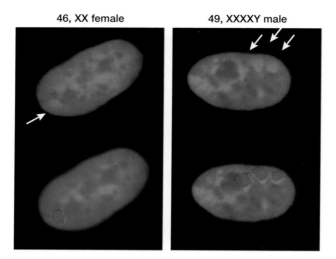

Figure 3-3. Barr bodies in interphase nuclei from a normal human female (left) and from a 4XY male (right) with one and three inactive X chromosomes, respectively. Top, DAPI stain; bottom, *XIST* RNA (red). Arrows show the position of the Barr body in DAPI-stained cells, which is difficult to visualize. Note that the Barr body is almost completely covered by *XIST* RNA, the silencing noncoding RNA in cells of eutherian mammals.

Xp

14q

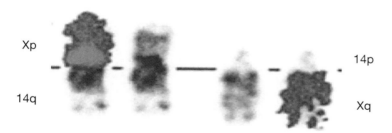

14p

Xq

Figure 5-3. Translocation between chromosomes X and 14 (X/14 translocation), shown by "painting" the X chromosome. The break in both chromosomes occurred near the centromere. Shown are the two translocation chromosomes either banded with Giemsa or painted with X chromosome unique DNA (red). The positions of short (p) and long (q) arms of both X and 14 are indicated. Adapted from figure 1D of Morrison and Jeppesen [423], with permission.

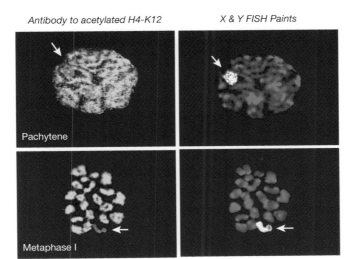

Antibody to acetylated H4-K12   **X & Y FISH Paints**

Figure 5-5. XY inactivation during spermatogenesis. The chromatin of the X and Y chromosomes is repressed during spermatogenesis. Left: Chromosomes from mouse cells, at pachytene and metaphase I stages, labeled with an antibody to acetylated histone H4–K12 (green label indicates acetylation). Repressed chromosome regions are red (unlabeled). Right: Same cells labeled by X (pink) and Y (aqua) FISH chromosome paint to identify the sex chromosomes. Note: X and Y (arrows) are underacetylated (red) from pachytene to round spermatid stage. Photomicrographs courtesy of Ahmad Khalil and Daniel Driscoll.

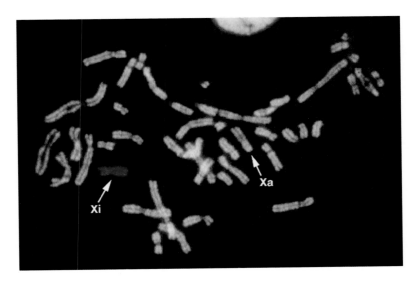

Figure 6-2. The inactive X has unacetylated histone H4: metaphase spread from a human female, labeled by an antibody to acetylated histone H4 (green), showing that the active X (Xa) is labeled (green) whereas the inactive X (Xi) is unlabeled (red because it lacks sufficient acetylated H4). Photomicrograph courtesy of Peter Jeppesen.

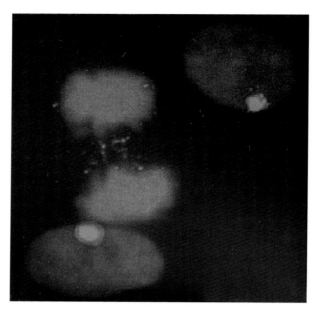

Figure 6-6. *XIST* RNA coats the human inactive X chromosome in adult fibroblasts, except in mitosis. Shown is the FISH analysis of human fibroblasts labeled with an *XIST* DNA probe that hybridized to *XIST* RNA. The RNA that coats the Barr body in interphase disappears from the chromosome when the cell divides, and then reforms by new transcription. This may not occur in mouse cells [118]. Photomicrograph from figure 9E of Clemson et al. [425], with permission.

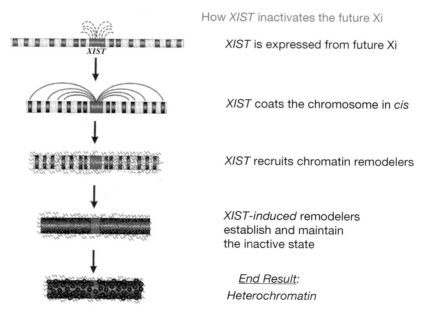

Figure 6-7. Diagram showing how Xist RNA inactivates the future inactive X (Xi). Adapted from figure 5 of Avner and Heard [167], reproduced with permission from *Nature Reviews Genetics*, 2001, Macmillan Magazines Ltd.

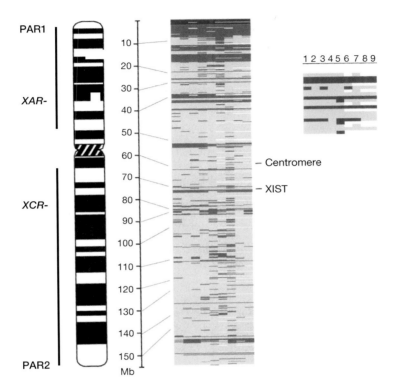

Figure 7-3. Genes that "escape" X inactivation: X inactivation profile of the human X chromosome (624 genes were examined). Pseudoautosomal (PAR1, PAR2), conserved (XCR), and added regions (XAR) of the X chromosome are indicated. Expression based on RNA analysis is shown for nine hybrid cell lines containing a normal inactive X chromosome, and no active X (each hybrid represented by a vertical row). Silent genes are yellow, PAR1 genes are purple, and genes with >5% activity are blue. Untested genes are white. Inset on the right shows the variability in expression among the nine hybrid clones. Adapted from figure 3 of Carrel and Willard [63], with permission of Macmillan Magazines Ltd.

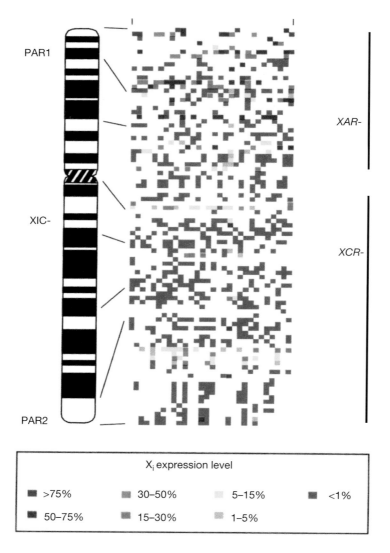

Figure 7-4. Expression levels of genes that "escape" X inactivation: expression based on RNA analysis of the inactive X in human fibroblasts, which express the same X in every cell (each sample is represented by a vertical row). Regions of the X are indicated as in figure 7-3. Note: The highest expression levels are seen in genes in PAR1 and the distal XAR. Adapted from figure 2 of Carrel and Willard [63], with permission of Macmillan Magazines Ltd.

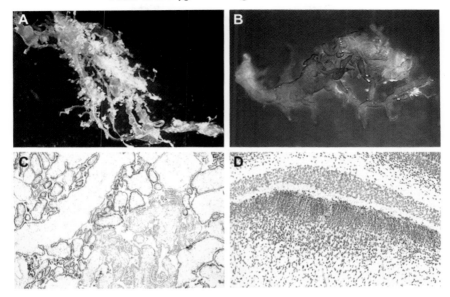

chorionic villi (A-C) and brain (D)

Figure 10-3. Random inactivation in the chorionic villi of the human placenta: tissues from a placenta (A–C) and brain (D) heterozygous for the fragile X mutation (*FMR1*). The *FMR1* protein is stained brown. The villi expressing the mutant X are unstained. Note: Both mutant and normal villi are present, as seen grossly (A and B) and in microscopic sections (C). There is closer commingling of the two kinds of cells in the brain (D), where the patch size is smaller. From figure 2 of Willemsen et al. [260], with permission.

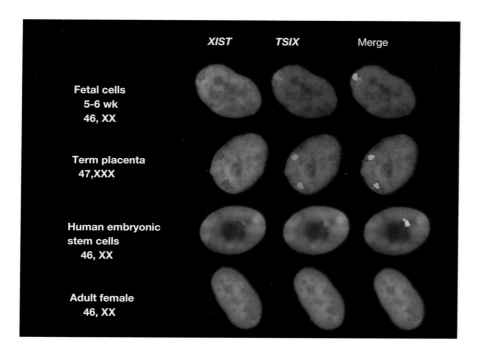

Figure 10-6. Human *TSIX* is coexpressed with *XIST* from the inactive X in human 46,XX fetal cells, but not in adult females. From top to bottom are fibroblasts from a 5–6 wk fetus, chorionic villi cells from a newborn with X trisomy, embryonic stem cells, and adult fibroblasts. Each specimen was fixed on slides, and the RNA was hybridized to a mixture of differentially labeled *XIST* (red) and *TSIX* (green) DNA probes. Merging the two images shows the area of overlap (yellow). The *TSIX* signal (seen in all the fetal specimens) is smaller than the *XIST* signal but always overlaps it, indicating that both are being expressed from the same X chromosome, which is the inactive X because it expresses *XIST*. *TSIX* does not repress *XIST*, because the *XIST* signal is not reduced in size. Note two *TSIX* signals in the 47,XXX placenta corresponding to the two inactive X chromosomes in that specimen. Adapted from figure 2 from Migeon et al. [67].

9.3. SUMMARY AND SPECULATIONS

The role played by DNA methylation in maintaining the silence of genes on the inactive X varies considerably among mammalian species and even among tissues from the same species. The maintenance of X inactivation is notoriously poor in all tissues of marsupials and in female germ cells of all mammals. However, some genes that are stably inactivated in adult tissues are expressed to some degree in human placental tissues, and some genes inactivated in one species are partially expressed in others. Even in tissues where inactivation is relatively stable, some genes are expressed from the inactive X. Most of the expressed genes are in the pseudoautosomal region, or have active Y homologues, or are recent arrivals to the X chromosome. In any case, the level of transcription is usually less than that from the allele on the active X, reflecting leaky rather than full expression.

This poor maintenance of the silent state is in all cases associated with scanty methylation of, or lack of, CpG islands in the relevant genes. Not all mammals require a lock-in mechanism to stabilize X inactivation through mitosis, as leaky or incomplete X inactivation is not a problem for some species.

Such remarkable species variation in the details of X inactivation reflects modifications acquired during mammalian evolution. These variations are adaptations that reinforce but do not interfere with the basic theme. Variations in stability of X inactivation have provided insights into the role of DNA methylation not only in X inactivation but also in other developmental processes as well, and will continue to do so. In accordance with a common genetic aphorism, such exceptions are treasures, because they tell us about the rules.

10

Variations 3

Choice of Active X

The concept of *random inactivation* is inherent in the Lyon hypothesis [46, 56]. Based on her observations of cellular mosaicism in mice, Mary Lyon assumed that "the heteropyknotic (*inactive*) X-chromosome can be either paternal or maternal in origin, in different cells of the same animal" [46, p. 372]. And, because inactivation occurs early in development, she said, "In adult life this leads to patches of cells some with one and some with the other X chromosome inactivated and hence to the mottled [mosaic] appearance characteristic of female mammals heterozygous for sex-linked color genes" [56, p. 145]. Certainly, the inactivation process is random in most female cells, although the proportions of active paternal or maternal X chromosomes may vary from the hypothetical 50:50 among various tissues of individuals, as expected by chance. Yet, the inactivation patterns are extremely nonrandom in all tissues of marsupials and in placental tissues of mice, where the active X is always the maternal one. Therefore, another major variation on the theme of X inactivation has to do with the choice of active X.

10.1. PRIMARY NONRANDOM X INACTIVATION

Defining Nonrandom Inactivation

First, we must consider what the term *nonrandom inactivation* really means; that is, how much deviation from the expected 1:1 ratio of expressed parental alleles is beyond the sphere of random choice? Because of the very small numbers of progenitor cells at the time it occurs, Ohno suggested that inactivation—even if random at onset—might be subject to subsequent chance variation, and that this could result in unequal distributions of the two cell populations in the mosaic female [1]. In fact, in various tissues of 90% of human females, the distribution can be called random, because it follows the bell-shaped curve around the mean of 50% (see figure 12-8). The remaining 10% of females are outliers, and these individuals certainly have what could be called *nonrandom* inactivation patterns. The most extreme skewing of inactivation patterns is found in heterozygous females who manifest the male versions of X-linked diseases, which is why they come to our attention. The explanation for full-blown manifestation in these females is that they express the same parental X chromosome in all of their cells, and any X-linked mutation on this chromosome will be fully expressed; the normal allele is always silent as its expression is repressed on the inactive chromosome (discussed fully in chapter 12). Because the same parental allele is expressed in all her cells, such a heterozygote is not a mosaic. In this case, her unequal distribution of cell populations clearly is not random.

Yet, the term *nonrandom* should not imply that the skewed inactivation pattern results from the preferential choice of the active X. The existence of unbalanced patterns of X inactivation does not tell us if they were caused by events occurring at the onset of inactivation, or subsequently. On the one hand, it is conceivable that the original choice was nonrandom; only one of the parental X chromosomes was earmarked or otherwise designated to be the active X. On the other hand, it is just as likely—and in fact more likely—that the choice was made in a random fashion but that the skewing occurred subsequently. Because the origin of X inactivation patterns observed after birth is uncertain, I will refer to the unequal distribution of cell populations in the mosaic female as *skewed patterns of X inactivation*. I reserve the terms *nonrandom inactivation* and *preferential inactivation* for events known to affect the original choice of active X at the onset of the choice process.

Primary Nonrandom Inactivation Due to *Xist* or XIC Mutations

What could be responsible for nonrandom choice of the active X? Any X chromosome with a mutation that interferes with its being chosen as the active X is likely to always end up as an inactive X. Conversely, if a chromosome has a mutation that interferes with its ability to inactivate, then the only cells that survive are those with that chromosome as the active X. Clearly, mutations that interfere with the ability to be active or inactive will lead to the choice of one X chromosome over the other. Therefore, primary nonrandom inactivation is caused by mutations affecting the choice of active X or the ability of an X chromosome to be silenced.

The mutations responsible for nonrandom choice are those occurring in the *Xist* gene itself, or elsewhere in the X inactivation center (XIC). For example, if *Xist* were defective or missing, there would be no transcripts to initiate the silencing process, so the chromosome on which it resides would be incapable of *cis* inactivation. Because choice of the active X is independent of—and occurs prior to—the *cis* inactivation event, any cells with the normal X chosen to be the active one would have two active X chromosomes and would be nonviable (figure 10-1).

We know that tiny X chromosomes without an *XIST* gene cannot be silenced [120–122]. Such chromosomes are associated with severe congenital abnormalities (see figure 5-2), because both the tiny X with the *XIST* deletion and the normal X are active in the same cell. The problem is that both alleles are transcribed at any loci that remain on the tiny X. In cases of *functional X disomy* such as these,

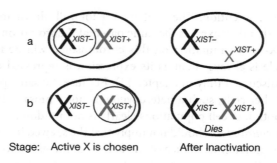

Stage: Active X is chosen   After Inactivation

Figure 10-1. Diagram showing the fate of cells with a heterozygous *XIST* mutation. (a) The X with the *XIST* mutation is chosen as the active X (black X, circled). The X with the normal *XIST* locus (gray X) is inactivated. This cell survives. (b) Alternatively, the X with the normal *XIST* allele is chosen to be active (gray X, circled). The X with the mutant *XIST* allele (black X) cannot inactivate and remains active. This cell has two intact active X chromosomes and does not survive. Consequently, all surviving cells have the same active X (black X).

the abnormal X is always a very small chromosome and therefore lacks many vital genes. Both X chromosomes are active because (1) the tiny X cannot be silenced and (2) the inactivation of the gene-rich normal X would cause the death of the cell. Girls with tiny *XIST*-deficient chromosomes can survive with two active X chromosomes only if the second X chromosome is tiny enough, hence minimizing the effective functional disomy. Such females are considered in detail in Chapter 11.

The *Xist* locus does not need to be completely compromised to influence the randomness of inactivation. Any mutations that *decrease Xist* expression will decrease the ability of *Xist* to induce inactivation, and hence they *increase* the probability that the relevant chromosome will be the active X in the cells.

On the other hand, any X chromosome that cannot respond to the signal to turn off its *Xist* expression would be inactive in every cell. Such mutations are also expected to affect the *Xist* locus, or another locus within the XIC involved in the choice process. They could affect one of a variety of *Xist* control elements, such as enhancers, and chromatin insulators or boundary elements that establish and maintain active and repressed chromosome domains. Functional mutations—all affecting a single nucleotide within the promoter of the human *XIST* gene in normal females—were identified in three unrelated families with skewed X chromosome inactivation [135, 136, 137]. We now know that the *XIST* mutations in these families affect a binding site for a conserved protein (CTCF) that is thought to mediate specific chromatin modifications [137] and has been postulated to have a role in *Xist-Tsix* interactions in the mouse [138]. The common mutation in two families [135] increases the binding of CTCF, and the one in the third family [136] decreases it. The skewing also occurs in opposite directions: The X with increased CTCF binding was more often the inactive X, whereas the one with decreased binding was more often the active X. That the effects of the two –43C mutations on CTCF binding correlate with the direction of skewing suggests that the differences in this binding affinity may indeed influence the skewing in these families. Although such mutations might exert a strong effect on inactivation patterns, in these families the influence is more subtle. In all three families, other individuals had the same *XIST* mutations, but their X inactivation patterns were not skewed, or skewing occurred in absence of the mutation. Nonetheless, they serve as an example of how mutations in *Xist* might lead to choice of one X chromosome over the other.

Although *Xist* may be the only gene in the XIC needed for *cis* inactivation, other genes or elements within the region could affect the probability of being chosen the active X. One X chromosome may be more or less likely to be the target of the *trans*-acting factors that choose the active X by silencing its *Xist* gene. The *Xce* locus in the mouse XIC is considered a prototype for such a model, because alleles at that locus seem to influence the probability of being an active X. On the other hand, because the initial choice of active X resides within the XIC, mutations elsewhere on the X chromosome are unlikely to affect the primary choice process. Mutations affecting an autosomal *trans*-acting factor could affect the process, but are unlikely to choose one parental *Xist* allele over the other. Attempts to identify autosomal mutations involved specifically in the initiation of X inactivation by mutagenizing mice have not yet given definitive results [252]. In addition, the search for factors involved in skewed allelic expression in the mouse is complicated by the *Xce* locus, which influences the choice of the mouse active X [99] and has no counterpart in humans. The evidence, discussed in great detail in chapter 12, suggests that most of the skewed inactivation patterns observed in human females are not due to primary nonrandom inactivation. Instead, they occur after *random* X inactivation, due mainly to cell selection, which favors alleles that provide a relative growth advantage. I will refer to this as *secondary* skewing of X inactivation.

10.2. PATERNAL X INACTIVATION

This having been said, there is indisputable evidence that in some cases the choice of active X is influenced merely by the parental origin of the chromosome. The maternal X is always the active one in all marsupial tissues and in placental tissues of mice [221] and bovines [253]. Studies of the expression of *PGK* and *G6PD* in a few marsupial species show that the paternal X chromosome is always the inactive one [254]. Although random inactivation is the rule in the tissues of the mouse embryo proper, this is not the case in tissues derived from placental lineages where the paternal X is always inactive. Hybrid mice with two distinctive X chromosomes were used to show that the paternal X in these tissues is always late replicating, as expected for an inactive X [221].

Yet, paternal X inactivation is not a feature of the placental tissues of all mammals. The paternal X is often the active chromosome in human placental tissues [215, 255–257][1] (figures 10-2 and 10-3), most likely related to the fact that X

1. The situation in the human placenta has been controversial—perhaps a semantic problem with the meaning of the word *preferential*. Ropers et al. [255] found that the G6PD isozyme

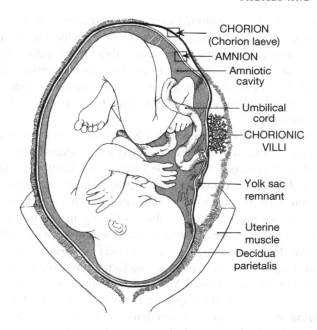

Figure 10-2. Diagram showing human fetus and placenta at the end of gestation. The chorionic villi (indicated) are derived solely from the fetus and are the tissues sampled in figure 10-3. From figure 1 of Migeon and Do [289].

FMR1 heterozygote showing cellular mosaicism

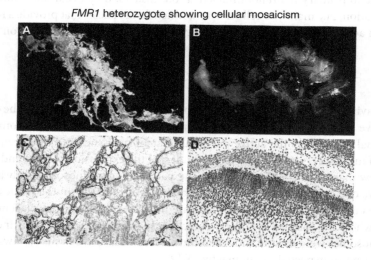

Figure 10-3. Random inactivation in the chorionic villi of the human placenta: tissues from a placenta (*A–C*) and brain (*D*) heterozygous for the fragile X mutation (*FMR1*). The *FMR1* protein is stained brown. The villi expressing the mutant X are unstained. Note: Both mutant and normal villi are present, as seen grossly (*A* and *B*) and in microscopic sections (C). There is closer commingling of the two kinds of cells in the brain (*D*), where the patch size is smaller. From figure 2 of Willemsen et al. [260], with permission. [See color plate.]

inactivation in this tissue occurs relatively later in humans than in mice. Although there may be a few more cells with an active maternal X than with an active paternal X, the differences in no way resemble the situation in marsupials or in mouse placental tissues, where the maternal X is always the active one.

Because the only alleles expressed in mouse placenta are the maternal ones, mutations in X-linked mouse genes that are important for normal placental function, such as *choroideremia* [258] and *cited 1* [259], may cause embryonic lethality when carried on the maternal X. As expected because X inactivation is random in human placental cells, the human counterparts of these maternally transmitted mutations are not lethal to embryos. The clearest evidence that X inactivation is random in the human placenta comes from studies of chorionic villi (figure 10-3) from a female newborn heterozygous for the *FMR1* mutation responsible for the fragile X syndrome [260]. Figure 10-3 (A-C) shows the biallelic expression at the *FMR1* locus in this placental tissue. The FMR1 protein is expressed in some villi but not in others: The presence of both normal villi (paternal X active) as well as mutant ones (maternal X active) documents the mosaic expression of this X-linked gene in trophectoderm-derived cells of the human placenta.

10.3. RELATIONSHIP OF PATERNAL X INACTIVATION TO GENOMIC IMPRINTING

For reasons discussed in the next section, paternal X inactivation is often referred to as *imprinted* X inactivation. Genes are said to be imprinted if only one of the alleles is expressed and the choice of which allele to express is based on its parental origin. Several autosomal genes are transcribed from only the paternal or only the maternal chromosome, and the process by which a chromosome remembers its parental origin is referred to as *genomic imprinting*. The reason for this uniparental expression has not yet been fully explained. It does serve to prevent *parthenogenesis* in mammals.[2] Often, the genes subject to this kind of imprinting are those that influence the growth of the fetus, and many of these genes function in placental tissues; this has

pattern reflected more of the maternal isozyme than the paternal one. Based on G6PD analysis, Harrison [256] reported that the paternal X was more often expressed in cytotrophoblasts. On the other hand, Migeon and Do [257] found random inactivation in newborn and fetal placentas. And studies of X reactivation in chorionic villi cells clearly show that the inactive X can be maternal or paternal [65, 215]. See figure 10–3, which shows the extensive mosaicism in the human placenta. It also shows the large size of the mosaic patches, in contrast to the brain, where the two populations of cells intermingle. It is the large patch size in human placenta that has led to sampling errors that can be misleading. Nonetheless, all of the papers with ample observations of inactivation patterns in human placenta (at least ten papers) report expression of the paternal alleles as well as maternal ones [155].

2. In the case of some genes, it does matter which parent contributes the allele. It seems that both maternal and paternal chromosomes are required for normal embryonic development. The reason is that some genes inherited from the father are programmed to be silent so that only mother's genes function, and vice versa.

led to the rather teleological speculation that imprinting is the result of competition between mother's and father's genes to control the size of the fetus [261]. That some genes are parentally imprinted is usually not a problem, because normally the fetus receives contributions from both parents. Problems do arise, however, when one of the imprinted alleles has a mutation that renders it inactive. If this happens in the gene that is normally silent, then there is no problem, but if it occurs in the gene that needs to be expressed, then the fetus will have no functional gene.

How are such genes earmarked so that they remember which parent they came from? Imprinted genes are marked epigenetically by DNA methylation and histone modifications. This mark or *imprint* is believed to be acquired during oogenesis or spermatogenesis and may take the form of an allelic difference in DNA methylation, which you recall from the discussion in chapter 7 can serve as a memory device in replicating cells. Most cell differentiation requires some kind of cell memory device.

Therefore, some form of genomic imprinting is a part of many developmental processes—although not always dependent on parental origin. Maintaining the silent status of the inactive X also requires cell memory to transmit the silent state from one cell to its progeny. In this case, DNA methylation—primarily within the CpG islands—serves as a kind of genomic imprint to molecularly mark the chromosome as being inactive, so that it can be transmitted as the silent X to all of its cellular descendants (see section 7.2, "Maintaining Inactivation by DNA Methylation of CpG Islands"; for reviews of genomic imprinting, see [262, 263]). Imprinting of the paternal X chromosome—a specialized kind of genomic imprinting—is used in some organisms and in some tissues and is another variation on the theme of random X inactivation (figure 10-4).

10.4. The Paternal X Imprint in X Inactivation

In each species where nonrandom X inactivation has been shown to occur, it is the paternal X that is consistently silent. Because X inactivation has to do with choosing the single active X in each cell, it seems more appropriate to say that in the imprinted form of X inactivation, the maternal X chromosome (X^m) is invariably selected to be the active one. Monk and McLaren [264] suggested that the paternal X (X^p) is prone to inactivate because it retains the memory that it was previously inactive. And, there is convincing evidence that at least some genes on the paternal X are inactivated during spermatogenesis [88, 265] (see figures 6-3 & 6-4). Based on changes in histone modifications [90], we know that, during some stages of spermatogenesis in the mouse, the chromatin of the paternal X is globally inactive (see figure 5-5), suggesting that most X-linked genes are probably not expressed at that time. Also, the paternal *Xist* allele is expressed during meiotic sex chromosome inactivation (MSCI) [265, 266], but *Xist* expression is not needed for MSCI to occur [130].

The nature of the imprint responsible for paternal X inactivation has not been identified, but the evidence suggests it is acquired during spermatogenesis.

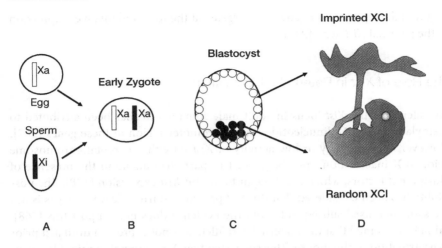

Figure 10-4. Imprinted and random X chromosome inactivation (XCI) in mice. *A*. Oocyte with active maternal X and sperm with an X that was inactivated during spermatogenesis, with some loci still repressed but undergoing reactivation. *B*. Early zygote with two X chromosomes, both expressing some genes. *C*. Blastocyst with outer trophectoderm cells, which will give rise to placental tissues, and inner cell mass from which the embryo is derived. *Cis* X inactivation begins in the trophectoderm at 3.5 days, when the paternal X is still partially repressed. It begins in the inner cell mass derivatives after 6 days, when the paternal X has lost its imprint and can be chosen as an active X. *D*. X chromosome inactivation (XCI) is imprinted in the earlier differentiating placental tissues (paternal X always inactive) and is random in the later differentiating cells of the embryo (either X is inactive). Adapted from figure 1 of Huynh and Lee [426], with permission.

Although the chromatin of the paternal X chromosome is transcriptionally competent prior to fertilization, studies of gene expression indicate that not all loci on the chromosome are fully reexpressed during the early cleavage stages in the zygote [88, 89] and that these loci are gradually reactivated (see figures 6-3 & 6-4). The reactivation is complete prior to the stage when random inactivation occurs in cells of the embryo proper [89]. The genes that are reactivated earliest are those farthest from *Xist* [88, 89] (see section 6.2, "Time of Initiation in the Embryo")—as if there were an imprint around the *Xist* locus. The fact that several genes on the paternal X are expressed during the early cleavage divisions and that these map relatively far from *Xist* [88] suggests that any paternal imprint must emanate from a small region of the chromosome—in the vicinity of the *Xist* locus. Therefore, the imprint that modifies the paternal X during spermatogenesis, marking it for inactivation in cells subject to paternal X inactivation, may affect only the XIC region and may be limited to the *Xist* locus. Further support for this comes from elegant studies of mouse embryos carrying a mouse XIC transgene inserted into an autosome; in the early stages of embryogenesis, the *Xist* locus in the transgene is always expressed if inherited from the father and never expressed if inherited from the mother. This suggests that the imprint is acquired during spermatogenesis, is targeted at the XIC, and involves expression of the paternal *Xist* gene [237].

The Role of *Xist* in Paternal X Inactivation

The silence of the *Xist* locus in adult male somatic cells has been attributed to methylation of CpG dinucleotides in the promoter region of these genes [267]. However, the inactivity or low activity of *Xist* on either parental chromosome prior to X inactivation must be at least in part attributable to the presence of pluripotent factors, which are thought to inhibit *Xist* expression [128]. The possibility has been considered that the *Xist* promoter during cleavage stages is not the same one used subsequently, but the evidence does not support this [268]. Initially, it seemed that the maternal *Xist* allele was not expressed until just prior to gastrulation in the mouse. This suggested that *Xist* expression might be regulated by a novel, imprinted, maternally expressed gene [113]. However, more sensitive assays indicate that, like the human gene, mouse *Xist* is expressed at low levels from both X chromosomes from the earliest cell divisions [125]. Yet, the expression of the paternal *Xist* allele is greater than that of the maternal one during the early cleavage stages (see figures 6-3 and 6-4). It seems to me that the imprint responsible for paternal X inactivation could be the active status of the paternal *Xist* allele—a holdover from spermatogenesis when the *Xist* locus is well expressed. In any case, the paternal imprint, whatever it is, needs to be released before the paternal X can fully participate as an active X chromosome. Paradoxically, this seems to be true even though many genes on the paternal chromosome certainly can and do function at that time. Therefore, one must distinguish between transcribability and ability to be designated an active X. The latter seems to require being responsive to a *trans*-acting signal, which will silence its *Xist* locus.

Why Is the Maternal X Chosen as Active X?

The active X is chosen by repressing its *Xist* gene. In the earliest differentiating tissues the paternal X seems to be imprinted in such a way that, if inactivation is initiated too early, its *Xist* gene cannot be silenced. The other alternative is that the maternal X cannot inactivate because other factors repress its *Xist* locus. It may be a combination of such events. But, I suggest that the maternal *Xist* locus is easier to repress in earlier differentiating tissues than the paternal one, because the paternal *Xist* allele, having been up-regulated during spermatogenesis, is still being expressed. In any case, epigenetic modifications on one or both of the parental X chromosomes prior to the process of *cis* inactivation must be responsible for the preferential inactivation of the paternal X.

   The hypothesis that the imprint for paternal inactivation is an irrepressible *Xist* locus requires that we consider the possibility that the embryo loses some cells at the time of *cis* inactivation. Although the paternal X chromosome can function in placental tissues of mice with a 45,X^p karyotype, subsequent development of these mice is retarded (compared to 45,X^m mice), consistent with the possibility that the paternal X is not fully functional when X inactivation is first initiated in the placental tissues, and some cells are lost from these embryos (discussed in [269]). It may be that paternal X inactivation results from the selective loss of a cell population with a partially functional paternal X. On the other hand, the relevant *trans* molecules may bind to both chromosomes and the one to repress *Xist* first is the active X—in which case, the maternal X would certainly have the advantage. The two X chromosomes appear to come close to one another prior to *Xist* up-regulation in mouse embryonic stem (ES) cells [270]. This suggests the possibility of communication between the two chromosomes during the choice process, via either a direct association or a common nuclear subcompartment. We know so little about the details of the choice process that all these possibilities are worthy of consideration.

10.5. DOES ANTISENSE TRANSCRIPTION HAVE A ROLE?

In addition to the paternal imprint that precludes an active paternal X, some kind of maternal imprint may protect the maternal X from inactivation. There is some experimental support for the notion that it is the X^m that is imprinted and that this imprint, acquired during oogenesis, permits it to resist inactivation until the imprint is erased (discussed in [271]). Indirect evidence suggests that the X^m chromosome of mature oocytes—but not immature ones—is resistant to inactivation and that resistance is acquired during oogenesis [272]. Jeannie Lee and her colleagues [150, 273, 275] report evidence that X^m is protected by the *Tsix* antisense transcript, which represses the maternal *Xist* allele. This gene produces a noncoding RNA that is antisense to *Xist* (see "The *Tsix* Antisense Transcript Locus" in section 6.5, "Silencing the Inactive X Chromosome," and figure 8-1). Induced genomic deletions that interfere with the function of the maternal *Tsix* allele result in inactivation of the maternal X in mouse cells [140, 147, 150].

How *Tsix* Functions in the Mouse

The *Tsix* locus in the mouse spans a 40 kb region downstream of *Xist*; because it is transcribed in the opposite direction of *Xist*, it completely overlaps the *Xist* gene, even extending a kilobase farther upstream. Like *Xist*, *Tsix* is transcribed from all X chromosomes very early in mouse embryogenesis, prior to the onset of X inactivation. In ES cells, the up-regulation of *Xist* on the future inactive X chromosome is accompanied by the transcriptional repression of *Tsix* on that chromosome. However, *Tsix* continues to be expressed during a short window of development from the future active X, and this serves to repress *Xist* on this chromosome, until DNA methylation can permanently silence the locus [276]. The experimentally induced loss of *Tsix* in female mouse ES cells is associated with reexpression of *Xist* on that chromosome. Mice with a complete deletion of *Tsix* on both their X chromosomes undergo what Lee [149] refers to as chaotic choice: What is observed is a loss of 60–80% of homozygous females, with the survivors exhibiting random inactivation. So despite the loss of *Tsix* from both chromosomes, surviving female mice can in some way carry out appropriate X inactivation.

It seems that the *Tsix* transcripts must cover the entire *Tsix–Xist* unit in order to repress *Xist*. Because the experimental disruption of *Tsix* modifies the chromatin structure at the *Xist* locus—making it less repressive—the *Tsix*-mediated silencing of *Xist* may be induced by epigenetic modification of its chromatin [275]. Of importance here is that the *Tsix* promoter has binding sites for the pluripotency factors, Rex1, Klf-4 and c-Myc [277]. Implicit in all of this is that *Tsix* is the *Xist* repressor, the molecules needed to choose the future active X. Both parental *Tsix* alleles are expressed at very low levels prior to inactivation, but only the maternal allele is up-regulated in placental tissues; the paternal allele is always repressed. What is not yet understood is the means to choose which of the parental *Tsix* alleles is to be up-regulated. Other X-linked elements such as *Xite* have been suggested as enhancers of *Tsix* (see "The *Xce* and *Xite* Loci" in section 6.5). However, it is difficult to envision how X-linked genes or *cis* elements could independently choose between homologous X chromosomal genes.

Another proposed function for *Tsix* in the mouse is as the focus of transient pairing of the two X chromosomes at sometime prior to their differentiation into active and active X chromosomes [270]. Live cell imaging of tagged *Tsix/Xite* followed by detection of *Xist/Tsix* transcripts suggests that the two *Tsix/Xite* loci pair transiently during early ES cell differentiation – an event that is followed by downregulation of one *Tsix* allele. A *Tsix* locus seems to be required for colocalization of X chromosomes in mouse ES cells [132]. As both *Tsix* and *Xite* loci are essential for the crosstalk, it remains to be seen if similar events occur in species that lack functional *Xite* or *Tsix* loci.

Human *TSIX* Does Not Repress *XIST*

TSIX, the human counterpart to *Tsix* [67, 153], is antisense to *XIST* but lacks the CpG island in its promoter region that is present in the mouse gene (figure 10-5). This was lost during mammalian evolution. A comparable deletion in the mouse *Tsix* gene has been shown to interfere with its function [147].[3] Also, the human *TSIX* transcripts do not completely overlap the human *XIST* gene, and in the mouse this overlap is needed to silence *Xist*. Most important, *TSIX* is cotranscribed in cis with *XIST* from the inactive X in human embryonic stem cells, fetal cells, and placental cells throughout gestation [67] (figure 10-6)—so it obviously does not repress *XIST*

---

3. There is evidence that CpG islands, like the one missing from human *TSIX*, are needed for imprinting [278, 279]—consistent with lack of imprinted X inactivation in the human placenta.

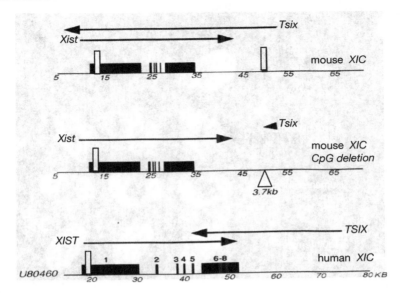

Figure 10-5. Comparing human *TSIX* with mouse *Tsix*. Top, Mouse XIC. *Tsix* is antisense to *Xist*, and its transcript initiated at a CpG island (indicated by vertical white bar) entirely overlaps that of *Xist*. Middle, mouse XIC with an induced 3.7 kb deletion of the *Tsix* CpG island [147]. This deletion eliminates the *Tsix* transcripts. Bottom, Human XIC. *TSIX* transcripts begin downstream of *XIST*, but overlap only the 3′ end of *XIST* presumably because the CpG island in the *TSIX* promoter region was deleted during primate evolution.

expression, or prevent *cis* inactivation of the chromosome from which it is expressed. It is conceivable that human *TSIX* has another role in X inactivation, perhaps acting *in trans* to help mediate the communication between X homologues, if that occurs in our species. Or, it may enhance the transcription in the region of *XIST*. But, it is not able to repress *XIST* and thus cannot be the *cis* repressor of *XIST*.

The Role of *Tsix* in Imprinting

The *Tsix* gene is an example of an important species difference that may have arisen from other variations on the theme of X inactivation. The species difference in *TSIX/Tsix* may be related to the fact that X inactivation is imprinted in mouse placentas but not in human placentas [280].

Mouse *Tsix* may be needed to reinforce the paternal imprint in the mouse extra-embryonic tissues. Yet, *Tsix* may not be required for imprinted X inactivation in other species. In bovine placenta, X inactivation is imprinted [253], but imprinting in this case does not involve *Tsix*. Evolutionary changes in the region 3′ to the bovine *Xist* gene [103] show that, despite the paternal X inactivation, bovine *Tsix* may have also lost sequences essential for repressing *Xist*.

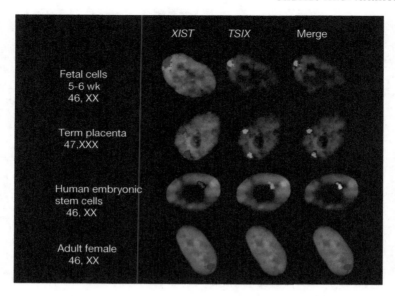

Figure 10-6. Human *TSIX* is coexpressed with *XIST* from the inactive X in human 46,XX fetal cells, but not in adult females. From top to bottom are fibroblasts from a 5–6 wk fetus, chorionic villi cells from a newborn with X trisomy, embryonic stem cells, and adult fibroblasts. Each specimen was fixed on slides, and the RNA was hybridized to a mixture of differentially labeled *XIST* (red) and *TSIX* (green) DNA probes. Merging the two images shows the area of overlap (yellow). The *TSIX* signal (seen in all the fetal specimens) is smaller than the *XIST* signal but always overlaps it, indicating that both are being expressed from the same X chromosome, which is the inactive X because it expresses *XIST*. *TSIX* does not repress *XIST*, because the *XIST* signal is not reduced in size. Note two *TSIX* signals in the 47,XXX placenta corresponding to the two inactive X chromosomes in that specimen. Adapted from figure 2 from Migeon et al. [67]. [See color plate.]

Preliminary studies suggest that, in female somatic cells as well as in testes of bovine embryos, *Tsix* transcripts are cotranscribed with *Xist* transcripts [281] as they are in humans. In fact, because the sequences homologous to the mouse *Tsix* major promoter are only detected in vole and rat, Shevchenko et al. [145] has proposed that this region of the XIC emerged *de novo* in the order *Rodentia*. Noting that transcription antisense to *Xist* is also not well conserved among mammals, they suggest that regulation of inactivation by *Tsix* may have arisen quite recently and is unique to rodents (mice, rats, and voles).

The newly discovered *XACT* gene (introduced in Chapter 8) may be a human counterpart to mouse *Tsix* as it is a long noncoding RNA that is expressed only in pluripotent cells from active X chromosomes (the chromosome not expressing *XIST*). Like *Tsix*, it is restricted in where it is expressed and is present in only a couple of closely related species (man and chimpanzee). These long noncoding RNAs inform us that they can evolve swiftly and be rapidly pressed into service to reinforce or otherwise support developmental processes species by species.

They are excellent examples of evolutionary tinkering.That X inactivation is imprinted in marsupials has led to the assumption that paternal X inactivation is the ancestral form. The case for this has yet to be made. What is clear is that both kinds of inactivation take place within different tissues of the same organism. Most likely, whether X inactivation is imprinted or random is determined by the timing of this developmental process—or interactions between one developmental pathway with another—that differ among species or among tissues of a single species.

10.6. Evolution and Tinkering

Evolution behaves like a tinkerer, who
During eons upon eons
Would slowly modify his work....
Cutting here—lengthening there,
Seizing the opportunities to adapt it progressively
To its new use.... Unlike engineers,
Tinkerers who tackle the *same* problem
Are likely to end up with *different* solutions.

Francois Jacob
adapted from [37]

According to Francois Jacob [37], the origin of divergences between organisms has many components: New proteins are produced by gene duplication, reshuffling pieces of genes to make new ones, and recruiting proteins used for one function to another [37, 238]. Borrowing gene-silencing factors used elsewhere in the genome for the purpose of heterochromatinizing the inactive X and adopting the ubiquitous CpG islands for the purpose of stabilizing the silence of inactive X-linked genes are good examples of recruitment. Yet, as Jacob points out, there are fewer differences in protein content from one organism to another than there are phenotypic variations between species. Therefore, much of this variation is not attributable to the nature of the proteins themselves. Instead, it is due to species differences in the way these proteins interact with proteins in other regulatory circuits in development. The critical factor is when and where the components of a regulatory circuit are produced during embryonic life. The way an active X is chosen might differ depending upon the time in development when the choice is made and the effects of other developmental events that occur simultaneously in one mammal but earlier or later in others. Most likely, imprinted X inactivation results from the earlier onset of X inactivation in marsupials and in rodent trophectoderm.

10.7. EFFECT OF INACTIVATION TIMING

The evidence suggests that the timing of inactivation is an important factor in the choice of active X. Mary Lyon was one of the first to suggest that eutherian mammals have a random (nonimprinted) and more stable form of X inactivation because X inactivation occurs later in them than it does in marsupials—at a time when the paternal imprint has been erased [282]. From the little we know about the timing of developmental events, it seems that the onset of X inactivation is subject to variation. Comparing the timing of specific events in one mammal with that in another is almost impossible, because the lengths of cell cycles and gestation are highly variable, and even the naming of developmental stages is inconsistent. Nor do we know precisely when X inactivation occurs in any species—that is, the number of cell generations that occur between fertilization and the choice of active X. *Xist* transcription, albeit at a low level, occurs too far in advance to be a useful marker, and the best indicator up to just recently has been the presence of an allocyclic or late-replicating X chromosome. The time of inactivation varies with respect to the developmental staging—using the times of conception and implantation, the maturation of the blastocyst, and the onset of gastrulation as guideposts.

Table 6-1 shows that the time when an inactive X is first detected differs in the various tissues of an individual and from one species to another. Hence the evidence based on when X inactivation is complete shows species variation. A recent study by Edith Heard's laboratory presents evidence of similar variation in the time that eutherian mammals *initiate* X-chromosome inactivation during development [66]. They confirm that in humans and rabbits, the *Xist* gene is not subject to imprinting, and X inactivation begins later than it does in mice—consistent with the data based on the appearance of an inactive X. Based on *Hprt* silencing, in mouse embryos, X inactivation begins in the blastocyst about 96 hr p.c., and was complete in trophectoderm by 120 hr p.c.; in rabbit embryo cells it begins a day later at 120 hr p.c.; in analogous cells of human embryos there was no evidence of silence up to the day 7 blastocyst stage—the latest stage analyzed. A recent study of the rhesus monkey shows biallelic expression of X-linked genes in the 11-day hatched blastocyst, indicating that inactivation had not yet occurred [283].

Earlier Onset of X Inactivation Relative to Time of Fertilization

Therefore, the evidence suggests that if one uses the time of conception as a measure, X inactivation occurs much earlier in tissues with paternal X inactivation than in those where inactivation is random (see table 6-1). Marsupials undergo inactivation much earlier than do other mammals; in some marsupials, X inactivation has already occurred in female unilaminar blastocysts at a stage when these cells are still undifferentiated and totipotent [284].

Based on the presence of a late-replicating X (see table 6-1) and supported by *Hprt* inactivation [66], X inactivation in the mouse begins in the trophectoderm and primitive endoderm cells, where inactivation is paternally imprinted, at approximately embryonic day 3.5, at least 36 hr and several cell generations earlier than in the differentiating tissues of the embryo proper, where inactivation is random (embryonic days 5–6.5) [79, 285]. The fact that the onset of inactivation in the trophectoderm occurs significantly earlier than it does in the embryo proper could explain the paternal inactivation in rodent placental tissues. This could also account for the imprinted X inactivation in the bovine placenta because X inactivation starts in preimplantation blastocysts (elongated-hatched blastocyst stage, days 7–9; presumably in trophectoderm, the earliest differentiating tissue in most mammals), and it is not complete in the embryo proper until days 14–15 [286].

Consistent with the random inactivation in human placental tissues is the fact that inactivation in this tissue occurs later than in mice, and later than in bovine even though the length of gestation is the same for humans and cows. The late-replicating X chromosomes observed at the time of implantation in mouse trophectoderm (embryonic day 4) are not seen in human trophectoderm until after implantation (embryonic days 12–14) [287, 288]. In the human embryo proper, sex chromatin is not seen until the beginning of the somite stage at about 20 days of gestation. The slight excess of cells with a paternal inactive X in human placental cells suggests that the onset of X inactivation in that tissue occurs close to the time when the paternal imprint, acquired during spermatogenesis, is lost so that X inactivation can be random [289].

Taking all the evidence into consideration, I suggest that it is the intersection between the events of spermatogenesis and X inactivation that influences choice of active X in early-differentiating tissues. It is the persistent expression of the paternal *Xist* allele in the early embryo [88, 89] that makes the locus harder to repress than the maternal one at the stage when the active X is chosen. Most likely, differences in the timing of the initial events also are responsible for many of the other variations that are observed.

X Inactivation Is a Multistep Process, Subject to Variation at Every Step

The single active X hypothesis has been the subject of intense investigation since it was proposed more than 50 years ago. From a large number of studies, we have learned that X inactivation occurs during the embryonic development of most mammals and is a very complex process. From the DNA analysis of the X and Y chromosomes of several mammals, including humans, we know that the process is dynamic—continually evolving in response to changes in the genetic content of both sex chromosomes. Most important, these studies show that the mechanisms underlying the single active X were subject to chance variation during the evolution of mammals. Some of the divergence no doubt reflects the species differences in the nature and timing of developmental events, and interacting pathways. It is likely that any modifications that reinforce the essential steps of X inactivation have been favored, whereas other modifications that could interfere with the blueprint were eliminated. We have also learned that some components of mammalian dosage compensation were borrowed from other developmental pathways. The mechanisms of silencing chromatin have many components that are not unique to dosage compensation. In the first edition I suggested that the means to uncover the role of *trans*-acting factors in maintaining the activity of the single active X was to look at features that are conserved in most mammals. Now that I am more aware of the extent of evolutionary tinkering, I expect that we will discover that mammals also may have solved this problem in more than one way.

10.8. SUMMARY AND SPECULATIONS

Mammalian X dosage compensation usually occurs without regard to the parental origin of either active or inactive X. However, there are variations on the theme of random inactivation, namely, paternal X inactivation in marsupials and in placental tissues of some mammals. Whether inactivation at onset is random or paternal seems to depend on the time when this developmental program is initiated. No doubt, the reason that the paternal X cannot be chosen as an active chromosome in marsupials and in mouse placental tissues is causally related to its having been inactivated during spermatogenesis. In early-differentiating tissues, the *Xist* locus on the paternal X of eutherians (or the *rsx* locus on the paternal X of marsupials) might not be as easily repressed as the maternal one. This would be expected if the time that the active X is chosen precedes the time when an imprint acquired during spermatogenesis can be released. The precise nature of that imprint is not known, but the evidence suggests that it has something to do with expression of the *Xist* locus.

PART THREE

Medical Consequences of X Inactivation

11

The Single Active X

The preceding chapters have dealt with the biology of X inactivation. We have considered the means of equalizing the expression of X-linked genes in males and females of our species, and how it differs from other mammals. The major feature of X dosage compensation in all mammals is the creation of a single active X chromosome in diploid cells of both sexes. Men have one X because the Y lost most of the X homologous genes during its evolution. Women have effectively a single X because only one is functional in each of their cells. Having only one working X chromosome in each cell has implications for the health of males and females. This chapter and the next deal with the medical consequences of the single X in both sexes and of the cellular mosaicism in females. Chapter 11 considers how the single active X affects the phenotype of normal individuals and those with chromosome abnormalities that change the dosage of X- and Y-linked genes (*sex chromosome aneuploidies*). Chromosome mutations such as duplications or deletions of entire sex chromosomes perturb the genetic program for sex in both males and females. Also included are the deletions and rearrangements of chromosomal segments that are detectable from the standard *karyotype*, because they change the shape of the chromosome. The effect of smaller deletions and nucleotide mutations is considered in chapter 12.

11.1. COPING WITH A MONOSOMY X

The first thing to consider is the intriguing question of how we tolerate a single working X chromosome, and therefore only one set of our X-linked genes. This is especially enigmatic when we remember the history of our sex chromosomes and their evolution from a pair of ordinary autosomes. At that time, there were two copies of each of the future X-linked genes. What kinds of adjustments were required to change from two copies to one? Does the evolution of dosage compensation require a prior adjustment in the activity level of the future X-linked genes? Does the basic unit of transcription for the X chromosome differ from that for autosomes? And when does such an adjustment occur?

It was Ohno [1] who first suggested that there had to be an increase in the transcription level of genes on the X chromosome in both sexes *prior to* the event that created X inactivation. How else could a single copy of these genes suffice when two copies were needed previously? How else could genes that had been expressed

Table 11-1. INDIVIDUALS WITH ABNORMAL NUMBERS OF CHROMOSOMES (ANEUPLOIDS)
LOST MAINLY BEFORE BIRTH.

Subjects	Triploidy and Tetraploidy	Autosomal		X0	XXY	XXX	XYY
		Monosomy	Trisomy				
Spontaneous abortions	9.8	0.0	26.8	8.6	0.2	0.1	0.0
Stillbirths	0.6	0.0	3.8	0.25	0.4	0.3	0.0
Live births	0.0	0.0	0.3	0.01	0.05	0.05	0.05

The frequency of each abnormality is given as a percentage of the total number of individuals (including those with normal chromosomes) in each population studied. Approximate number of subjects studied: 3,000 abortions, 1,000 stillbirths, and 57,000 live births. Adapted from Jacobs and Hassold [309], with permission.

NOTE: The absence of autosomal monosomies (which occur as frequently as trisomies) is misleading as such specimens are lost prior to the time when pregnancies are recognized. (See "Why Is X Chromosome Monosomy Tolerated When Autosomal Monosomy Is Uniformly Lethal?" in section 11.4.)

from two chromosomes produce enough of their proteins when reduced to only a single copy by loss of its Y homologue? How else could X-encoded proteins interact with autosomal ones? How else could the effective monosomy for X-linked genes be tolerated, when we know that autosomal monosomy is so lethal? The data in table 11-1 attest to the inviability of autosomal monosomies, because none have ever been observed even among first-trimester miscarriages. Mary Lyon considered the possibility that the transcriptional output of the X was increased by duplicating individual X-linked genes [291]. Although she found some genes with duplicated functions, such as the two clotting-factor genes for hemophilia A and B, two color vision genes, and the two muscular dystrophy genes *DMD* and *EMD* (see *Appendix A*), duplicate genes were not more frequent on the X chromosome than on autosomes.

11.2. DOSAGE COMPENSATION OF THE ACTIVE X

Most likely, the transcriptional activity of genes on the single X chromosome was up-regulated in both sexes before or concomitant with the establishment of X inactivation. And there is evidence to support this kind of transcriptional up-regulation. The chloride ion channel gene *Clc4*, by virtue of a chance evolutionary translocation, is X-linked in one species of mouse and autosomal in another. *Clc4* is expressed in the brain in both species. The X-linked gene is subject to X inactivation but nonetheless produces twice as many transcripts as each of the autosomal genes. In contrast, another chloride ion gene, *Clc3*, that is autosomal in each species is expressed equally in both species [290]. Such results are consistent with Ohno's hypothesis that the expression of genes on the active X chromosome is greater than it would have been on an autosome in order to maintain the balance with the expression of autosomal genes. Other supporting evidence has come from studies of Nguyen and Disteche [292], who used expression microarray analysis of many mouse and human tissues to calculate the X:autosome expression ratio. They found that it was close to 1:1 in both species, implying a generalized transcriptional up-regulation of X-linked genes. However, similar studies using RNA sequencing to quantify the number of transcripts were inconsistent (see reference [293]). It seems that when quantitating transcripts one needs to take into account the variable expression profiles of X-linked genes, as the frequency of genes with no expression is significantly higher on X chromosomes than autosomes.[1] Data that consider only the *expressed* X-linked genes support the hypothesis of upregulation, not only for the human and mouse genomes but also for worms and flies [293]. We must conclude that the need to maintain balance between sex chromosomes and autosomes occurs in all individuals that require some kind of X dosage compensation, no matter the method used.

Figure 11-1 shows the two-step dosage compensation in human cells. To compensate for the loss of genes from the Y chromosome, the transcripts from the active Xs increase *in both sexes*. This does not eliminate the sex difference

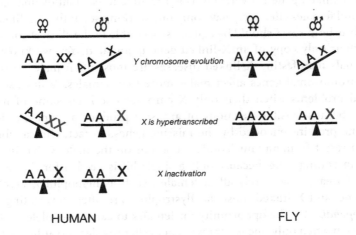

HUMAN   FLY

Figure 11-1. Comparing dosage compensation in human and fly. In humans, dosage compensation for the active X necessitates X inactivation. Top row: Degeneration of the Y chromosome causes autosome–sex chromosome imbalance. Middle row: Up-regulation of X chromosomes in *both* males and females again creates imbalance. Bottom row: Balance is restored by inactivation of one X in females. In flies, degeneration leads to imbalance between X and autosomes, but is corrected by doubling the transcription *only* from the male X. This single event also serves to compensate for sex difference in the number of X chromosomes.

1. Many of the unexpressed X-linked genes are multicopy genes expressed only in testes.

in number of X chromosomes, and so a second step is needed—one that would silence one of the two X chromosomes in females. When in evolution these events occur and in what order remain to be elucidated. Lahn and Page [18] proposed that when the genes on the X were up-regulated as an adjustment to the loss of the homologous genes on the Y, they subsequently became subject to X inactivation. Only the genes in the process of being eliminated would be subject to up-regulation and subsequent inactivation, and these adjustments would be repeated with each subsequent wave of Y chromosome rearrangement. From studies of recent events of such evolution in plants, we know that such adjustments can occur quite rapidly, at least in plants [25].

Figure 11-1 also compares our compensatory methods with those of flies. By increasing the transcription of the X *only in males*, flies have achieved the most efficient way to accomplish both sex and autosomal balance, requiring only this single step for both processes.

11.3. SEX DIFFERENCES IN SUSCEPTIBILITY TO DISEASE

Males are predisposed to disease by virtue of their single X chromosome. Even if each X-linked gene is overtranscribed relative to each autosomal gene, both males and females effectively have only one working set of their X-linked genes. Therefore, both sexes should be equally susceptible to the clinical consequences when their only copy of an X-linked gene is mutated. Yet, we know that the individuals manifesting X-linked diseases are most often male, so mutations in X chromosomal genes affect males more than females. Males usually have medical problems when their only X chromosome loses some of its genetic content because visible deletions of any size produce a complete deficiency of all the proteins encoded by the missing genes. In fact, clinical abnormalities can result from any nucleotide mutations on the male X that incapacitate a protein-coding gene, because only a single hit is needed for the severe deficiency. Diseases that rarely affect females, such as hemophilia, Lesch Nyhan syndrome, and X-linked muscular dystrophies are often devastating in males (see *Appendix A*). The opportunity for females to carry two alleles at the same locus, even when only one is expressed per cell, provides versatility not possible in *hemizygous* males. Although some of their cells may be deficient, females have other cells that make the normal protein. Having some cells that can do the job is often enough to carry out the function. However, even if the number of competent cells is not sufficient, the disease can be ameliorated by interactions between the normal and mutant cells (discussed in detail in chapter 12). Therefore, cellular mosaicism in normal females—or, for that matter, in males with extra X chromosomes—not only protects them from the deleterious effects of two active X chromosomes but also helps mitigate the effects of X-linked mutations, duplications and deletions.

11.4. VIABILITY OF TURNER SYNDROME, KLINEFELTER SYNDROME, AND X CHROMOSOME ANEUPLOIDY

The single active X imposes some degree of vulnerability for males, even if they have the proper number of sex chromosomes. It also influences the phenotype of individuals of both sexes who are born with extra sex chromosomes. On one hand, the mechanisms responsible for the single active X can eliminate the deleterious effect of additional X chromosomes—enough for aneuploid fetuses of both sexes to survive the perils of embryogenesis. On the other hand, X inactivation cannot eliminate all the clinical abnormalities. The residual problems are due to the overexpression of the genes transcribed from the pseudoautosomal region or other regions on inactive X chromosomes not subject to inactivation (see section 7.3, "Escape from Inactivation," and figures 7-3 and 7-4). *Appendix B* provides a brief description of many of the chromosomal aneuploidies considered below.

Turner Syndrome: Is the Single X in Turner Syndrome Comparable to That in Normal Males and Females?

Turner syndrome is the genetic disorder caused by the accidental loss of one of the sex chromosomes (either X or Y) during gametogenesis in either parent, or in the embryo during early development (reviewed in [294]). In either case, the result is an embryo with 45 chromosomes and a single X chromosome (45,X).[2] Such individuals have contributed to our understanding of some of the components of femaleness, because they tell us that a single X may be sufficient for many female features, but not all of them. Turner females have the external genitalia and body habitus characteristic of prepubertal females, but their gonadal development is very abnormal. Instead of an ovary with follicles and oogonia, they have poorly developed fibrotic gonads, called *streak gonads* as they lack germ cells and even ovarian follicles. Because their streak gonads are not functional, Turner females do not synthesize estrogens. Figure 4-2 shows a girl with Turner syndrome and some of the somatic abnormalities associated with the syndrome. Although female in appearance, they require exogenous estrogen hormone in order to develop the sexual features associated with femaleness, such as breasts and menses. In addition, usually they are extremely short (less than five feet at full growth) and may have a variety of somatic (nongonadal) abnormalities, including excessive skin folds in the neck region (webbing), limb and chest malformations, and sometimes renal and cardiac abnormalities.

You may wonder why Turner females with a single X chromosome have any problems at all. After all, males also have a single X, and normal females express only one X in each of their cells. The answer is that one X is not equivalent to having two of them, even if one is not working. The reason for their streak gonads is

---

2. Loss of the X chromosome in an XY individual would be lethal, because 45,Y males do not survive past the early cleavage stages.

that one X chromosome is not sufficient in female germ cells, which unlike somatic cells need the activity of two of them (see section 7.4, "Transient X Inactivation in Germ Cells"). It seems that two active X chromosomes are needed because both alleles of some X-linked gene or genes have to be functional in order to maintain the germ cells, and ultimately the ovary itself. From the study of the 45,X embryos aborted spontaneously during the first trimester of gestation, we know that a single X chromosome is sufficient for the development of a perfectly normal ovary containing normal female germ cells. At three months of gestation, the ovaries and oocytes of 45,X and 46,XX fetuses look the same, but this changes when the programmed loss of oocytes begins. All human females undergo an orchestrated loss (attrition) of their germ cells during embryogenesis. Normally, the ovary has the most germ cells (~7 million) at about 5 months of gestation—the time when the programmed attrition begins. At birth, female infants have 1–2 million germ cells, significantly less than *in utero*. Germ cells continue to undergo programmed cell death all through the life of the female, but this usually is not problematical because only about 400 oocytes are needed during her reproductive lifetime, and she starts with tremendous excess. This normal attrition is grossly exaggerated in the 45,X Turner female such that although she has normal numbers of oocytes at 3 months of gestation, by birth few if any oocytes remain in the ovary. And this loss of oocytes leads to a virtual destruction of the ovarian architecture, with loss of follicles and subsequent fibrosis leading to the characteristic streak gonad. The X-linked genes that maintain ovarian structure have not yet been identified; clearly, the germ cells themselves are needed to induce follicles and maintain the ovary.[3]

The lack of two working X chromosomes in germ cells explains the gonadal abnormalities associated with Turner syndrome, but what is the explanation for their congenital malformations in tissues other than the ovaries? In addition to the hallmark short stature, at least one-fifth of patients with Turner syndrome have some kind of congenital heart defect, and one-third have a kidney malformation. And these liveborn individuals are survivors of a much larger population of 45,X fetuses that are lost during gestation. The incidence of the syndrome among spontaneous abortions is 8.6%, compared to 0.01% of live-borns (table 11-1).

The evidence that so many 45,X fetuses are lost *in utero* and that many who are born have congenital malformations tells us that the single X chromosome in girls with Turner syndrome is not equivalent to the single male X chromosome. Most of the time the single X chromosome originates from the mother (70–80%), but some are of paternal origin (20–30%). Survival *in utero* is not determined by the parental origin of the X, at least among recognizable pregnancies; the ratio of maternal to paternal X in specimens from miscarriages is the same as that in newborns [295]. The fact that more have a maternal X could mean that more of the fetuses with the paternal X die before implantation. More likely, it simply reflects the 2:1 ratio of

---

3. In the absence of germ cells, ovarian follicles—which give the architectural structure to the ovary—never form, and follicles formed before the loss of germ cells rapidly degenerate.

maternal to paternal X chromosomes expected, because in cases where the Y is lost from an XY fetus, the X that remains must be the maternal one.[4]

Some have suggested that Turner females with only the paternal X might be poorer survivors because of some imprinted gene(s) on the paternal X chromosome. However, the only X-linked genes among the more than 75 known parentally imprinted genes in the mouse genome are a cluster of three related genes, *Xlr3b*, *Xlr4b*, and *Xlr4c*, that function in lymphocytes and brain, and these do not seem to be present in the human genome. In fact, inconsistent with imprinted X-linked genes, the phenotypes of Turner females with paternal or maternal X do not differ regarding most parameters (i.e., birth weight, height, gonadal function, or other clinical abnormalities) [433], and the evidence of small differences in social cognition that has been reported [296] is not yet compelling.

The Somatic Abnormalities of Turner Syndrome Are Due to Abnormal Dosage of Pseudoautosomal Genes

The short stature and other congenital abnormalities are better explained by the pseudoautosomal region of the X and Y chromosomes—or other genes expressed from the Y and the inactive X. Unlike escape genes in other regions of the X that are poorly expressed, genes in PAR1 may be fully expressed from these chromosomes. Having only one of the two sex chromosomes means that Turner females have lost at least 24 genes from PAR1 that normally function on the Y chromosome in males, and on the inactive X in females (see tables 2-1 and 2-2, and figures 2-5 and 2-6). Most likely their somatic abnormalities are due to the gene dosage problem created by the loss of these XY-homologous genes. The genes from PAR1 encode proteins involved in many processes, including dentition and stature. One of them is the short-stature homeobox gene *SHOX*, which is thought to play a major role in growth. Mutations in this gene cause short stature in individuals whose short stature is their only clinical abnormality, or is one feature in a group of abnormalities (referred to as a syndrome). In addition, the normal *SHOX* gene is expressed in the limb buds of embryos, and mutations in the gene produce a syndrome that includes the same kind of skeletal abnormalities affecting the limbs of Turner females [297]. Therefore, having only a single copy of this gene might explain the short stature and limb abnormalities associated with the 45,X karyotype or other karyotypes that include only one copy of PAR1.

Some Turner females have 46 chromosomes; one X chromosome is normal, and the other is not, having a deletion or duplication of X chromosome segments (figure 11-2). For reasons discussed later, the abnormal X is always inactive. Therefore, the clinical manifestations result from the loss or gain of

---

4. Only females can lose a maternal X chromosome. If the male maternal X were the target of nondisjunction the result would be an inviable fetus, as 45,Y embryos do not survive.

pseudoautosomal regions—or the other genes expressed from the inactive X chromosome. Correlating chromosomal deletions with clinical manifestations is difficult because many Turner individuals are chromosomal mosaics, having a 45,X cell line as well as the one with a partially deleted X chromosome, 46,X,del(X), and it is difficult to know if the relevant tissues are mosaic, and if so, the proportion of 45,X cells. Fortunately, methods are now available to examine the question of whether individuals carry minor populations of cell lines with different genetic compositions [298].

Why the majority of 45,X fetuses are lost *in utero* remains to be explained. Studying human embryonic stem (HES) cells, Urbach and Benvenisty [299] found that among the genes most highly transcribed in normal 46,XX cells but not in 45,X cells are pseudoautosomal genes expressed in the placenta. They suggest that one of these pseudoautosomal genes, *CSF2RA*, which encodes the receptor for macrophage stimulating factor, may be responsible for the loss of 45,X fetuses as it is essential for placental differentiation. Clearly, haploinsufficiency for *CSF2RA* or some other pseudoautosomal genes needs to be considered as a possible cause of such fetal loss. That a deficiency of placental gene products might be lethal for most of the 45,X fetuses makes one seriously consider the possibility that the few survivors are 45,X/ 46,XX mosaics, at least while *in utero*. Alternatively, the single X in the Turner female may be transcribed at higher levels than the single X in an XY male. (See section 13.3.)

Klinefelter Syndrome

It is likely that pseudoautosomal genes and other genes transcribed from inactive X chromosomes are also responsible for the somatic abnormalities in males with Klinefelter syndrome (see *Appendix B*). These individuals are phenotypically male despite the one or more extra X chromosomes in each of their cells. Although the only abnormality in some Klinefelter men is infertility (XXY males usually do not produce sperm), many of them have somatic abnormalities, including increased stature with disproportionately long legs, sparse body hair, mild mental retardation, and skeletal abnormalities. Because of X inactivation, only one of their X chromosomes is fully functional in each of their cells. Yet, they have extra doses of the X- and Y-linked genes that are not subject to inactivation. Overexpression of the *SHOX* gene, transcribed from every sex chromosome, may be responsible for the increased height of males with this syndrome. As one might expect, the congenital abnormalities in Klinefelter syndrome become more numerous and severe as the number of X chromosomes increases. With each additional X chromosome, cognitive abilities decrease [300]. On the other hand, there is variability in clinical and cognitive functioning among men with the same karyotypes. No doubt this reflects skewed X inactivation, or the presence of unrecognized mosaicism, as well as the nature of the specific X-linked alleles they carry.

Triple X Syndrome

The female counterpart of Klinefelter syndrome is trisomy for the X chromosome—47,XXX (see *Appendix B*). About one woman in 1,000 has an extra X chromosome. Diagnosed in chromosome surveys, these women are largely lost to medical follow-up because as two of the three X chromosomes are inactive in each of their cells, they have relatively few medical abnormalities attributable to their trisomy X, and many do not come to the attention of physicians. Yet, some of them have serious language and learning problems with a generalized depression of both verbal and nonverbal abilities [301]. They tend to be tall because of their increased leg length [302], and their tooth enamel is thicker [303]. Both features might be predicted for individuals with three doses of the *SHOX* gene in PAR1 and of the X-linked *AMELX* gene encoding a component of tooth enamel. *AMELX* may be expressed from all sex chromosomes, because it is located close to the pseudoautosomal boundary. Triple X females sometimes come to attention because of premature ovarian failure; although the majority are fertile, reproductive fitness may be reduced in some of them. Studies of their long-term health [304] reveal an increased mortality rate (about twice normal), with excess deaths due particularly to cardiovascular and respiratory disease. The incidence of mental retardation and heart defects is especially notable in those with more than three X chromosomes.

Thus, we see that the medical problems in Turner, Klinefelter, and multiple X syndromes are likely to be directly attributable to the loss or gains of genes, expressed from the inactive X or Y. In addition, Turner females are also prone to a host of diseases that usually affect only males. Among them are muscular dystrophy, hemophilia, color blindness, and structural abnormalities of the aorta that are present for the same reason as they are in males. Having the same active X in all of their cells makes them vulnerable to single-hit mutations. They express every abnormality present on their single X.

In contrast, Klinefelter males with additional X chromosomes are protected from some of the male-only disorders. Like females, they are mosaics, having some cells that express a second repertoire of X-linked genes, and therefore they are spared the diseases that affect XY males with the same X-linked mutations. However, males with two or more X chromosomes in addition to their Y chromosome have too many sex chromosomes and therefore an overdose of pseudoautosomal genes.

Why Are Extra Copies of X Chromosomes Tolerated Better Than Those of Autosomes?

Studies of the human products of conception miscarried during the first trimester of pregnancy tell us that chromosomal abnormalities have a large role in fetal loss. At least 50% of all miscarriages detectable during the first trimester have abnormal chromosomes, with most of them being trisomic—that is, having three copies of the same autosome instead of the two copies expected. A small proportion of them have trisomy for a sex chromosome, but only Klinefelter males are found in excess among miscarriages. Table 11-1 gives the frequencies of numerical chromosome abnormalities in various populations and shows that among >50,000 liveborns the numerical abnormalities of the sex chromosome are more frequent than those of autosomal ones. That is, X chromosomal aneuploidies are better tolerated than are those of autosomes in both sexes. No doubt this is because only one X chromosome is active in each diploid cell—no matter how many are present. Although the presence of extra sets of pseudoautosomal genes or other genes expressed from the inactive X may be detrimental and even cause congenital malformations, it is compatible with survival of the fetus.

Why Is X Chromosome Monosomy Tolerated When Autosomal Monosomy Is Uniformly Lethal?

Table 11-1 shows that although the incidence of Turner syndrome (monosomy X) is relatively rare among liveborns (1/10,000 live births), it is the commonest of the chromosomal monosomies, because none of the autosomal monosomies is found among liveborns. The lack of autosomal monosomies among recognizable pregnancies is unexpected because the errors in cell division that create monosomies (referred to as *nondisjunction*) are the same ones that produce trisomies. The absence of autosomal monosomies among first-trimester miscarriages means that they are more lethal than trisomies and that none of them survives long enough to be recognized as a pregnancy. In fact, tests that detect early pregnancy show that for every fetus that survives long enough to be clinically recognized, two others are lost at very early stages [10].

Therefore, like trisomies, it seems that X chromosome monosomies are better tolerated than autosomal ones. However, Table 11-1 also shows that even if X monosomies can be viable, most of them are not. We know this because the frequency of X0 newborns is about 0.01%, far less than those found among spontaneous abortions. Although most do not survive to term, those that are born do rather well subsequently; the survivors have the nonfunctional streak gonads and short stature, which are not usually life-threatening abnormalities, and they do not even have mental retardation. Recent findings suggest that the survivors are actually mosaic for the 45,X abnormality, having some cells with a normal 46,XX karyotype (see above and section 13.3). In any case, the fact that all of us have a single active X is why some individuals with an X monosomy can survive while those with autosomal monosomies cannot.

11.5. X DELETIONS, RING X CHROMOSOMES, X DUPLICATIONS, AND FUNCTIONAL DISOMY

X Chromosome Deletions

No matter the sex, deleting part of an X chromosome usually removes essential genes. We know that every embryo has to have at least one X chromosome because embryos without one do not survive beyond the earliest embryonic stages. Therefore, most deletions large enough to be visible in a standard karyotype are lethal or, at best, cause severe congenital abnormalities in males. In contrast, the same deletions in females are likely to be less detrimental because the deleted X is usually the inactive X in most cells (see figure 11-2). It is true that either the deleted X or the normal one can be chosen as the active X; however, when the deleted X is the active X, the cell dies because of the missing genes within the deleted segment and the deficiency of all the proteins encoded by those genes. Such cells are lost early in embryogenesis. Fortunately, at that stage the embryo can tolerate the loss of a relatively large number of cells because many cells present in early stages of development are not needed in subsequent ones. The loss of as much as half the blastocyst is well tolerated and does not compromise survival of the embryo. Certainly, twins and even quadruplets originate from a single fertilized ovum, attesting to the surplus of cells in the early embryo. The existence of females with X deletions shows the protective advantage that X inactivation provides for such embryos. But not all deletions are well tolerated. Those occurring within the X inactivation center produce severe effects in females because they interfere with the inactivation process—for example, tiny ring X chromosomes with XIC deletions.

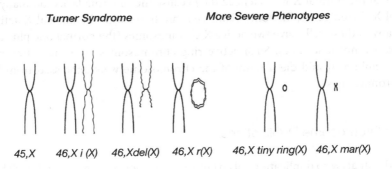

Figure 11-2. Chromosomes associated with typical Turner syndrome and more severe phenotypes. From left: X monosomy, isochromosome Xq, deleted Xq, large ring X, tiny ring X, small linear X. Inactive chromosomes are indicated by wavy lines.

Ring X Chromosomes

Ring chromosomes are chromosomes that were broken at two sites and became circular when the broken ends rejoined. Rings have been found for all the human chromosomes, and their size varies greatly depending on how much of the chromosome was deleted in the breakage and reunion process. Most autosomal rings produce very deleterious effects because the deletions they carry often result in monosomies for a large number of autosomal genes. In contrast, most X rings are more benign because they are usually the inactive X, so the deletions are never expressed. Ring chromosomes tend to be unstable, because they are often torn apart and lost during replication. Therefore, most individuals with X rings have some cells lacking the ring, and so their karyotype is often mosaic—45,X/46,Xr(X). In most cases, the ring chromosome is the inactive X, and their phenotype is Turner syndrome (figure 11-2).

However, some females with a very small ring X have a more severe phenotype. These girls not only have features of typical Turner syndrome (short stature and failure to maintain normal ovarian structure and function) but also have severe mental retardation, developmental delay, growth retardation, and multiple congenital anomalies not usually seen in Turner syndrome, including facial dysmorphism (coarse features, epicanthal folds, upturned nares, long philtrum, wide-set eyes, strabismus), fused fingers and toes, and heart defects. Such constellations of abnormalities have been called the severe phenotype of Turner syndrome (reviewed in [305]; see figures 5-1 and 5-2). Small ring X chromosomes are more harmful than large ones because they cannot inactivate, and therefore some genes (those within the ring) are expressed from both ring and normal X chromosomes. Such genes are functionally disomic; that is, both copies are transcribed [121]. In fact, the tiny ring X chromosomes in girls with such severe phenotypes invariably lack XIST DNA, or, if the locus is present, it is compromised in some way and not expressed [120–122]. As a consequence, the ring chromosome remains active. Any cells in which the normal X was silenced die because the tiny ring lacks too many essential X-linked genes. The only viable cells are those with the normal X active. Yet, many of these cells have two active X chromosomes (the normal one plus the ring that cannot inactivate). Such active ring chromosomes are usually tiny because the embryo would die if more of the chromosome were expressed from both X chromosomes.

X Chromosome Duplications

Individuals with duplications of an entire X chromosome do relatively well because much of the effect of the extra X chromosomes is nullified by the X inactivation process. However, there are individuals—both male and female—who have duplicated segments within one of their X chromosomes. In the case of females, such duplications are detrimental to cell survival and so will result in that chromosome consistently being the inactive X in all the surviving cells. The functional disomy is mitigated because the normal X is always the active one. Rare exceptions are very small duplications that do not affect cell selection; however, if the duplication has any deleterious effect at all, it is likely that such cells will eventually be overgrown by cells with a normal active X. Clearly, X inactivation helps to eliminate the problem of intrachromosomal duplications of X-linked genes in females. Therefore, such chromosomes are ascertained mainly in abnormal males—yet another example of the greater male vulnerability. The effects of the duplicated segments are related not to their size but to their gene content. Even relatively small duplications in males can have devastating effects [306]. Although data are limited, studies of males with duplications on the long arm of the X chromosome suggest that growth retardation, learning, and speech problems as well as craniofacial anomalies are significant issues.

11.6. X/AUTOSOME TRANSLOCATIONS AND SPREADING OF INACTIVATION

The outcome of chromosomal translocations involving X chromosomes is also influenced by X inactivation. X/autosome translocation chromosomes are formed when breaks occur in both an X chromosome and a nearby autosome during cell division; the broken pieces reunite such that a piece of X chromosome becomes attached to an autosome (see figure 5-3). Often the process is reciprocal: Fragments may break off from two different chromosomes and swap places such that both halves of the broken X reattach to different segments of the broken autosome. This produces two rearranged chromosomes: One has the centromere of the X chromosome (the derivative X, or *der* X); the other has the centromere of the autosome (see figure 11-3). Often, this kind of reciprocal translocation is balanced—that is, all the genes are present, but they are now split between two rearranged chromosomes. Translocations of this kind in somatic cells are usually benign—and it is the rare one that initiates a cancer.[5] However, if the translocation occurs in one of the germ cells—egg or sperm—there are several potential problems. The first is that both products of the translocation may segregate independently from each other during meiosis and not end up in the same germ cell; in that case, the karyotype of the zygote is unbalanced because this results in deletions or duplications of a large number of genes. No wonder unbalanced translocations of this kind are rarely seen in liveborns. Even when an individual receives both translocation chromosomes and the right number of genes, there is a problem relating to dosage compensation. Only the translocation chromosome that has an XIC can inactivate. Yet, if it does, there is a good chance that some of the genes on the attached autosomal segment will be inactivated as well, because the inactivation

---

5. Some leukemias and other tumors result from translocations in blood cells that place a quiescent oncogene on one chromosome next to active chromatin of the other, and this turns on the oncogene and initiates the cancer.

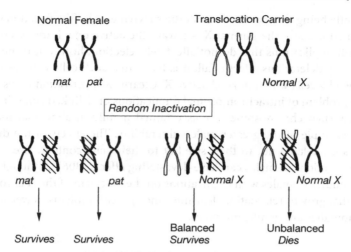

Figure 11-3. X inactivation in X/autosome translocations. Top: X chromosomes (black) in normal female and in a carrier of an X/autosome translocation (X segments, black). Bottom: After random inactivation, either parental chromosome can be the inactive X (shaded). However, in the case of the translocation carrier, only the cells in which the normal X is inactive survive. Inactivation of the *XIST*-bearing translocation chromosome would result in cell death because of spreading of inactivation into some autosomal genes, and disomy for the distal part of the X short arm that cannot be inactivated.

can spread into the autosomal portion of the translocation chromosome, silencing some autosomal genes. The extent of the spreading varies from one translocation to another and could interfere with the function of some autosomal genes. (See section 7.1, "Spreading Inactivation by Modifying Chromatin".)

Figure 11-3 shows how X inactivation affects the X/autosome translocation chromosomes. Because either normal or translocated X can be chosen as the active one, initially there will be mosaicism, as expected. However, cells that silence one of the translocation chromosomes are usually nonviable because (1) adjacent autosomal genes are silenced and (2) the other part of the translocation X chromosome remains active because it has no XIC. This means that the only cells that can survive in the long run are those in which the two translocation chromosomes are active. Therefore, it is not surprising that in most individuals with balanced X/autosome translocations, the normal X is the inactive chromosome in every one of their cells. Although at first glance this looks like preferential inactivation of the normal X, in fact, it is the result of cell death following random X inactivation. We know this because cells that inactivate the rearranged X have been detected in the fetus but are rarely seen after birth. When they are seen, it is usually in individuals with medical problems.

Schmidt and Du Sart [307] reviewed the outcomes in more than 100 females with balanced X/autosome translocations regarding the X inactivation pattern and their clinical phenotype. The normal X was late replicating (inactive) in three-quarters of them. As a consequence of this inactivation pattern, most of the females were either clinically normal or had only Turner syndrome. Less than 10% of them had congenital malformations and/or mental retardation; in the remaining 25%, one of the translocation chromosomes (the one with the XIC) was inactive in a proportion of cells, resulting in inactivation of some autosomal genes (see figure 11-3). In addition, such cells have a functional disomy for all the genes on the X segment of the translocation chromosome that lacks the XIC. As expected, the presence of such unbalanced cells was always associated with more severe phenotypes, including mental retardation and other congenital malformations. The conclusion of this study is that the X inactivation pattern was the major determinant of the clinical status in most patients with balanced X/autosome translocations.[6]

Most females with balanced X/autosome translocations are perfectly normal—provided their normal X chromosome is inactive in all their cells. However, there is a significant risk that some of their offspring will be unbalanced if they inherit only one of the two translocation chromosomes. An additional caveat: X inactivation may create a problem for the rare heterozygote with an X-linked mutation on either of her translocation chromosomes. Because the normal X is consistently inactive, such females are no longer mosaics. Therefore, the wild-type allele on their normal X is never expressed, fully exposing the mutations.

11.7. POLYPLOIDY AND THE CHOICE OF ACTIVE X

Studies of individuals with X chromosome aneuploidy tell us that every diploid cell has a single active X—no matter the number of X chromosomes. Even diploid cells whose two X chromosomes have the same parental origin, such as *ovarian teratomas* ($46,X^mX^m$, with two maternal X chromosomes) or *hydatidiform moles* ($46,X^pX^p$, with two paternal X chromosomes), have a single active X[7] (see "Parthenogenetic Conceptuses," *Appendix B*). Even when the two X chromosomes in these germ cell tumors are duplicate copies, originating from the very same X chromosome, one of the identical copies is inactivated.

Yet, there is an exception to the single active X rule, because cells of polyploid embryos may have more than one active X. Among the cytogenetically abnormal fetuses that survive gestation are those with duplications of their complete set of chromosomes, referred to as polyploids. Most polyploid embryos die early in pregnancy and are miscarried (see table 11-1). Most often they are triploid (three copies of each chromosome), but some of them may be tetraploid (four copies of each).

---

6. Despite remarkable variation among specific autosomal segments in their ability to spread X inactivation, Sharp et al. [188] found a good correlation between the pattern of gene silencing and the clinical phenotype.

7. These germ cell tumors arise because because 1) the developmental program leading to embryo formation is initiated parthenogenetically in a nonfertilized egg, or, 2) the zygote has only the paternal chromosome complement because of loss of the maternal genome from a fertilized egg. Because of parental imprinting of some essential genes throughout the genome, the resulting uniparental conceptus is very abnormal and does not give rise to a normal embryo.

Tetraploidy

Tetraploid embryos have 96 chromosomes, and four sex chromosomes, most often XXXX or XXYY. In either case, two X chromosomes are active. All of these embryos are lost very early in gestation, and any survivors are usually diploid/ tetraploid mosaics with malformations of many organ systems. Tetraploid embryos are thought to result from a mitotic error in a diploid embryonic cell, rather than from meiotic errors. If this were true, then the tetraploidy occurred after X inactivation as a result of duplication of all the chromosomes in a diploid cell. In this case, the two active X chromosomes would merely be the result of duplicating the entire diploid set of chromosomes in a female cell. If the error occurred before the time when the active X chromosomes was chosen, there must have been enough of the *Xist* repressor for two active X chromosomes, presumably because of the two extra sets of relevant autosomes.

Triploidy

In contrast to tetraploids, triploids are relatively common products of conception, occurring with a frequency of 1%. However, being one of the major causes of spontaneous abortions, they are rarely seen among liveborns. Such embryos have 69 chromosomes in each cell, with three copies of each chromosome. Most triploid fetuses are lost during the first trimester and have a developmental age of less than 9 weeks. Some triploids survive longer, but most are lost before term (table 11-1). The rare liveborn triploids are usually mosaics, having diploid cells as well as triploid ones (see *Appendix B*). Complete triploids are most often produced when an ovum is fertilized by two sperm that penetrate the egg simultaneously or by a diploid sperm that because of a meiotic error has 46 chromosomes instead of 23. Occasionally, triploidy results from fusion of the ovum with the polar body. Triploid cells have three sex chromosomes rather than two, and these can be XXY, XXX, or XYY; YYY triploids are never seen. The origin of the X chromosomes can differ, so the sex chromosomes may be X^mX^mY or X^mX^pY (see figure 11-4).

With respect to the rules of X inactivation, although only one X chromosome is designated an active X in diploid cells, two X chromosomes can be active in triploid cells [158–162, 427] (see figure 6-8). Based on analysis of *G6PD* variants in one liveborn 69,XXY triploid, both X chromosomes can be fully expressed in all cells, and the two-active-X phenotype can be stably maintained from one cell to its clonal progeny [160]. Based on studies of late replication [159] or *XIST* expression [161], most 69,XXY triploids have no inactive X, whereas a few may have one, or a mixed population, and this difference does not correlate with the parental origin of the chromosome [159]. Similarly, most of the 69,XXX triploids also have two active X chromosomes, and, again, only the minority have two inactive X chromosomes, or a mixture of both types of cells. However, the presence of a mixed population does not reflect instability in the maintenance of the active X phenotype because cell lines breed true. Although one inactivation pattern may

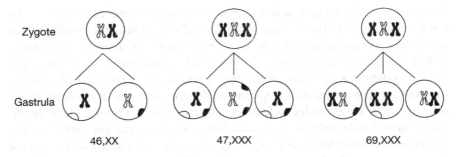

Figure 11-4. Random choice of the active X. Diagram shows sex chromosomes in the zygote, and active and inactive X chromosomes at the gastrula stage of embryogenesis in normal female (46,XX), left; diploid female with X trisomy (47,XXX), center; and triploid female with X trisomy (69,XXX), right. The paternal X is white, the maternal Xs are black, the inactive X is a Barr body. Note the single active X in both 46,XX and 47,XXX cells; it is the number of inactive Xs (Barr bodies) that differs. Also note the single active X in 47,XXX cells and the two active Xs in the 69,XXX cells despite the same set of sex chromosomes.

be favored over the other in mixed cell populations, the inactivation pattern of a given cell (whether zero, one, or two active X chromosomes) does not change during growth in cell culture, as the number of active X chromosomes in all the cells within a clone is the same [160, 162]. Therefore, it seems that any variation in the number of active X chromosomes arises at the onset of X inactivation. That cells of 69,XXY triploids have two active X chromosomes tells us that X inactivation does not invariably occur in cells with more than one X chromosome. The fact that triploid cells with two active X chromosomes survive as long as they do suggests that the extra autosomal set in some way balances the effect of the additional active X. It is likely that this additional set of autosomes is responsible for the activity of two X chromosomes in triploid cells, presumably because more of the autosomal repressor of *XIST* is available. Based on these human triploid embryos, it seems that if enough of this *trans* factor is available, no X chromosome need be inactivated.

In contrast, the variable numbers of active X chromosomes in triploid cells supports the notion that the choice of active X is subject to a good deal of probability. As discussed in section 6.7 ("Choosing the Active X Chromosome"), the process of choosing an active X is highly dosage sensitive. Most likely, only a small number of these signaling molecules are needed and their function is subject to cooperativity. In diploid cells, it seems that once one X chromosome receives the signal, the other cannot, and there is sufficient *trans* factor to repress only one *Xist* locus. However, triploid cells have more molecules available by virtue of the extra set of autosomal chromosomes and can often repress two *Xist* loci. Yet, it seems that even in triploid cells, the amount of *trans* factor is not always sufficient to fully repress both of them. Jacobs and colleagues [159] suggested that in some cases the variable inactivation status might reflect the process of cell selection favoring perhaps less active X chromosomes in placental tissues and more in the fetus proper. The relatively small number of 69,XYY triploids (<2% of all triploids

[162]) supports the suggestion that two active X chromosomes better balance the three autosomal sets. The findings in triploid cells again raise the possibility that the choice process also might be perilous for human 46,XX embryos, and that this probability decision might lead to the loss of cells, and even some embryos, very early in gestation. It may well explain the distortion of sex ratio at birth. Despite the likely equal sex ratio at conception and the greater loss of males *in utero*, the sex ratio of newborn males to females is approximately 1.05–1.07:1. If significantly more female embryos than male embryos were lost at the time of choice, this preimplantation loss could help explain the excess of males at birth. Because they have only one X, the choice of active X in XY males is bound to be less dosage sensitive, and hence the risk of errors would be less.

11.8. SUMMARY AND SPECULATIONS

Despite the fact that only a single X is active in cells of males and females, and that extra X chromosomes are inactivated in both sexes, it is apparent that gains or losses of entire X or Y chromosomes still may create clinical abnormalities. Often, the problems can be attributed to overexpression or underexpression of those rare XY homologous genes that are transcribed from the inactive X chromosomes and the Y chromosomes—because such genes are not subject to rigorous dosage compensation. The gain or loss of such genes can contribute to the abnormal somatic phenotypes seen in Turner, Klinefelter, and triple X syndromes. The very existence of individuals with sex chromosome abnormalities serves to remind us of the role that X dosage compensation plays in their survival *in utero*. By comparison, the same kinds of abnormalities occurring in autosomes certainly do not fare as well.

For me, the greatest lesson learned from the studies of individuals with extra X chromosomes is the realization that X dosage compensation is not female specific. Many of my colleagues who study mice consider X inactivation a developmental program for females only—probably because they do not think about Klinefelter males. However, because of patients with X chromosome aneuploidy, we know that irrespective of the sex, or numbers of X chromosomes, there is a program for maintaining the activity of a single active X in diploid cells. One does not need to count the chromosomes, because only one X remains active in 49,XXXXY males with four X chromosomes just as it does in females with two of them (46,XX). The simplest way to explain it all is to consider the designation of one active X per diploid cell, by repressing its *Xist* locus, to be the first step in X dosage compensation in both sexes. Up-regulation of the *Xist* locus on any and all remaining X chromosomes is the default pathway.

The other important lesson is that the rules of X inactivation differ in diploid and triploid cells, but the basic process is the same. The reason that two X chromosomes are usually active in 69,XXY and not in 47,XXY cells is most likely related to the additional amount of gene product(s) provided by the extra set of autosomes.

Mosaicism

There are two major medical consequences of X inactivation. The first, the single active X in somatic cells of both sexes, was the subject of chapter 11. This chapter considers the second: the cellular mosaicism.

12.1. THE X-LINKED PHENOTYPE IS DOMINANT AT THE CELLULAR LEVEL

Historically, genetic diseases have been classified as being either *dominant* or *recessive*, depending on whether one mutated allele or two of them are needed for clinical manifestations or whatever phenotype one is examining. As we learn more about what genes do, it becomes increasingly difficult to classify diseases in this way, because the nature of specific mutations plays a large role in determining clinical phenotype. The clinical outcome is greatly influenced by the extent of the functional loss. Also, the outcome of mutations that cause loss of the normal function usually differs from that of mutations in the very same gene that result in the acquisition of a novel function. Classifying diseases as dominant or recessive is especially arbitrary in the case of X-linked diseases because of the hemizygosity in males and the cellular mosaicism in females. (For a full discussion of this issue see Dobyns et al. [311]). What is relevant and important to our consideration of the clinical effects of cellular mosaicism is that any allele on the active X of males or females is the dominant one—in any cell in which it is expressed. No matter whether an X-linked disease is called dominant or recessive, the protein encoded by any expressed X-linked allele is always dominant at the cellular level. That is, whatever allele is on the active X chromosome will be the only one, or at least the major one expressed in that cell.[1] In contrast, the cellular phenotype determined by autosomal genes is a joint venture of the two parental alleles—often a blend of both of them. But, for X chromosomal genes subject to X inactivation, one allele is most often the sole determinant.

How well a tissue carries out its functions depends to a large extent on the competence of the cells within the tissue. In the case of females with X-linked mutations, the additive effect of all the individual cellular phenotypes in the tissue

1. There may be minor expression from escape alleles on the inactive X.

is what determines if disease occurs and its severity. The ultimate function of a tissue may depend on the interactions between cells expressing the normal allele (the haves) and the mutant cells (the have-nots).

12.2. FEMALES ARE MOSAICS

Females are mosaics because X inactivation creates two populations of cells that differ with respect to their active X (figure 12-1). A woman is mosaic because the same X chromosome is not expressed in every cell. In each of her somatic tissues, she has a mixture of cells, some expressing her maternal alleles, the others expressing the paternal ones. The bottom line is that although females have only a single working copy of their X-linked genes in each cell, they have a backup copy of these genes in reserve, even though the copy resides in neighboring cells.

Having two populations of cells would be meaningless if the alleles carried on one X were the same as those on the other. However, human females are highly heterozygous, and many of the alleles on maternal and paternal X are not the same. We are indebted to Harry Harris [312] for first showing how variable our proteins are. His observations suggested that any single individual is likely to be heterozygous at about 6% of the loci coding for enzyme proteins (for the X, this would mean that more than 60 alleles are not the same on the two X chromosomes). Because his analysis was based on electrophoresis, which could not detect all the differences in protein structure, the level of heterozygosity is undoubtedly greater and may approach 20%. Based on the frequency of changes affecting a single nucleotide (one single nucleotide polymorphism, or SNP, every 1,000 base pairs), most likely no allele is precisely the same as its homologue. Most of this variation does not interfere with—or even influence—the function of the gene but merely enables us to distinguish one allele from another. However, a good

RANDOM X INACTIVATION

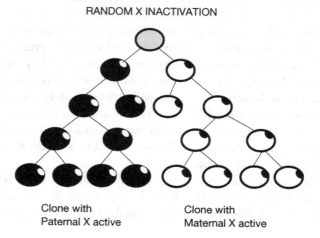

Clone with
Paternal X active

Clone with
Maternal X active

Figure 12-1. **Random X inactivation creates two clonal populations of cells:** one with paternal X active (black) and the other with maternal X active (white).

number of variations do influence the activity of the gene, and some of these may significantly compromise its ability to function at all.

Because females have a single active X, a deleterious mutation in an allele on that chromosome will have the same detrimental effect, at the cellular level, as it would if it occurred on the male X. However, the heterozygous female has the advantage that such a mutation will not affect all of her cells. The intermingling of normal and abnormal cells during embryonic development is extensive so that both kinds of cells are present in very small patches of tissue. And the normal cells within the tissue protect her from many of the deleterious effects of any mutation.

Patch Size

You may wonder how the two cell populations are distributed in tissues. One might expect to see a salt-and-pepper distribution, but in fact the patch size differs from one tissue to another depending on the migration patterns of individual cells and their clonal descendents. In most human females, both cell types can be found within a 1 mm skin biopsy that samples all dermal layers. However, the size of clonal patches of melanocytes in the skin of female mice is very large (see figure 4-4). Because the pigmented patches in mice heterozygous for the X-linked *mottled* mutations were so large, the German geneticist Hans Gruneberg questioned the validity of the Lyon hypothesis [313]. The patch size was explained subsequently by observations of chimeric mice made from aggregating the blastocysts of two mice differing in skin pigment genes [314]. The size of the patches in chimeric mice was identical to those in mosaic females heterozygous for the *mottled* mutation. The large patches in both cases are the result of the tendency for the clonal population of skin cells to stay together rather than to intermingle as they do in many other tissues. Therefore patch size depends on the patterns of cell migration and the degree to which the clones intermingle.[2]

An X-linked mutation that affects the embryonic development or function of human skin is usually reflected by a linear, patchy, or otherwise mosaic pattern. Shortly after birth, girls with *NEMO* mutations that produce incontinentia pigmenti (see section 12.5, *Appendix A* and figure 2 in Happle [315]) show vesicular eruptions arranged along the lines of Blaschko, reflecting the admixture of normal and mutant cells and the transverse outgrowth of clonal descendants from the primitive streak during embryogenesis [315]. These lesions evolve to a pigmented stage, and eventually, a hypopigmented and hairless stage when the mutant cells die.

---

2. This is consistent with all pigmentary ontogeny; each hair-bulb melanocyte descended mitotically from a single cell, one of only 34 precursor cells. As the embryo grows, these cells proliferate laterally (and to some extent longitudinally), as if a sheet of cells were spreading in the loose junction between epidermis and dermis.

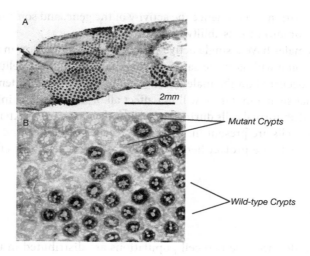

Figure 12-2. *G6PD* staining in a +/- heterozygote showing large patch size in colon tissue.
Low-power (A) and high-power (B) views with crypts cut in cross section. Note: Mutant
crypts are unstained, whereas wild type are positively stained. *Scale bar: 2 mm.* From Novelli
[316] with permission.

Figure 12.2 shows the large mosaic patch size in colon tissue. The tissue
obtained from a heterozygote for severe *G6PD* deficiency was stained for enzyme
activity. The mutant crypts are unstained, whereas wild-type crypts have G6PD
activity. The patch size in tissues from a female heterozygous for the fragile
X syndrome is shown in figure 10-3. In the placental villi (figure 10-3A–C),
the patches are quite large because each villus is a clone made up of cells that
originated from a single progenitor cell. Cells of both types are also present
in the brain (figure 10-3D), but the pattern is like salt and pepper, reflecting
greater intermingling of progenitor cells. Treating glomeruli from the kidney
of a heterozygote for Alport syndrome with an antibody to the mutant protein
COL4A5 reveals striking mosaic patterns, with clusters of immunolabeled
cells, (normal clones), and unlabeled clusters, (mutant clones) ([317], figure 1B). This suggests that each glomerulus is composed of progeny of several
progenitor cells, and is often mosaic with respect to the composition of its
basement membrane.

The tremendous range of patch size can be seen in female mice whose two
X chromosomes are marked with different Cre-activated, nuclear-localized
fluorescent reporters. Notable is the variation between littermates, and left and
right sides of retina, reflecting stochastic events, differences in cell migration
and the fine grain intermixing in neural tissue [432].

No matter how her two cell populations are distributed, the heterozygote has
a greater variety of gene products. The more limited repertoire of X-linked genes
expressed by males places them at a relatively greater risk of genetic diseases.

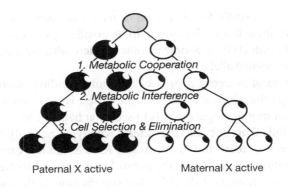

1. Metabolic Cooperation

2. Metabolic Interference

3. Cell Selection & Elimination

Paternal X active   Maternal X active

Figure 12-3. Interactions between mosaic cell populations: Cells can (1) share products, (2) interfere with the wild-type function, or (3) compete with one another for predominance.

12.3. INTERACTION BETWEEN MOSAIC CELL POPULATIONS

For many metabolic functions, it may not be necessary that all cells within the relevant tissue are functional. After all, there is a great deal of redundancy in tissues. We have two lungs and two kidneys, but one might do in a pinch. From studies of enzyme replacement in X-linked diseases we know that as little as 5% normal enzyme activity in some cases may be enough to ameliorate the disease. As little as 5% normal enzyme might be sufficient for mutant cells to carry out essential functions.

And in case more than 50% wild type cells within the tissue is required for adequate function, the population of normal cells may play another role: maintaining normal function by sharing their essential products with the mutant cells. In a mixed population of wild-type and mutant cells, the protein lacking in mutant cells can be furnished by the neighboring cells that make the essential protein.

Although the clonal cell populations appear discrete, no cell is an island, and there are myriad ways that cells from one cell population can interact with those of the other (figure 12-3). Cell-to-cell communication is important for many biological processes. Interactions that permit exchanges of materials from one cell to another are the means that multicellular organisms use to maintain homeostasis and to coordinate and even regulate the cellular activities. Sometimes, intracellular communication requires intimate physical contact—cells must touch one another to mediate the transfer. Alternatively, secreted cell products are transferred by means of extracellular fluids such as blood. Such interactions include cell-to-cell communication through intercellular channels, such as gap junctions, and the uptake of lysosomal enzymes by the process of endocytosis.[3] Communication

3. Endocytosis is the process by which extracellular molecules are captured and enclosed within membrane vesicles derived from invagination of the plasma membrane. Cells use endocytosis to feed and defend themselves.

of gene products usually fosters a kind of *metabolic cooperation* between cells. Unfortunately, there is also the more remote possibility of *metabolic interference* when mutant products from abnormal cells interfere with the function of the cells expressing the normal allele.

One of the most powerful approaches to understanding normal biology is to view it through the window of disease. The easiest way to understand the interaction between mosaic populations is to see what happens when one cell lacks a particular X-linked product and the other is wild type (normal). To put things in proper perspective, recall that most mosaic females are not carriers of harmful X-linked mutations. Nonetheless, the points I wish to make are best illustrated by such mutations. *Appendix A* describes the specific genetic diseases and includes details that may not be provided in this discussion. For those readers who want more information about specific disorders, *Appendix A* also includes the reference numbers for each disease in the Online Mendelian Inheritance in Man (OMIM) database.

Sharing Gene Products by Metabolic Cooperation

The benefits of having two cell populations are most evident in females who carry deleterious X-linked mutations. Women heterozygous for the same mutation that is harmful and even lethal to their sons often show no effect of the mutant gene. One explanation for this is that the normal cells in the mosaic heterozygote often provide enough of the essential gene product to the deficient cells to correct their defect—or at least enough to circumvent the lethality of the mutation. Cell-to-cell transfer of gene products masks the genotype because the mutant cells are not really deficient [318]. A good example of this is provided by the mutations affecting enzymes involved in the metabolism of large intracellular proteins. Such enzymes freely enter and leave the lysosomes, the site of their digestive activity, and can be transferred from one cell to another by mannose-6-phosphate–mediated endocytosis (figure 12-4). There are a number of devastating diseases caused by the deficiency of one of these lysosomal enzymes such as X-linked Hunter syndrome and Fabry disease (see *Appendix A*). The consequence of such enzyme deficiencies is that undigested products accumulate and plug up, or otherwise disrupt, the normal function of the lysosomes. The defective enzyme in Hunter syndrome is *iduronate sulfatase*, which is synthesized in some cells of carrier females but not in others. The cells that synthesize and secrete this enzyme (wild-type cells) can transfer it to those cells that cannot (mutant cells); in this way, the defect in the mutant cells can be corrected (figure 12-4). This is also true to some extent for carriers of Fabry disease, but the enzyme transfer is not as efficient because the α-galactosidase A enzyme is not taken up by mutant cells as well as is iduronate sulfatase. As a consequence, Fabry heterozygotes may manifest some of the deleterious effects of this mutation—but their disease is usually much milder than that of affected males [319].

A similar advantage is seen in women heterozygous for Lesch Nyhan mutations, which cause a severe deficiency of the enzyme hypoxanthine phosphoribosyl

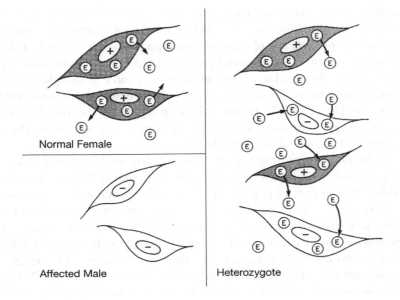

Figure 12-4. Transfer of X-linked lysosomal enzymes (E) from wild-type cell to mutant cell in mosaic heterozygotes. In normal females, the transfer of enzymes has little or no import. The cells in affected males are entirely enzyme-deficient.

transferase (HPRT). In males, these mutations causes mental retardation, spastic cerebral palsy, uric acid deposits in joints (gout), and self-destructive biting of fingers and lips; in contrast, the carrier female who has both deficient and normal cells (figure 5-7) manifests none of these symptoms—not even gout. In most of her tissues, inosinic acid, the small product of the HPRT metabolic reaction, is transferred from the normal cells in which it is made to her mutant cells by means of the intercellular channels called gap junctions. These channels connect the cytoplasms of neighboring cells. Gap junctions carry small molecules such as inosinic acid across the lipid bilayer of the cell membranes, mediating their transport between cells. In this way, the wild-type cells provide the essential product to the mutant ones.

Cellular Interference

During normal embryonic development, there is a great deal of interaction between cells of different lineages. One type of cell may induce function in another or may actually repel the physical movement of another. This has been observed in the development of the skull, where the growth of bones must be constrained in some way so that they do not prematurely fuse with one another, constricting the growth of the brain. Some insights into this kind of cellular interaction come from studies of the craniofrontonasal syndrome (CFNS) that results in premature fusion of the coronal suture separating frontal from parietal bones (see *Appendix A* and section 12.5). CFNS is caused by a deficiency of an X-chromosome–encoded member of the ephrin family of transmembrane proteins—very important signaling molecules in many developmental processes [320, 321]. One role of the *CFNS* gene is to define the position of the coronal suture, and it is thought to do this by repulsing cells from crossing the normally sharp neural crest/mesoderm tissue boundary [321, 322]. The transmembrane receptors on the neural crest cells recognize the ephrin proteins, which serve to restrict their migration; wherever ephrin proteins are, neural crest cells do not go.

From the phenotypes of males and females carrying a mutant *CFNS* gene, we have learned about another way that cells in the mosaic female interact with each other. Having a mixed population of cells differing in function—instead of a homogeneous one—seems to disturb some cellular functions. Hence, these mutations produce more severe defects in heterozygous females than in hemizygous males. Males with the deficiency of the ephrin B1 protein have minimal, if any, congenital abnormalities; in contrast, the carrier females have full-blown craniosynostosis and other skeletal abnormalities. Why do mutations in *EFNB1* lead to craniosynostosis only in females? It has been shown the patterns of X inactivation in affected females are random, and therefore these heterozygotes have a mixture of mutant and normal cells. The prevailing thought is that their craniosynostosis results from the presence of this mixed population of ephrin B1-positive and -negative cells. The mixture of mutant and normal cells in some way perturbs the signaling process and the subsequent sorting required for the formation of the future coronal suture, and as a consequence of faulty signaling, the bones prematurely fuse.

To explain why males with the mutation are so minimally affected, it has been suggested that other functionally redundant members of the ephrin family substitute for ephrin B1 in completely deficient cells in males but not in females—again, because of the admixture of mutant and wild-type cells. Recently, Twigg et al. [298] studied exceptional males who presented with the more severe phenotype characteristic of females; all six of them were mosaic, having a population of cells that lacked the *CFNS* mutation. This observation confirms the association between severe outcome and mosaic cell populations. Although only a few examples of this kind of interaction are known, they suggest that the outcome of cellular interactions during the development of heterozygotes may sometimes cause problems not seen in the hemizygous male.

Less well understood is the case of infantile epilepsy that is also restricted to females. This disorder, which results from mutations in the X-linked protocadherin-19 gene is thought to be another example of cellular interference [323]. The same nonsense and missense mutations that produce epilepsy in girls are not deleterious to their fathers who transmit the mutation, suggesting that the fathers are spared in some way—perhaps similarly to what happens in males hemizygous for ephrin B1 deficiency [324]. In support of this hypothesis, the only affected male found so far is one who is mosaic for the *PCDH19* mutation [324]. (See Epileptic Encephalopathy, Early Infantile in *Appendix A*) On the other hand, cellular interference of this type may not always be detrimental to the heterozygous female. Studies carried out to explain why *G6PD* deficiency is so prevalent in malaria-infested areas of the world suggest that one reason is that the heterozygotes for *G6PD* deficiency—are protected to some extent against infection with malaria [325, 326]. The parasite, when grown in *G6PD*-deficient cells, undergoes adaptive changes that gradually improve its ability to multiply in these deficient cells; this does not occur in cultures of heterozygous cells [327]. These results were interpreted to mean that the parasite can grow in deficient or in normal cells but has difficulty in a mixed culture. Although the evidence for this conclusion is not yet compelling, certainly the possibility that some pathogens might become a bit schizophrenic trying to adjust to conditions in a mixed population of cells cannot be ignored.

Cell Competition

Another interaction between the two cell populations in the mosaic female is adversarial: They compete with one another, and one can outgrow the other. One cell population may better utilize nutritional resources or respond better to growth signals and so may be able to proliferate faster than the other.

Clearly, some X-linked mutations adversely affect the growth of cells. In the mosaic female, the presence of two kinds of cells—differing in their proliferative capacities—sets up a competition between them; the cells that reproduce faster outgrow the other ones. Even small differences in growth rate can have an effect. Cells expressing an X-linked mutation that interferes with its proliferation are likely to be eventually eliminated by overgrowth of the cells expressing the normal allele. In fact, the best evidence that an X-linked mutation influences the rate at which cells proliferate *in vivo* is the presence of unbalanced or *skewed X inactivation* in the heterozygote. Unbalanced X inactivation is a powerful means to ascertain X-linked genes that affect cell proliferation.

Cell Selection at the Level of the Chromosome

Chapter 11 considered the fate of cells whose X chromosome carries a large deletion or has translocations involving an X and an autosome. No doubt, the fate of such cells is determined by cell selection. Studies of chromosome replication indicate that X chromosomes lacking large blocks of genes are almost always inactive X chromosomes. This is not surprising, because if the normal X were inactive, the cells, having no copy of the deleted genes, could not survive. We can exclude the alternative explanation—that is, that the abnormal X is in some way recognized as aberrant and is preferentially inactivated, because it is the normal X that is consistently silenced in carriers of balanced X/autosome translocations. In this case, cells do not proliferate well when the translocated chromosome is inactive; inactivation spreads into the autosomal portion of the chromosome, creating monosomies for autosomal genes (see figure 11-3). Therefore, the best explanation for nonrandom X inactivation patterns observed with such abnormal chromosomes is not preferential inactivation but cell death and subsequent overgrowth of cells that can survive. Selection of this intensity implies an extensive loss of cells from the embryo. Yet, cell losses of this magnitude occur during the development of monozygotic twins, and studies in mice show that mice of normal size result even when half of the early blastocyst has been removed.

Cell Selection at the Level of the Gene

The cells subject to elimination are those expressing an X-linked allele that adversely affects cell proliferation. *Appendix C* summarizes the results of cell competition for many X-linked disorders. Among the best examples of this are those cells from Lesch Nyhan heterozygotes that lack the HPRT enzyme (see figure 5-7). When these cells have gap junctions (e.g., skin cells), they can take up inosinic acid—the product of the enzyme reaction—from their wild-type neighbors. However, this kind of transfer is precluded for the heterozygous cells that lack gap junctions, such as blood cells. Fortunately, in blood cells, another mechanism is available to ameliorate the effect of the deleterious mutation. Having the normal enzyme gives the normal blood cells a proliferative advantage, and this leads to the gradual elimination of the HPRT-deficient blood cells (figure 12-5, top) [318]. In this case, the precise reason for the selective advantage is not known, but HPRT is one of the energy sources for the cell. Because affected males are only mildly anemic, it was not suspected that the heterozygous female would eliminate all of her enzyme-deficient blood cells (both leukocytes and red cell lineages) by the time she is 10 years of age. The loss of mutant cells is gradual—telling us that even a small difference in the growth rate of such cells can lead to their eventual elimination. Of interest, chimeric mice derived from HPRT-deficient cells have mutant cells in all tissues but blood [328], and

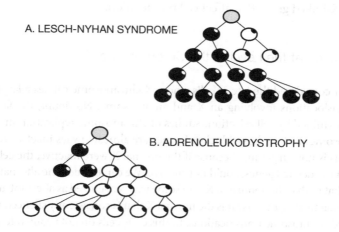

Figure 12-5. Skewing of X inactivation. In the case of Lesch Nyhan syndrome (a), the wild-type allele (black) has the selective advantage. In the case of adrenoleukodystrophy (b), the mutant allele (white) has the selective advantage.

they lack HPRT-deficient blood cells for the same reason as human Lesch Nyhan heterozygotes. Even the rare heterozygote who, because of severely unbalanced X inactivation, manifests the full-blown Lesch Nyhan syndrome has no mutant blood cells (see section 12-6, "'Manifesting' Heterozygotes"). How cell selection occurs in a Lesch Nyhan heterozygote can be understood by examining two dishes of her skin cells, one cultivated in nutrient medium, which permits the growth only of cells with HPRT activity (HAT medium), and the other in medium containing 6-thioguanine (6-TG), which permits only the growth of HPRT-deficient cells [329]. Figure 5-8b shows that only heterozygotes have cells that proliferate in both media. In contrast, cells from noncarrier females grow only in HAT, whereas cells from Lesch Nyhan males only grow in 6-TG. Selective cell growth occurs because of genetic differences in the two kinds of cells' ability to utilize the nutrient media.

For cell elimination to occur, the mutation must produce a severe loss of the enzyme. It does not occur in the case of X-linked gouty arthritis (Kelley-Seegmiller syndrome, *Appendixes A* and *C*), resulting from less severe mutations in the *HPRT* gene. The residual enzyme activity, which is less than 1.5% of normal in classic Lesch Nyhan mutations, is no more than 8% of normal in HPRT-deficient males whose only manifestations are nonsyndromic gout and kidney stones. Carriers of the less severe mutation are asymptomatic and their normal blood cells have no growth advantage because of the greater amount of residual enzyme; they remain mosaic because this seemingly small amount of activity is sufficient to abolish any growth disadvantage of the mutant blood cells. Also, to have a growth advantage, the normal cell must keep the wild-type gene product to itself—not sharing it with other cells. When inosinic acid—the end product of the HPRT enzyme reaction—is transferred from the normal cell via gap junctions in skin cells, the mutant cell is no longer at a disadvantage. Although the mutant cells have less inosinic acid than do the normal cells, they have enough to proliferate normally. As you see, the phenotype associated with HPRT deficiency in heterozygous females is determined independently in each tissue, based on the severity of the mutation and the availability of intercellular communication. As a consequence, mutant cells may receive essential products in one tissue and be eliminated in another tissue.

An even more impressive demonstration of cell selection is the elimination of abnormal cells in heterozygotes for X-linked immunodeficiencies such as Wiskott Aldrich syndrome or Bruton agammaglobulinemia (see *Appendix A*). The genes deficient in these diseases affect the ability to make antibody-producing cells. In this case, the mutant gene, when it is on the active X, precludes the development of that cell type from progenitor cells. Therefore, the heterozygote will be nonmosaic in the immune tissues where the mutation is expressed because she has only a single population of B- or T-cells, the normal one. Yet, in all the tissues other than those of the immune system, she still has cellular mosaicism. Cell elimination is so complete in these cases that the absence of mosaicism in the relevant tissue (reflecting the loss of the mutant T-cells and/or B-cells) is used as a diagnostic test to detect carriers of these diseases.

Cell selection occurs in X-linked diseases, whenever the mutation affects cell proliferation. Some of these diseases are listed in table 12-1 and many more are included in *Appendix C*. Most often, it is the mutant cells that are lost because the growth of

Table 12-1. INACTIVATION PATTERNS IN HETEROZYGOTES FOR X-LINKED DISEASES

Pattern of Inactivation	Disease
1. Random inactivation is usually associated with normal phenotype at birth.	Adrenoleukodystrophy Duchenne muscular dystrophy Emery-Dreifuss muscular dystrophy Hemophilia A and B Hunter syndrome Lesch Nyhan syndrome X-linked hemolytic anemia
2. Random inactivation leads to manifestations, more or less. Normal phenotype requires skewing, favoring wild type, in expressing tissue.	Craniofrontonasal syndrome Fabry disease Fragile X syndrome Hyperammonemia Incontinentia pigmenti Orofaciodigital syndrome 1 Otopalatodigital group Rett syndrome
3. Skewing always extreme as mutant cells die, fail to develop, or fail to migrate to destination.	ATRX syndrome Bruton's agammaglobulinemia Fanconi anemia B Incontinentia pigmenti Severe combined immunodeficiency Wiskott Aldrich syndrome
4. Skewing gradual because of cell selection due to a proliferative advantage of wild-type (or mutant) cells in the expressing tissue.	(Adrenoleukodystrophy) Lesch Nyhan syndrome X-linked hemolytic anemia

Parentheses indicate that skewing favors mutant cells.

the normal cells is favored. However, on rare occasions, the deficient cell has the proliferative advantage (see figure 12-5b and "Adrenoleukodystrophy" in section 12-5). The loss of cells from the heterozygous female can be rapid or slow, depending on the severity of the growth disadvantage. Even if the measured effect of these mutations on cell growth is minimal, slight differences in the rate of proliferation eventually lead to predominance of one cell population over the other. This is seen especially in tissues that undergo the most replication, such as blood cells. As pointed out by Belmont [330], even mild selective advantage can lead to severe unbalanced mosaicism in blood cells because they are continuously being replaced throughout the life of the individual. Any imbalance is often tissue specific, occurring only in expressing tissues. The skewing attributable to growth advantages of this type is usually unidirectional (i.e., favoring the normal allele in all families segregating the mutation). Almost all Lesch Nyhan heterozygotes select against their mutant *HPRT* allele in blood cells, to similar degrees [329, 331]. However, a few of them do not, presumably because they have other alleles on their X chromosomes that also influence the proliferation of their cells. The lesson to be learned from Lesch Nyhan heterozygotes is that the interaction between cell populations differs in various tissues and that proliferative outcomes are influenced not only by the nature of the mutant allele but also by all the other alleles on the X chromosome on which it resides.

12.4. SKEWING OF X INACTIVATION PATTERNS

Primary versus Secondary Skewing of X Inactivation

Nonrandom patterns of X inactivation are those where the ratio of the two cell populations deviates significantly from what one might expect for a standard random (1:1) distribution. Such deviations are referred to as skewing of X inactivation patterns, or skewed inactivation (see "The Role of Stochastic Events in Skewing" below). Severe skewing (>90:10) usually results from differences in the rate of cell proliferation, hence is secondary to cell selection, such as the elimination of mutant cells from Lesch Nyhan heterozygotes. The choice of active X was random at onset, but the mutant allele in expressing cells adversely affects their proliferation—leading to the overgrowth of the wild-type cells. But skewing can also occur when the choice of the active X during embryogenesis is biased because of mutations that affect the choice process (figure 12-6).

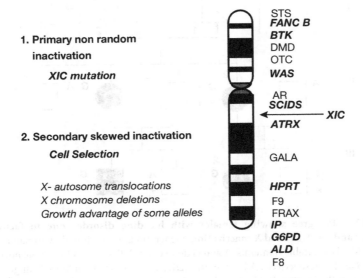

Figure 12-6. **Primary versus secondary skewing of X inactivation.** The X chromosome, showing the XIC region responsible for primary non-random X inactivation (1) and other relevant X-linked loci, with those subject to cell selection (2) shown in bold italics.

Primary Skewing

One expects that the choice of active X would be influenced by mutations residing in the region of the genome shown to be essential for choice—that is, in the *Xist* gene, or elsewhere in the X inactivation center (XIC; figure 12-6). Because choice and *cis* inactivation are independent events, mutations that prevent *Xist* from silencing the chromosome would lead to cells with two active X chromosomes, the designated active X and the X with the *Xist* mutation (see figure 10-1). The only surviving cells are those in which the mutant *Xist* allele resides on the chromosome chosen to be the active X. Cases of primary skewing are rarely found because the number of *Xist* mutations is small compared to the large number of mutated genes elsewhere on the chromosome that affect cell proliferation. Even families with mutations in the XIC are sometimes segregating other mutations that also might cause proliferative disadvantages [135]. And in some cases, human *XIST* mutations thought to be responsible for skewing have been found in other family members with random inactivation patterns [135, 136]. The effect of the *XIST* mutations in these families is rather subtle and may require the coincidence of other factors that help skew inactivation. Yet, studies of a family (shown in figure 12-7) suggest that the hemophilia A in three females is probably due to nonrandom choice of active X [332]. The three women in this family have only one mutant *F8* allele but all suffer from hemophilia. With only one defective allele, they were not expected to manifest a clotting disorder. But in each of them, the hemophilia is associated with complete skewing of X inactivation,

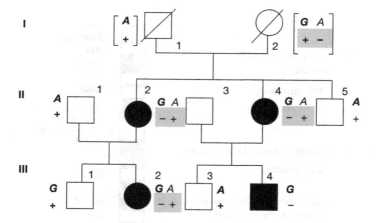

Figure 12-7. **Pedigree showing females with bleeding disorder due to factor VIII deficiency and >95% skewed X inactivation.** Generations are indicated by roman numerals and individuals by Arabic numerals. A and G denote *XIST* alleles; + and − denote normal and mutant *F8* alleles, respectively. Alleles on the active X are shown in bold to distinguish them from those on the inactive X. Hemophilia in these heterozygous females segregates with the *XIST* G allele that is always on the active X, most likely because it cannot induce inactivation. Note that the A allele can be on either an active or inactive X. Adapted from figure 1 of Bicocchi et al. [332].

and the mutant allele is expressed in all of their cells in all of the tissues analyzed. What these affected heterozygotes also have in common is the *XIST* allele, inherited on their maternal X chromosomes. It is likely that this *XIST* allele or another relevant gene in the XIC, has a defect that interferes with its chromosome's ability to undergo inactivation, and so is never seen on the inactive X.

Analysis of Mosaic Cell Populations as a Test of Randomness of Inactivation: Assays for Skewed X Inactivation

The assays designed to show the skewed distribution of the two cell populations were briefly considered in chapter 5. Such assays are referred to by several names, depending on the reason the assay is being performed. They are called *clonality* assays by those who use them to determine if a given tumor arises from a single cell or multiple cells. If the tumor is a clone, it will not be mosaic but will express only one of the parent's alleles, unlike the normal tissues from that individual that express both of them.

These assays are called X inactivation assays when they are used to determine the proportion of each cell type in the heterozygote (the ratio of cells with active maternal X to cells with active paternal X). Any expressed variation can be used as an assay. One needs a marker—either a variant protein such as G6PD A (discussed in chapter 5) or a common DNA sequence variant (polymorphism)—to distinguish one allele from another. If the allelic difference is in the expressed (exonic) portion of a gene, then which parental allele(s) is being transcribed in that tissue can be determined by RNA analysis, and the proportion of each transcript can be determined and quantified. In fact, this is the most direct way of determining relative numbers of cells whose active X is the maternal one. Only those cells with an active maternal X express the mother's allele, whereas only cells with an active paternal X express the father's allele. Expression assays at the level of the RNA are the very best ways to look for skewing, because they depend only on the level of gene expression.

Yet, X inactivation patterns are usually assessed using a less direct assay, called HUMARA because the gene most often used for the assay is the human (HUM) androgen receptor (AR) gene [333] (see *Appendix A*); it is also called the methylation assay for X inactivation (figure 12-8). The advantage of methylation assays is that the common DNA polymorphisms in *nontranscribed* areas of the genome (more common than transcribed ones) can be used, and DNA is the target of analysis rather than the more fragile RNA needed for expression assays. The composition of the mosaic populations is determined from the proportion of parental alleles that are methylated (inactive) because the assay can distinguish methylated from unmethylated alleles. The assay is based on the fact that CpG islands on the inactive X are usually methylated, whereas those on the active one are unmethylated (see section 7.2, "Maintaining X Inactivation by DNA Methylation of CpG Islands"). It is also based on the presumption that an allele on the inactive X is always methylated and the one on the active X is always unmethylated. Then, it follows that if (1) all inactive alleles are methylated and (2) inactivation is random, then one would see equal numbers of methylated maternal and paternal alleles.

The *AR* gene is used as the means to distinguish between the parental alleles because it is highly polymorphic—in most women (~90%), one allele differs from the other. The two *AR* alleles differ in length because of variable numbers of CpGs within the CpG island in the gene, and these length differences can be used to distinguish one allele from the other. Once a parental allele is identified, then its activity status can be examined by determining the methylation status of its CpG island. The proportion of each parental allele that is methylated (inactive) is ascertained by digesting it with a methylation-sensitive restriction enzyme such as HPAII. The allele will be digested only if it is unmethylated, and in this case digestion makes it disappear. Therefore, only the methylated alleles from the inactive X remain after digestion. And so the proportion of the methylated alleles from each parent can be determined by the ratio of the two undigested alleles (see figure 12-8).

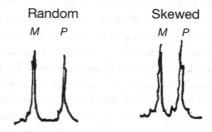

A. *Predigestion, showing equal amounts of maternal (M) and paternal (P) alleles*

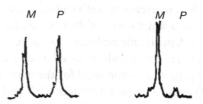

B. *After digestion with HpaII, showing undigested (inactive) alleles*

Figure 12-8. The HUMARA assay for X inactivation patterns. The maternal and paternal *AR* alleles can be distinguished from one another based on size differences on gels. *Top*: Before digestion, there are equal amounts of maternal and paternal alleles. *Bottom*: The inactive (methylated) allele can be distinguished from the active (unmethylated) allele by digesting the sample with methylation sensitive enzyme HPAII. The active alleles will be digested, and only the inactive alleles remain. The ratio of maternal to paternal undigested alleles gives the percent skewing. When inactivation is random (left), equal amounts of paternal and maternal alleles are inactive (methylated) and so will not be digested by HPAII. Therefore, the ratio of M:P alleles is close to 1:1 In this case of skewed inactivation (right), most of the inactive alleles are maternal, with about 5–10% inactive paternal alleles.

One caveat: This assay, like most methylation assays, is based on the assumption that CpGs within an island on the active X are completely unmethylated whereas those on the inactive X are entirely methylated. The problem is that inactive alleles may not always be adequately digested or sufficiently methylated in all cells to resist digestion. Because DNA methylation at any particular cytosine may change, methylation patterns may be variable from individual to individual, from tissue to tissue, from cell to cell, and from gene to gene. Therefore, methylation status may not always correlate with inactivation status. In the case of severe skewing, such errors are of little consequence. However, the assay is not sensitive enough to determine small quantitative differences and at times may indicate more skewing than really exists. And often the assay is carried out not in the relevant tissue but in blood cells because they are most accessible. Blood cells are replenished more than most other cells, and the faster turnover provides more opportunity for cell selection. Therefore, the degree of skewing may be exaggerated in that tissue. In any case, it may not always reflect cells ratios in brain and other less accessible tissues. In the first edition, I predicted that as more polymorphisms are found in expressed genes, and assays of RNA become less tedious, and with quantitative improvements in microchip analysis, all assays of this kind would be based on gene expression and not on DNA methylation. In fact studies of the RNA sequence are now widely used to quantitate single allele expression [334, 335]. The patterns of X inactivation are frequently used as a means of obtaining insights into the pathogenesis of an X-linked disease, whether or not the causative gene is known. Finding random inactivation in heterozygous cells suggests that the mutation does not cause cell lethality, and perhaps the gene product can be transferred from one cell to another. Skewed patterns in normal heterozygotes suggest that the normal phenotype is possible only if the majority of cells express the normal allele, or that mutant cells are disadvantageous. The composition of cell populations has prognostic implications and has been used to detect carriers for some of the immunodeficiency diseases, based on the elimination of mutant cells. In addition, X-linked genes involved in mental retardation syndromes have been discovered by ascertaining skewed X inactivation in mothers of affected males [336] (see *Appendix C*).

The Role of Stochastic Events in Skewing

When are deviations in the patterns of X inactivation considered sufficient to reflect skewing? There is a bell-shaped curve around the mean of 50:50 such that even 30:70 ratios may merely reflect normal variation around that mean.[4] Figure 12.9 shows that 30:70 is within one standard deviation from the mean and that many normal women would fall within that distribution. Even 20:80 ratios

---

4. About 68% of values drawn from a normal distribution are within one standard deviation away from the mean, about 95% of the values lie within two standard deviations, and about 99.7% are within three standard deviations.

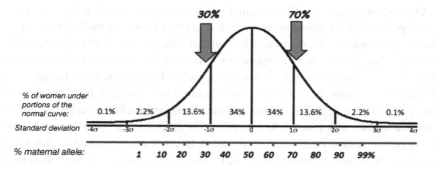

Figure 12-9. The normal distribution of random X inactivation. Shown is the percentage of women under portions of the normal curve for each percentage of cells with the maternal allele expressed. The arrows show that many women with random choice of maternal X would fall between 30–70%, as these values are within one standard deviation of the mean.

of parental alleles may be within the range of the normal distribution, especially when one considers stochastic deviations from the mean in a biological process such as this one. In addition, there can be some skewing even when inactivation occurs randomly because the cell population at the time of inactivation may be relatively small. The underrepresented cell population may then undergo further loss because of additional stochastic events.

The literature on the subject of what constitutes a significant deviation is inconsistent, because the cutoff point that is used to distinguish deviant from normal values may range from 70–95% skewing, depending on the investigator's perspective, control population, and experience with the assay. The control values for the same assay in different laboratories vary widely. As one might expect, the most variable assays are those that depend on the methylation status of the CpG island in the *AR* gene, because it is subject to methylation variation. I used G6PD protein variants in blood from normal mothers of newborn males to determine the number of women who completely excluded the allele expressed by their son. My results indicated that approximately 5% of these heterozygotes had completely skewed (>95%) patterns.[5] This estimate is at the low end of the 5–20% range reported in the literature for normal individuals, based on the HUMARA assay in blood cells.

What is the cause of extreme skewing in these populations of ostensibly normal women? It is usually attributed to chance deviations from random and is said to be a consequence of the limited number of embryonic precursor cells present in the embryo when the active X is chosen. However, normal stochastic events are rarely responsible for cell populations in which the minor population is less than one-tenth of the whole, that is, >90% skewing. At least some of the extreme

---

5. This estimate took into account the cases where the mothers might be homozygous, and so allelic exclusion could not be detected.

skewing in presumed controls may be due to small degrees of proliferative advantages of alleles carried on either X chromosomes. And the control group may include normal females who are unidentified carriers of one or more deleterious alleles, that is, those without an affected son.

Other Causes of Skewed X Inactivation

The distribution of the two mosaic cell populations may be skewed whenever the number of cells in the blastocyst is reduced. Perhaps this can explain the association between skewing and human monozygotic (MZ) twins [337]. These are the kind of twins that develop from a single ovum, in contrast to fraternal (dizygotic, DZ) twins that arise from the simultaneous fertilization of two ova. MZ twins heterozygous for mutations causing X-linked diseases are sometimes discordant in the clinical expression of their mutations. One twin of the pair will have hemophilia, Duchenne muscular dystrophy, Lesch Nyhan syndrome, or another X-linked disease, whereas the co-twin will have no manifestations at all. The reason for the discordant phenotype may be (1) differential environmental exposure *in utero* (least likely), (2) epigenetic variability in imprinting their genes, or (3) or skewing of X chromosome inactivation (most likely).

In the case of MZ twins with discordant phenotypes, only one twin may show skewing. Such discordant phenotypes are directly attributable to the inactivation patterns, because usually skewing occurs in the twin who manifests the disorder, and most of her cells are mutant. Rarely, the opposite occurs—usually in cases where skewing is required for a normal phenotype. In all reported cases, the composition of the mosaicism in the affected twin favors the expression of the disease. The reason for the skewing is believed to be associated with a reduced cell pool because of cleavage preceding X inactivation. Although not well documented, skewing is observed most often in MZ twins with separate *chorions* (see figure 10-2)—an indicator of relatively early cleavage. The time when MZ twins cleave apart (5–9 days after conception) is earlier than the time when *cis* inactivation occurs in the embryo (~20 days after conception). If cleavage occurs before the onset of choice, the reduced pool size in each embryo may increase the probability of skewing for stochastic reasons. No doubt there will be other explanations. In any case, discordant twins of this kind may be overreported because of a bias in ascertainment: The female who manifests a disorder usually seen only in males is an attention getter, especially if her twin is not affected. In any case, these are exceptional twins because the majority of MZ twins show random X inactivation patterns, and there is no skewing in either of the co-twins (reviewed in [338]).

At times, cell selection may underlie what seems to be a stochastic event. Skewed X inactivation is common in fetuses or newborns whose mosaicism was limited to placental cells [339]). This confined placental mosaicism is most often associated with the most frequent trisomy—that of chromosome 21 in individuals with Down syndrome—although it also has been seen in other trisomies. In the case of Down syndrome, the placental cells are a mixed population, either trisomic for chromosome 21 (Down syndrome) or disomic (normal). The disomy occurs when one of the cells from a trisomy 21 fetus loses one of its three copies of chromosome 21; no longer being trisomic, the cell with only two copies of chromosome 21 flourishes, eventually giving rise to an extensive clonal population of cells. The result is a disomic fetus and a placenta that is mosaic for trisomy chromosome 21. It seems that in a mixed trisomic/disomic population, trisomic cells may be tolerated in a terminally differentiated tissue such as the placenta but eliminated from the fetus proper. If the event that restores the 21 disomy occurs after X inactivation, then all the cells derived from it (all the clonal progeny) would have the same active X. If only disomic cells found their way into the fetus, then the fetus would have only the disomic population of cells, all having the same active X.

For similar reasons, the X inactivation patterns in most tumors—whether the original tumor or a metastasis—are most often completely skewed. The reason for the skewing is that these tumors are ultimately clonal, having been derived from mutations with an effect on cell proliferation, which occurred initially in a single somatic cell; because the single cell had a fixed pattern of inactivation, all its descendants have the same inactive X. Disomic cells in trisomic embryos as well as tumor cells can be thought of as bottleneck effects; the progeny of one cell are overrepresented in the individual or tumor or tissue that is being analyzed, because although a minuscule part of the original population, they are the ones with the growth advantage.

Age-Related Skewing of X Inactivation Patterns

Several studies report that the frequency of skewed patterns of inactivation is greater with age [340–343]. However, further investigation suggests that the increase is not a gradual one, but is more catastrophic—occurring quite late in life. Repeat samples of women taken approximately 20 years apart suggest that little change occurs during that interim [341]. However, several females who were older than 60 at the time of the first sample acquired significant changes in the X inactivation ratio subsequently. Twin studies support this observation because elderly twins have a higher frequency of skewed X inactivation (34%) than do young twins (15%; $P < .001$). Yet, the fact that both MZ and DZ twins show the same increase suggests that the increased skewing with age is not genetically programmed. The parental origin of the predominantly active X chromosome was not a factor. The results of these studies suggest that both stochastic and genetic factors contribute to the increased skewing. The biological reason for the increased skewing with age in some cases may have something to do with cell selection. Certainly the frequency of normal cells in HPRT and G6PD heterozygotes increases with age, as does the frequency of mutant cells in adrenoleukodystrophy (ALD) heterozygotes.

In addition, expression of silent genes from the inactive X has been observed with aging in mice, and it is likely that reactivation is responsible for some of the leaky expression of escape genes on the human X chromosome. What effect instability of maintenance has on the methylation assays for X inactivation patterns remains to be seen.

Inheritance of Skewed Inactivation

Contrary to expectations for primary X inactivation, where defective function of the XIC is expected to be inherited from one generation to another, the mutations responsible for cell selection in one generation may not have the same effects when transmitted to the next generation. It is important to remember that it is the alleles on *both* X chromosomes that determine whether there will be competition. The dynamics of interactions between cell populations may differ from one generation to the next because the paternal X chromosome in a mother's cells is not the one in her daughter's cells. Hence, there are different paternal alleles to influence the outcome of the competition. The outcome can also differ between generations because of recombination between homologous X chromosomes in the mother that removes the selectable marker from one chromosome and puts it the other, such that even when the paternal X is the same, identical mutations inherited from mother may reside on different maternal X chromosomes in her daughters.

One more caveat: It has also been tempting to use cellular mosaicism in adult females to determine the size of the pool of precursor cells at the time inactivation occurs. Because of the influence of cell selection on the composition of cell populations in human females, it is not possible to determine this with any accuracy. The population of cells after birth is not likely to be the same as the one at the time of inactivation, because of cell selection. Estimates of pool size must be carried out in less heterozygous laboratory animals where the influence of cell selection is not as prominent.

12.5. EFFECT OF X INACTIVATION ON CLINICAL PHENOTYPE

Up to now I have discussed how cellular mosaicism comes about and how these cell populations interact in the mosaic female. Cell-to-cell communication of gene products can serve to correct deficiencies in mutant-type cells; if this is not possible, and the deficiency is severe enough, then the mutant cells are often eliminated. In this section I consider some of the X-linked diseases listed in *Appendix A* to illustrate the points in this chapter. Table 12-1 summarizes the X inactivation patterns for some of these diseases. *Appendix C* summarizes the sex differences in phenotype and results of studies of cell selection. I hope this discussion further illuminates the many complex issues that influence the ultimate phenotype and the health status of the female carriers of these disorders. Remember that in most cases females are protected against most of the manifestations seen in males, but there are a few exceptions.

X-Linked Hemolytic Anemia Due to G6PD Deficiency

In this disorder, the selective advantage of the normal cell is rather subtle and is mainly evident in older heterozygotes. There are many different mutations in the *G6PD* gene, especially in the African, Mediterranean, and Asian populations because these mutations convey some degree of protection against infection by the malarial parasite that is rampant in that part of the world. In most males, the amount of G6PD deficiency is not enough for clinical manifestations, and hemolytic anemia needs to be induced by the ingestion of fava beans or drugs such as sulfa and primaquine. But males with mutations leading to more severe enzyme deficiencies do not need an inducer. Women heterozygous for the severe mutations rarely have anemia because inactivation is slightly skewed in favor of the normal allele as it conveys a relative growth advantage. The only women with anemia are those who happen to be homozygous for the mutation or those whose mutant alleles are favored for reasons unrelated to the *G6PD* locus. For example, they may have a deleted X chromosome (always the *inactive* X), which unmasks a *G6PD* mutation on the normal X (always the *active* X). Of significance, more than 90% of heterozygous females have normal G6PD activity at birth, indicating that most mutations are not severe enough to reduce enzyme levels in the mosaic embryo. In contrast, severe G6PD deficiency is lethal to male mice, as the enzyme is required in placental cells. This is also the case in female mice who inherit the *G6PD* mutation from their mothers because the normal allele on their imprinted paternal X is never expressed in placental tissue. The difference in survival of female mice and humans heterozygous for severe G6PD deficiency is an excellent example of how the species differences in details of X inactivation can affect the clinical phenotype.

Incontinentia Pigmenti

Incontinentia pigmenti (IP) is an X-linked disease that is usually lethal in males. Females eliminate mutant cells; the degree of elimination correlates with the severity of their mutation and the manifestations of disease. Males with a mutation in the NEMO gene survive only if they are mosaic (somatic mosaicism or XXY Klinefelter syndrome), or have a non-severe mutation. Therefore, it is the heterozygous female who is affected. There is considerable overlap between manifestations of IP, many of which are due to deletions of the NEMO gene, and those of hypohidrotic ectodermal dysplasia (HED, OMIM #300291) that is attributable to less severe mutations in the NEMO gene. Both mutations causes highly variable abnormalities of the skin, hair, nails, teeth, eyes, and central nervous system, paradoxically less severe in IP than in HED. In the skin of IP heterozygotes, there is a distinctive pattern of hyperpigmentation followed by dermal scarring, reflecting the death of skin cells that express the mutant gene from their active X. These mutant skin cells die shortly after birth, so females heterozygous for IP exhibit extremely skewed X inactivation in their skin cells and white cells [344]. In the case of IP, it is the disease process itself that causes the death of mutant cells—which explains their growth disadvantage. That is why the normal cells in the mosaic population outgrow and replace the dying mutant ones. The differences in severity of the disease among IP heterozygotes may be related to the extent and the rate at which the mutant cells are eliminated. One girl heterozygous for a less severe NEMO mutation that caused transient immunodeficiency [345] had a pattern of X inactivation in her granulocytes and T-cells that was random at birth but over a period of 4 years gradually changed to one in which all of the cells expressed the normal allele, presumably because of progressive death of mutant cells. The percentage of cells expressing the normal allele was 55% at age 24 months, 58% at 30 months, 73% at 38 months, and 100% at 4 years, at which time all signs of immunodeficiency had disappeared. The relatively late and progressive cell selection and the transient immunodeficiency in this girl (not seen in most IP heterozygotes) was because her mutant NEMO allele was less detrimental than the ones responsible for the classic form of IP. Paradoxically, the less severe protein deficiency in this girl produced more severe disease because cell elimination was less efficient. This case illustrates how clinical manifestations can be ameliorated when mutant cells are eliminated, and replaced by normal ones.

Hunter Syndrome

In Hunter syndrome, the enzyme is transferred from normal to mutant cells bringing the essential product to the deficient cell. This not only prevents cell elimination but also usually protects the heterozygote from disease manifestations. The mutations in Hunter syndrome produce a deficiency of iduronate sulfatase, a digestive enzyme needed for the degradation of mucopolysaccharides. The deficiency results in an accumulation of undigested protein in lysosomes (see *Appendix A*). Males with the deficiency have more or less severe disease depending on the severity of their enzyme deficiency. Heterozygous mothers and sisters of affected males usually have no symptoms [346] because the enzyme is efficiently transferred from their normal cells—which synthesize and secrete iduronate sulfatase—to the mutant ones (figure 12-4). Because there is no basis for cell competition, the X inactivation patterns are perfectly random. The fact that mutant cells can be corrected by normal cells in heterozygotes has been exploited as a means to treat affected males by transfusing them with donor hematopoietic stem cells or recombinant enzyme, or transplanting them with normal tissues.

Fabry Disease

In Fabry disease, enzyme transfer from normal to mutant cells precludes cell elimination, but heterozygotes have some symptoms because the transfer is not adequate. A recent survey of European patients with this disorder showed that females heterozygous for the disease are often affected [319]. However, manifestations are much less severe than those in males and may be overreported. In females, symptoms begin later than in males, and affected females live significantly longer than affected males. And enzyme replacement therapy is more effective in relieving their symptoms. The incidence of females with full-blown disease is 1 in 200, but 10% of all heterozygotes eventually undergo dialysis or kidney transplants for renal failure. In any case, the symptoms, and circulating levels of alpha-galactosidase A (GLA), are more variable in females, and the disease appears to have a slower rate of progression. The milder disease is undoubtedly due to the effect of X inactivation. There is no evidence of cell selection favoring the mutant *GLA* alleles, but skewing of inactivation for stochastic reasons—or for reasons unrelated to this gene, such as twinning—does influence the clinical expression of the disease. The influence of X inactivation is striking in a pair of female MZ twins, who you will recall are uniquely prone to skewing. One of the twins had the classic form of Fabry disease, and her cells expressed predominantly the mutant allele. The other twin was asymptomatic—with a majority of cells expressing the normal X. Although few women with more serious manifestations have been examined for X inactivation patterns, it is likely that they have by chance, significant skewing in favor of mutant cells as they have zero levels of enzyme in many tissues [R. Desnick, personal communication, December 2005].

Yet, the fact that a majority of carriers have the same degree of benign opacities in the corneas of their eyes, as do males indicates that most carriers have at least one feature of the disease. This suggests that more than 50% normal cells are needed to supply enough enzyme to suppress all manifestations, and that the mutant cells in the cornea are not rescued by their normal cell neighbors. Clearly, Fabry disease differs from Hunter syndrome in this respect. The difference between the two lysosomal disorders is that iduronate sulfatase, the enzyme deficient in Hunter syndrome, is a higher uptake enzyme than is GLA. That is, the uptake of GLA from the lysosomes of one cell and its delivery to the lysosomes of another is relatively inefficient, compared to that of iduronate sulfatase. The difference between high- and low-uptake lysosomal enzymes has to do with the density of mannose-6-phosphate receptors or their position on the enzyme. Based on observations of enzyme transfer in heterozygotes, a high-uptake synthetic form of the enzyme instead of the natural enzyme is used to treat Fabry disease. The variable phenotypes of Fabry heterozygotes illustrate why the term *X-linked recessive* is misleading and should be discontinued.

Danon Disease

This is the third of the X-linked lysosomal disorders. Unlike Hunter and Fabry diseases, the mutations causing Danon disease affect the lysosomal membrane glycoprotein, LAMP2, and not a proteolytic enzyme. Because the mutated protein is part of the lysosomal membrane, it is cell autonomous. This means that the mutant gene product stays within the mutant cell and cannot be rescued by normal LAMP2 synthesized by the wild-type cells in the mosaic female. Mutations responsible for Danon Disease produce a severe deficiency of the protein, and so affected males have an early onset of cardiomyopathy, many dying during their second decade. On the other hand, depending on the proportion of normal cells, females have less morbidity, with onset of cardiomyopathy usually when they are adults. As expected, there is a great range of clinical phenotypes among carriers of the same mutation. To date, there have been no studies of cell selection in blood cells of heterozygous females, but their clinical phenotype suggests that many adult heterozygotes have a good number of mutant cells.

Lowe Syndrome

Although most Lowe Syndrome heterozygotes are asymptomatic, like carriers of Fabry disease they have lens opacities that usually do not interfere with visual acuity [347, 348]. This suggests that the mutant population of cells in the lens is particularly sensitive to the effects of the mutation, and that mutant cells are generally well represented in the mosaic lens, that is, not subject to cell selection or metabolic cooperation. In any case, lens opacities provide a rather sensitive assay for heterozygotes in both diseases. Historically, Lowe syndrome was defined as only affecting boys, in whom a mutation in the OCRL1 gene causes congenital cataracts, rickets, dysfunction of the kidney, and mental retardation. Heterozygous females often have only lens opacities, which are punctate, peripherally located, and distinguishable from the lens changes seen in carriers of adrenoleukodystrophy and Fabry disease. On the other hand, a few Lowe heterozygotes are as fully affected as males; this was explained in one case by severe skewing such that she had only mutant cells, with her normal OCRL1 allele mute on her inactive X [349]. The skewing was not related to the OCRL1 mutation, as five other females in the family, who had no OCRL mutation, also had complete skewing.

Hemophilia A

In the relatively common disorder of hemophilia A, heterozygotes do not manifest the disease unless there are complicating factors. Although the mutation does not affect cell proliferation, the clotting process will be adversely affected if the mutant gene happens to be expressed in the majority of cells. Hemophilia A is the commonest of the bleeding disorders caused by mutations in the metabolic pathway responsible for blood clotting. The gene responsible, *F8*, encodes clotting factor VIII. Another clotting factor, factor IX, is also encoded by an X-linked gene, *F9*, and deficiency of that protein is known as hemophilia B.[6] In each case, affected females may be homozygous for the mutation because affected males may be healthy enough to reproduce and pass on their mutant genes to every daughter. In heterozygous females, X inactivation is usually random, and half normal cells are sufficient for normal clotting function; therefore, carrier females are usually not bleeders.

Yet, some heterozygotes manifest hemophilia. Because both clotting factor genes (F8 and F9) are part of an extensive metabolic pathway, heterozygous mutations affecting any other gene in the clotting cascade may have an additive effect if they occurs simultaneously with the F8 or F9 mutations, and the result is a debilitating bleeding problem. Other reasons for manifesting heterozygotes are discussed in section 12.6, "'Manifesting' Heterozygotes."

Also, something you should know about hemophila A: Some severe mutations in the F8 gene are caused by flipping the tip of the X chromosome, in an attempt to pair with itself during male meiosis. Identifying mutations responsible for many cases of severe hemophila A was difficult until Lakich et al. [27] used Southern Blots to discover that the gene is often separated into two halves by a common inversion resulting from recombination between the real locus at Xq28 and two 9.5 Kb intronless copies of part of the gene—misaligned near the long arm telomere of the X. Such aberrant recombination happens because PAR2 at the long arm telomere of X and Y provides only a weak pairing segment during meiosis (8% crossing over) and instead, pairing occurs between two F8 inverted repeats, which causes the frequent inversion that bifurcates the gene.

Duchenne and Becker Muscular Dystrophies: The Distropinopathies

The effect of X inactivation in these two X-linked diseases that are allelic mutations in the dystrophin gene is complex because the gene is huge (>2.5 MB), and mutations range from nucleotide substitutions to giant deletions in the gene, which either reduce the amount of dystrophin or completely eliminate the protein, sometimes interfering with the function of other X-linked loci in the vicinity. Furthermore, assays to determine the patterns of X inactivation most often are carried out in blood cells, and not muscle. The literature is replete with papers reporting the results of such assays but these are generally unsatisfying because of failure to find a unifying conclusion. The problem is the heterogeneity of the populations assayed with respect to nature of the mutations, size of the deletions, and age and degree of manifestations in females studied. These days the two disorders are treated as one, "the distrophinopathies."

Nonetheless some conclusions may be drawn. In the case of X autosome translocations at any age, where the mutation is expressed in every cell, the affected

---

6. Even though many proteins participate in the clotting cascade, these two genes are the commonest causes of bleeding disorders, because being X-linked only a single mutation is needed. Hemophilia A is more common than hemophilia B, probably because its gene is 5-fold larger and hence a larger target for mutation.

Table 12-2. Characteristics of Manifesting *DMD* Heterozygotes[A]

Patient #	Age of diagnosis	XI Ratio in WBC	Muscle Biopsy
Duplications/deletions			
#5	9 yr	95:05	Mosaic
#6	7 yr	91:09	ND
#9	5 yr	57:43	ND
Point mutations			
#4	5 yr	70:30	ND
#8	2 yr	96:04	Mosaic
Translocations affecting DMD			
#2	6 yr	93:07	Mosaic
#7	5 yr	ND	Mosaic
DNA not sequenced			
#3	5 yr	100:1	Mosaic

[a] Data taken from Seemann et al. [350].

female will have manifestations similar to affected males. However, in case of deletions of the locus, the degree of manifestations will depend on the degree of loss of dystrophin, and the number of wild-type cells in the mosaic female. In many cases neither the size of the deletions nor the amount of residual dystrophin activity is known. Only in rare cases do manifesting heterozygotes have a high degree of skewing with the mutant allele predominating. Most likely, females like those in table 12-2 were the unlucky recipients of too many mutant-type cells for stochastic or other reasons. Table 12-5 shows precipitating causes—in addition to X autosome translocations—for heterozygotes who manifest muscular dystrophy. These include monozygotic twinning, Turner syndrome, and uniparental disomy (where they received two X chromosomes bearing the mutant gene, and no X chromosome with the wild-type gene). Clearly, there is no evidence of selection favoring or disfavoring the presence or absence of dystrophin in the white blood cell, or, in fact, muscle cells as they are often observed histologically to be mosaic. Table 12-2, showing data for young manifesting heterozygotes, tells us that skewed inactivation is not always seen in leukocytes of girls with muscular dystrophy. Yet, skewing is more likely to be seen in those who manifest the earliest. [350, 351].

The ATRX Syndrome of α-Thalassemia and Mental Retardation

Males have the severe form of ATRX syndrome, and females are ostensibly normal because of their extremely skewed X inactivation. ATRX is considered one of the chromatin diseases because the deficient protein—a helicase—has a role in remodeling chromatin. In this capacity, it regulates the transcription of the two loci, residing side by side on chromosome 16, that encode the alpha hemoglobin chains; it also helps maintain the neurons needed for normal cognitive function. Affected males have a disease called alpha-thalassemia (because of abnormal regulation of α-globin), and are mentally retarded, as well. Most of the females heterozygous for these mutations are entirely asymptomatic, although they may have a few cells with the same inclusion bodies seen in males with α-thalassemia. It seems that almost all of the mutant cells in the heterozygote must be eliminated for her to be asymptomatic. In fact, *all* of the asymptomatic women have extremely skewed X inactivation that favors expression of the normal gene, because the mutation confers a striking growth disadvantage to cells in which it is expressed. In the developing brains of these females, any neurons expressing the mutation could not survive.

However, some carriers have mild mental retardation, and their X inactivation patterns are less skewed, indicating that their mutant cells are not as disadvantageous as those from most *ATRX* heterozygotes. Why are mutant cells not completely eliminated in these females? In a few cases, other genes in their genomes may ameliorate the lethal effects of the *ATRX* mutation. In most cases, their mutations produce less of a deficiency and are less detrimental to cell survival, so they are not eliminated as completely (similar to what happens in incontinentia pigmenti). It is paradoxical that random inactivation is associated with disease manifestations—albeit milder than the disease in males— whereas skewed inactivation (attributable to death of mutant cells) is what prevents disease manifestations. Highly skewed X inactivation is also characteristic of most heterozygotes carrying *FANCB* mutations associated with Fanconi's anemia B deficiency in males. Female carriers are normal because they eliminate mutant cells.

Cullin Ring–Associated X-linked Mental Retardation

Another example of severe skewing that begins in utero *is the X-linked mental retardation syndrome associated with the deficiency of Cullin Ring E3 ubiquitin ligase. Females may have mild tremors but generally escape any manifestations because of selection disfavoring the mutant cells, starting during early development.* The adult heterozygotes who have been studied have completely skewed X inactivation in their blood cells, such that they express only the wild-type CUL4B allele [352]. Studies of heterozygous mouse embryos that carry Cul4b deficiency confirm the early loss of mutant cells in their tissues [353]. These studies also show that the rate of loss differs among tissues, being relatively slower in hippocampus (mutant cells still present at 4 months after birth) than in lung, which eliminates all of them in the developing fetus. In addition, the placentas of heterozygous mice are abnormal and this along with evidence of loss of female mouse embryos and developmental delay suggest that Cul4b plays a role in their placental development. There is as yet no indication of early female loss among human heterozygotes; the difference no doubt is related to the paternal X inactivation in mouse placenta, and the random inactivation in human placentas.

Rett Syndrome

Females are the affected individuals, but they express a milder disorder than the one that is fatal to males with the same mutations. In addition, although the clinical phenotype in females is determined to some extent by the nature of their specific mutation, it is modified significantly by the X chromosome inactivation pattern. Rett syndrome is caused by the deficiency of one of the proteins that binds to methylated DNA to mediate gene silencing. For reasons perhaps related to its interaction with RNA binding proteins, the MeCP2 protein is a key player in the maturation and modulation of mature neurons. Rett syndrome was originally thought to be a disease unique to females. Because it is rare and not clustered in families, there was no obvious history of male loss. When the mutation was identified, it became possible to identify affected males. A few males, perhaps those with less deleterious mutations, have the same features as most girls with the disorder but were not diagnosed because Rett syndrome was supposed to be a *female-only* disease. Other males have a more severe disease and die during infancy. Some males with the mutation also have Klinefelter syndrome (47,XXY), which protects them from the severe male form of the disease. Heterozygotes for an *MECP2* mutation (females and Klinefelter males) are the ones most commonly affected with the syndrome as Rett described it. Because the mutant gene is usually not present in more than half their cells, they are protected from death, but having 50% normal-type cells does not protect them against the neurological manifestations of the syndrome. How severe the disease is in females is determined by the type of mutation and site in the protein that is affected. However, the severity is strongly influenced by the X inactivation pattern. Because *MECP2* mutations do not usually affect the proliferation of blood cells and do not result in cell elimination, most heterozygotes have random patterns of inactivation in blood; however, there may be skewing favoring normal neurons. Mice with an induced *Mecp2* mutation show a proliferative advantage of the wild-type neurons in cell culture, and selective survival of neurons in which the wild-type X chromosome was active [354].

An important thing to remember is that any skewing of X inactivation that occurs independent of the Rett mutation can greatly modify the phenotype. If skewing favors cells expressing the wild-type Rett allele, then the heterozygote will be only mildly affected—if at all—depending on the extent of the skewing; however, if skewing happens to favor the cells expressing the mutant gene, then the phenotype can be more severe. The moderating effect of X inactivation on manifestations of Rett syndrome is found to some degree in many other X-linked diseases, such as X-linked hyperammonemia and fragile X syndrome (both discussed below). X inactivation occurs randomly in these diseases, and the mutation does not seem to influence the growth of blood cells. However, if X inactivation is skewed by a chromosome aberration, or by cell loss early in the embryo, then the skewing will modulate the severity of any diseases attributable to an X-linked gene. The severity depends on the direction of the skewing, but irrespective of whether skewing favors mutant or wild-type cells, the outcome of the disease will be affected. Although predominant expression of the mutant allele can enhance the severity, predominant expression of the wild-type allele will help normalize the phenotype.

Even considering that many loss-of-function *MECP2* mutations are lethal in male embryos, one would expect to see more males affected by less severe mutations. The predominance of affected females and sporadic occurrence of the disease is explained by the fact that most *de novo* Rett mutations, like most other mutations, occur in father's germ cells, and if X-linked, they are transmitted only to daughters. Unless the phenotype is modified by X inactivation, girls who are severely affected cannot reproduce. Only those rare females, whose phenotype is ameliorated by highly skewed X inactivation that favors their normal allele, can pass the mutation on to their sons—hence the relative paucity of males with Rett syndrome [355]. Another interesting feature of the sex-specific expression of diseases has to do with what happens when the *MECP2* locus is duplicated on one X chromosome. While the "loss-of-function" mutations of *MECP2* result in Rett syndrome, duplications of the locus also produce a mental retardation syndrome, but in this case, males are almost uniquely affected. The duplicated gene leads to overproduction of the protein, which in turn results in very severe cognitive defects in males, along with other abnormalities, some resembling those seen in Rett syndrome. However, in such families, the females who carry this duplication are perfectly asymptomatic. This is because the duplicated locus adversely affects their cell's proliferation relative to the wild-type cells. Because of this selective disadvantage, the mutant cells are almost completely eliminated (85–100% skewing), and carrier females end up with mostly normal cells.

Severe Combined Immunodeficiency

Severe combined immunodeficiency, an X-linked immunodeficiency disorder, differs from the others because the mutation in the IL2RG gene affects many cells in the immune system. However, because the effects differ from one cell type to another, not all cells are affected equally. The gene product is essential for the *growth* of T-cells but is needed only for the *maturation* of B-cells. Heterozygotes with this mutation are normal because only their normal allele is expressed, as they lack mutant T-cells. The mutant T-cells either were eliminated very early, or never developed at all. On the other hand, heterozygotes do have some mutant B-cells, but these tend to be immature and are the minority population in many carriers, their numbers reflecting the severity of the mutation. This is another good example of the fact that the selective disadvantage is proportional to the severity of the deficiency. And it may differ from tissue to tissue. The elimination of mutant T-cells has been used as a means to distinguish the X-linked form of the disease from a similar disease caused by an autosomal gene. It has also been used to determine whether the mother with only one affected son is a carrier and therefore at risk of having additional affected sons.

X-Linked Hyperammonemia (OTC Deficiency)

OTC deficiency, like Rett syndrome, is often associated with postnatal male lethality, and it is the heterozygote that is affected. X inactivation is usually random in heterozygotes, but the normal cells in the mosaic females ameliorate the disease to varying extents, depending on how many are present. Ornithine transcarbamylase (OTC) deficiency is the most common disorder of urea synthesis. Mutations in the *OTC* gene block the metabolic pathway that prevents accumulation of toxic levels of ammonia, so they produce hyperammonemia—that is, too much ammonia in the blood. Until recently when treatment became more effective, the disease was usually fatal for male infants. The clinical expression of OTC in heterozygous females is highly variable, ranging from no disease at all to recurrent episodes of hyperammonemic coma (encephalopathy) and, rarely, to the profound neurological impairment observed in affected males. However, because the disease is episodic, many women may be unaware of their risk. In fact, they may be diagnosed for the first time as adults during one of these infrequent episodes. Some of these women tell us that they avoid eating meat or other high-protein foods because it makes them feel sick. Hyperammonemic episodes can be induced by high-protein diets (or even the protein load administered as a means to diagnose the disorder) as well as physiologic stress such as bone fractures, pregnancy, and delivery.

The correlation of phenotypic severity with either the nature of the DNA mutation is imprecise because X inactivation plays a role in determining the disease severity. In this disease, the OTC deficiency does not influence cell proliferation, and many heterozygotes have an equal distribution of mutant and wild-type cells—not only in their blood but also in their liver, the tissue most affected by the disorder. Studies of the liver reveal cellular mosaicism in each of the histological sections analyzed. However, despite the random inactivation in liver cells, even having 50% normal cells does not fully protect against some manifestations of the disease. Because the enzyme is not transferred between cells, even if only half the cells are mutant, this metabolic function is perturbed. Because X inactivation patterns are not directly affected by the *OTC* mutation, any skewing of X inactivation in these heterozygotes has occurred for reasons independent of the *OTC* mutations. If such skewing is present, then it will influence the clinical phenotype significantly, in either direction. Those heterozygotes with the most severe disease have too many mutant liver cells, whereas those with a majority of wild-type liver cells are the asymptomatic women at the other end of the spectrum.

Fragile X Syndrome

Like Rett syndrome and OTC deficiency, fragile X syndrome has little if any effect on cell proliferation, and heterozygotes generally have random distributions of mutant and wild-type cells. However, 50% normal cells are not enough for completely normal function, so that many females have some clinical manifestations. Fragile X mutations are responsible for two distinct diseases. Neither causes skewed X inactivation, but both are greatly influenced by it. The full-blown fragile X syndrome is caused by the loss of an RNA-binding protein called FMRP (fragile X mental retardation protein). This protein regulates the transport and translation of a messenger RNA involved in the synapses of nerve cells, and ultimately in memory and learning, which explains the mental retardation in this syndrome. The mutation is an unusual one involving innumerable duplications of the CGG trinucleotide within the CpG island in the *FMR1* gene. Normal individuals have 40 or fewer of these CGG repeats, whereas fully affected males have more than 200 of them.

The mutation responsible for the classic fragile X syndrome in males has little effect on cell proliferation, and heterozygotes generally have random X inactivation. However, whereas most heterozygous females with the full *FMR1* mutation are usually not as severely retarded as the males, many have IQs lower than normal controls. This suggests that more than 50% of the neurons have to express the protein to ensure a normal phenotype in females [356]. Those women who are more severely affected have a preponderance of mutant-type cells either for stochastic reasons or because of cell selection favoring an allele at some unidentified locus.

Individuals of both sexes with >40 but <200 repeats are said to have a premutation and were thought to be normal until it was discovered that in old age both the hemizygous men and some heterozygous women develop another syndrome consisting of tremors and abnormal gait (ataxia). Carriers of the premutation are also susceptible to premature menopause. While the fragile X syndrome is due to a deficiency of FMR1 protein (also called FMRP), the premutation ataxia disorder is due to an abnormal *FMR1* RNA. Like the females with the full mutation, those with the premutation have a range of severity of their disorders, depending on the proportion of their cells that express the mutation. With either the full mutation or premutation, males have the more severe manifestations of the disease.

Adrenoleukodystrophy

Heterozygotes carrying adrenoleukodystrophy (ALD) mutations have skewed X inactivation because of cell selection but the selection favors the mutant gene. Before my analysis of females heterozygous for the *ALD* mutation [357], I thought that cell selection always acted to favor the normal cells and that it invariably gave women a biological advantage. Although this is true in most cases of X mutations, women carrying *ALD* mutations are the exceptions, providing compelling evidence that such cellular interactions can sometimes have deleterious effects. For reasons not yet understood, it is the mutant cells that have the selective advantage (figure 12-5b). As a consequence, many women who carry such alleles eventually develop some of the symptoms of the disease. Yet, even though the proliferative advantage of the mutant cells renders these females symptomatic with age, they almost never acquire the full-blown disease.

ALD is also unique because the expression of the disease among males is highly variable; the severity of the disease and age of onset may differ greatly even among brothers with the same mutation. One brother may have adrenoleukodystrophy with cerebral deterioration in the first decade of his life; the other may have the milder disease, called *adrenomyeloneuropathy (AMN)*, which affects only the spinal cord, with symptoms beginning in the second decade or later. Although the cause of this extreme variability is not yet known, it is believed that other genes or environmental elements influence the expression of the mutant ALD alleles. This kind of variability is also reflected in the expression of the disease in female carriers—because the age when clinical symptoms occur varies a good deal. In a recent study of 165 ALD carriers, half showed some degree of neurological involvement. Their symptoms develop later than in males with AMN, ranging in severity from mild loss of sensation to a phenotype resembling AMN [358].

Craniofrontonasal Syndrome

The pattern of X inactivation in CFNS is random, and, in fact, it is the mixed cell population that creates the clinical disorder because of cellular interference. It seems that X inactivation is responsible for the paradoxical reversal in phenotypic severity between the males and females affected with this disorder; affected females have multiple skeletal malformations and craniosynostosis (premature fusion of bones of the skull), whereas males with the same mutation have mild malformations (e.g., widely spaced eyes) or none at all. This may be best explained by (1) the promiscuity among the family of ephrin proteins in hemizygous males and (2) the effect of random X inactivation in females [321]. X inactivation has been shown to be random in blood and cranial periosteum (the fibrous lining of the bone) of affected females, so that the lack of ephrin-B1 protein does not compromise cell viability in these tissues. Ephrin-B1 normally has a boundary of expression in neural crest–derived tissue that precisely demarcates the future course of the developing coronal suture. Based on observations in heterozygous mice, there is abnormal sorting of cells into larger ephrin-B1 expressing and non-expressing patches. It has been shown that in heterozygous female mice, it is patchwork loss of ephrin-B1 protein that disturbs tissue boundary formation at the developing coronal suture; in males with the same deficiency, the normal boundary between neural crest and cephalic mesoderm is maintained by some alternative mechanism that does the job when ephrin B1 cannot [321]. Perhaps the ephrin receptors and their ligands engage in promiscuity[7] such that the function of ephrin-B1 can be replaced by another B-class ephrin. Yet, in females, it is the interaction between the mixed population of ephrin-B1–expressing and nonexpressing cells that ultimately leads to a more severe disturbance than if all the cells were nonexpressing. In heterozygous females, and males mosaic for the mutation [298], ephrin-B1–expressing and ephrin-B1–deficient cells lead to divergent cell sorting and migration, especially pronounced in the contact areas of EFNB1-positive and EFNB1-negative cells. Wieland et al. [320] has suggested the term *cellular interference* for what occurs

7. Mutations in EFNA4 have recently been shown to be responsible for coronal suture synostosis, and it could be one of the genes with redundant function that rescues males with the EFNB1 mutation [359].

between ephrin-B–receptor positive migrating cells and the mixture of ephrin-B1 mutant and wild-type cells in heterozygotes. How this cellular interference actually works must await a better understanding of the role of ephrin-B1, but failure to make gap junctions between mutant and normal cells seems to play a role [322].

Otopalatodigital Syndrome (OPD Group)

Mutations in the X-linked filamin A (FLNA) gene cause a variety of clinical disorders depending on the site of the mutation within the gene, whether normal function is lost or a novel one is acquired, and on the sex of the affected individual. X inactivation has an ameliorating influence, especially when skewing favors inactivation of the mutated allele. Loss-of-function mutations in the *FLNA* gene are lethal for male embryos but cause a localized neuronal migration disorder, called periventricular nodular heterotopia (PVNH1), in females (figure 12-10, table 12-3). On the other hand, the novel functions resulting from gain-of-function mutations are responsible for the OPD-spectrum diseases [360]. This group of four allelic

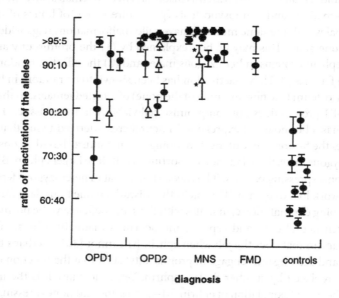

Figure 12-10. Skewed X inactivation in heterozygotes for OPD-spectrum disorders. Gain-of-function mutations in the X-linked filamin A gene are responsible for four allelic diseases affecting the cytoskeleton, shown on the horizontal axis in increasing order of severity: otopalatodigital syndrome (OPD1 and OPD2), Melnick-Needles syndrome (MNS), and frontometaphyseal dysplasia (FMD). Controls were shown to have two wild-type alleles. The values are mean ±SEM calculated for 3–7 independent measurements. Circles are individuals assayed. Triangles indicate that the direction of the skewing (in individuals where it could be determined) favors the wild-type allele. Reprinted with permission from figure 5 of Robertson et al. [360].

Table 12-3. SEX-SPECIFIC MANIFESTATIONS OF *FLNA* MUTATIONS IN OTOPALATODIGITAL SYNDROME AND RELATED DISORDERS(SEE REFERENCE [360])

	Males	Females	Mutation	Exon	X Inactivation
OPD1	Severe[ab]	Mild	Gain of function	3	Skewed
OPD2	Severe[abcde]	Less severe	Gain of function	3, 5, 11, 29	Skewed
FMD	Like MNS in females[b]	None	Gain of function	22, 29	N.A.
MNS	Lethal *in utero*	Manifest[b]	Gain of function	22	Skewed
PVHNI	Lethal *in utero*	Manifest[f,g]	Loss of function		Random

[a] Cleft palate.
[b] Short stature, bowed bones, abnormal digits.
[c] Perinatal death.
[d] Hydrocephalus.
[e] Omphalocele.
[f] Brain nodules, seizures.
[g] Cardiac malformations.

disorders is attributable to mutations in one of the *FLNA* alleles. Table 12-3 shows that all of the disorders are characterized by a generalized disturbance in skeletal growth, craniofacial anomalies and occasional extra-skeletal defects, but they differ widely in severity. The severest of them all is the Melnick-Needles syndrome (MNS), a rare disturbance of bone growth. Because males are stillborn or die *in utero*, only females suffer from MNS. However, MNS mutations affect the very same exon of *FLNA* as those classified as frontometaphyseal dysplasia (FMD), which affects primarily males (table 12-3). Although these diseases have been considered separate entities in the past, it is likely that they represent a continuous spectrum with males and females both manifesting clinical phenotypes, but males always more severely than females. Heterozygosity clearly ameliorates the phenotype. Such male-specific or female-specific features of mutations within the same gene are compelling examples of the influence of the single active X and cell mosaicism on sex differences in manifestations of genetic disease.

And what about the X inactivation patterns in these disorders? On one hand, carriers of the loss-of-function mutations (PVNH1) have random X inactivation patterns in peripheral blood cells (the only tissue studied). On the other hand, the X inactivation data suggest that the *gain-of-function* mutations causing OPD-spectrum disorders do disadvantage cell growth, as most heterozygotes show skewing [360]. In each case, the mutant gene is usually inactive—even in females who manifest the disorders (figure 12-8) so that even a predominant population of wild-type cells is associated with some clinical manifestations. Apparently, enough mutant cells were present during embryogenesis to account for the congenital malformations. This suggests that the mutant cells present earlier have been eliminated with time, or perhaps the skewing may be exaggerated in that tissue, and mutant cells persist in more relevant tissues such as bone or brain, a possibility that has not yet been studied.

Orofaciodigital Syndrome Type 1

The gene responsible for OFDI (CXORF5; [361]) is expressed to some extent from the inactive X, and this low-level expression is enough to protect heterozygous females from renal failure during infancy. Only females are affected with the syndrome (malformations of the face, oral cavity, and digits) because males die *in utero.* Half of these females have polycystic kidneys, especially those whose *CXORF5* mutation affects a splice site. Deficiency of the CXORF5 protein in the centrosome of the basal body of primary cilia causes ciliary dysfunction, which in turn causes developmental defects in the heart, neural tube, and kidney.

The severity of the polycystic renal disease in heterozygous females varies widely, undoubtedly influenced by their X inactivation status. An additional source of variation is the variable expression of the *OFDI* gene from the inactive X [63] ; most likely the locus escapes inactivation because of its location on the nonconserved portion of the X, near the short arm telomere (Xp22.3). In mice, the gene on the inactive X is completely silent; as a consequence, all affected female mice have polycystic kidneys, surviving only a short time after birth. Clearly, human heterozygous females are protected to some extent by the small amount of protein produced from the normal allele on their inactive X. In any case, the variability in severity of the renal disease among carriers can be explained not only by variation in the nature of the mutation, but also by variable expression from the inactive X or by variable numbers of mutant cells. Some women may have enough OFD1 protein for cilium assembly. Because the homologous locus on the Y chromosome is a nonexpressed pseudogene, affected males cannot benefit from the allele on their Y chromosome. However in females, the leaky expression of the normal allele from the inactive X weakens the influence of X inactivation on the severity of the polycystic disease [317]. There is no evidence of cell selection: Studies show that 7 of 23 patients had skewing, but in none was it extreme (>90%), and neither the normal nor mutant allele was favored [362].

The Effect of X Inactivation on Non-X-Linked Diseases

We have considered the effect of the single active X and cellular mosaicism on the sex differences in expression of diseases resulting from mutations on the X chromosome. However, the influence of X inactivation is not limited to the X chromosome. Obviously, any disease process that has an X-linked component might be influenced by patterns of X inactivation, and this possibility should be considered for any disorder that occurs more frequently in one sex than the other or has different manifestations in one sex than the other. *Appendix A* lists a few disorders that are not X-linked but may influence or be influenced by X-linked genes and/ or X inactivation. For example, mutations in the DNA methyltransferase *DMT3B* gene encoded by chromosome 20 (see *Appendix A,* "ICF Syndrome") have the potential to influence the regulation of some X chromosomal genes; the gene product is part of the epigenetic machinery and may indirectly cause leaky inactivation of X-linked genes as well as imprinted autosomal genes. Epimutations are discussed in greater detail in chapter 13.

Skewed patterns of X inactivation among women with diseases that are more frequent in females point to the possible influence of X chromosomes on genes no matter where they reside in the genome. In the case of autosomal imprinting disorders (i.e., Beckwith Wiedemann or Prader-Willi syndromes), skewing may occur because of rescue of trisomy in early pregnancy, leading to uniparental disomy, a frequent cause of such disorders. Both autosomes come from the same parent because of accidental loss of the other parent's chromosome from a trisomic cell, restoring the disomic state. The disomic cell has a proliferative advantage over trisomic cells so that, if created after X inactivation has occurred, its fixed inactivation pattern becomes the predominant one [365].

Another clue might be finding discordant phenotypes in female MZ twins expressing autosomal mutations, reminiscent of female MZ twins with discordant expression of X-linked mutations (both twins carry the mutation but only one twin has clinical symptoms). A case in point is the Beckwith-Wiedemann syndrome (BWS), which is most often of epigenetic origin and characterized by generalized overgrowth and predisposition to embryonal tumors (see *Appendix A*). This congenital malformation disorder, attributed to an *imprinted* locus, or loci, on chromosome 11 is inexplicably common in MZ twins; the twins are nearly always discordant for BWS, and nearly all twins are female. Intriguingly, some discordant twins are also discordant for skewed X inactivation. Yet because twinning alone seems to be associated with skewed X inactivation patterns, the skewing may not be related to BWS. On the other hand, skewing, MZ twinning, and BWS may be related events because of the chance interaction of all of them at the same time in development. It has been suggested that MZ twinning itself may be an epigenetic phenomenon. At the morula stage (the stage when most twinning occurs), the fetus may be perturbed by chance imprinting abnormalities that differentially affect one clone and not the other, and this difference could induce cleavage of the zygote [363] and separation of the cells with imprinted and nonimprinted BWS genes into different blastomeres [364]. This could also account for the skewed inactivation in one of the twins. All of this seems a bit like science fiction. Yet, the coincidence of MZ twinning, BWS, and X inactivation in this disorder provides at least a theoretical example of how developmental processes occurring at or about the same time in the embryo might influence one another.

Autoimmune Disease

A class of diseases that seems to be much more prevalent in females than males is the one resulting from failure of autoimmunity, paradoxically called *autoimmune disease.* Such diseases include type 1 diabetes, arthritis, and thyroiditis, where self-antibodies to the relevant tissues, found in the blood of the affected individuals, suggest an autoimmune origin (see table 12.4). Type 1 diabetes is the only major organ-specific autoimmune disorder not to show a strong female bias; in contrast, diseases such as thyroiditis, primary biliary cirrhosis, systemic lupus erythematosus, and systemic scleroderma have a 5- to 10-fold increase of affected females. For example, women comprise ~90% of those who develop systemic lupus. Although the high female:male ratios are often attributed to the effect of estrogen, as first pointed out by Jeffrey Stewart [366], the explanation for at least some of the greater propensity in females might lie elsewhere. Other sex differences might have as much or more relevance to autoimmune disease—for example, the cellular mosaicism induced by X inactivation.

The details of the immunological processes are beyond the scope of this discussion, but here I briefly present the argument. A unique feature of autoimmune disorders is the apparent loss of immunity to self-antigens (referred to as *tolerization*); that is, the individual does not recognize the antigen as part of itself and starts making antibodies to his or her own tissues. In the case of mosaic females, the self-proteins that are expressed and presented for tolerization will differ in the two populations of cells. Because this mosaicism is also present in the tolerizing cells of the thymus, the body's sampling process that is involved in establishing recognition of self might miss the antigens on one of the parental X chromosomes. In this way, X chromosome inactivation predisposes females to a loss of T-cell tolerance, especially when skewed X inactivation in the thymus leads to inadequate recognition of self. If the self-antigen is not "presented" in the thymus or in other sites that are involved in immunological tolerance, then it will not be recognized, which increases the risk of autoimmunity. The probability that a self-antigen encoded by the X chromosome might elude the recognition process would increase if one of the parental X chromosomes were not expressed in

Table 12-4. AUTOIMMUNE DISEASES WITH A FEMALE PREPONDERANCE[a]

Autoimmune Disease	Female: Male Ratio
Autoimmune chronic hepatitis	7
Graves disease	7
Hashimoto's disease	5–18
Idiopathic thrombocytopenic purpura	3
Myasthenia gravis	3
Primary biliary cirrhosis	10
Rheumatoid arthritis	2
Sjogren's syndrome	9
Systemic lupus erythematosus	9
Systemic sclerosis	5

[a] Adapted from table 1, Selmi et al. [371].

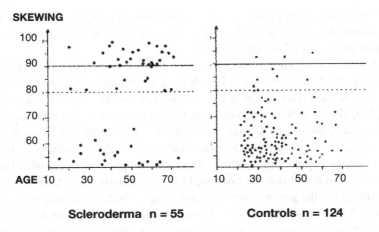

Figure 12-11. Skewed X inactivation in scleroderma: results of the HUMARA analysis
of blood in females attending a rheumatology clinic. Note that the relative percentage of
individuals in the 90–100% range is greater in patients than in the controls. Adapted from
figure 2 of Ozbalkan et al. [367], with permission.

many cells. The more extreme the skew in thymic cells (specifically, the dendritic
cells that present antigen), the more likely it becomes that antigens will evade the
tolerizing process. Therefore, highly skewed X inactivation provides the means
whereby X-linked self-antigens may escape adequate recognition.

Several studies lend support to this conjecture. Systemic scleroderma is a sporadic autoimmune disease of connective tissue whose cause is unknown. Because
the clinical features are reminiscent of a host-versus-graft response, it was suggested that perhaps systemic scleroderma was due to microchimerism resulting
from transplacental transfer of fetal cells to the mother during gestation. This may
account for some cases of scleroderma, but it cannot account for the individuals who were never pregnant. On the other hand, recent studies show that a significant number of females with scleroderma have skewed X inactivation in their
blood cells [367] (figure 12-11).[8] Although there is no evidence that scleroderma
involves an X-linked mutation, or for that matter, any mutation at all, this remains
a remote possibility in light of the skewed inactivation. But it is more likely that X
inactivation itself plays a role in producing the disease, at least in some women.
Skewing of X inactivation for one reason or another increases the chance that
antigens expressed on the minor population of cells may escape tolerization. One
should not expect all affected individuals to show skewing, because it is only one
of many risk factors for this disease. In the same study, skewing in blood cells
was not seen in individuals with rheumatoid arthritis, but perhaps the patient
population or the tissue analyzed was not the inappropriate one. As pointed out
by Chitnis et al. [368], it is the skewing in thymic cells that counts, so analysis

8. Skewing was not observed in the skin cells of these women [367].

of peripheral blood may not accurately reflect the population of cells sampled. Autoimmune diseases in general are heterogeneous, and most likely, everyone has his or her own unique form of a disease.

In addition, there is clear evidence of skewed X inactivation in a third or more of the women with Graves disease and Hashimoto's thyroiditis—two thyroid diseases that are associated with the presence of autoimmune antibodies to the thyroid gland [369, 370]. Cellular mosaicism and hidden antigens may explain the higher prevalence of autoimmune disease in individuals with Turner and Klinefelter syndromes, because they often are chromosomal mosaics with additional X chromosomes in minor populations of cells. And we cannot ignore the possibility that the small amount of gene products expressed from the inactive X or from reactivated genes throughout the genome also may have escaped the tolerization process [371].

Clearly X inactivation, cell mosaicism, or aneuploidy does not explain the majority of autoimmune diseases. However, the X chromosome may contribute to the unequal sex ratios in autoimmune diseases in other ways. More of the genes responsible for immunodeficiencies are encoded on the X-chromosome than anywhere else in the genome, and males are uniquely susceptible to the dozen or so X-linked immunodeficiencies. Also there are at least eight micro-RNAs that reside on the X chromosome that play a role in immunity [372]. Perhaps it's the extra amounts of some of these gene products that perturbs the immune system in females. Alternatively, long exposure to estrogen hormone may in fact induce excessive immune response in women with appropriate risk factors, or males may have some unique factor that protects them from such disorders.

12.6. "MANIFESTING" HETEROZYGOTES

Mosaicism provides a tremendous biological advantage to females because it serves to ameliorate many diseases. Yet, X inactivation can create problems for some women, when the mutation provides a growth advantage (reminiscent of cancer cells, or the *ALD* mutation) or creates mixed signaling (e.g., in CFNS). Women lose the benefits of cellular mosaicism when skewing because of an X chromosome abnormality fully exposes a deleterious mutation on the X that is consistently active, or when a detrimental mutation is unmasked by the skewing associated with twinning or stochastic events. Table 12-5 lists some of the diseases in which heterozygous females are reported to be as severely affected as the hemizygous male with the same mutation. Because such females have only one copy of the mutant allele, they are often referred to as *manifesting heterozygotes*. Also included in table 12-5 are the reasons—when known—for the existence of these manifesting heterozygotes.

The best examples of manifesting heterozygotes are the females with balanced X/autosome translocations. Such women have very skewed X inactivation because their normal X is always silent. Often, the break that creates the translocation chromosome also disrupts the function of a gene at the site of the breakage.

Table 12-5. Precipitating Cause of Rare Heterozygous Females with
Full-Blown X-linked Diseases

Disease	Gene	Cause[a]
Adrenoleukodystrophy	ALD	MZ, U
Duchenne muscular dystrophy	DMD	MZ, XA, TS, UPD, U
Hemophilia A	F8	MZ, TS, XA, U
Hemophilia B	F9	MZ, XA, HI, U
Hunter syndrome	IDS	XD, XA, U
Lesch Nyhan syndrome	HPRT	MZ, U

[a] Monozygotic twin (MZ); skewed X inactivation of unknown cause (U);
X-autosome translocation (XA); Turner syndrome (TS);
Uniparental disomy (UPD); heterozygous for an interacting allele (HI);
X-deletion (XD).

Unfortunately, the disrupted gene will be clinically evident because the wild-type allele on the normal X chromosome is always mute, as that chromosome is always inactive. The good thing is that their X/autosome translocation often identifies the gene responsible for their *de novo* disease. The culprit gene is most likely the one disrupted by the translocation, and so the gene can be localized to the breakpoint; this breakpoint can be mapped, facilitating the cloning of these relevant genes. For example, four unrelated females with *de novo* Duchenne muscular dystrophy (having no affected relatives) had an X/autosome translocation (see figure 12-12, top). Although the autosome differed in each of them, they all had a common breakpoint on the X chromosome at Xp21. This mapped the *DMD* locus to Xp21, and this assignment enabled cloning of the gene [369]. Yet, the mutation does not have to be at the breakpoint to cause disease manifestations. Any preexisting mutation on the translocation chromosome will be expressed in every cell. If a girl happens to inherit a *DMD* mutation and that mutant allele is anywhere on the translocation chromosome, she will also manifest DMD (figure 12-12, bottom). Among the translocation carriers manifesting DMD, there was another affected female whose X breakpoint was not at Xp21 but instead on the long arm of the chromosome. It turns out that she had a brother with DMD and was a carrier of the disease. In her case, the X/autosome translocation created a *manifesting* heterozygote simply because her DMD mutation was always expressed from the translocation chromosome, and her wild-type *DMD* allele on the normal X was never expressed.

Of course, heterozygous females can become truly *hemizygous* for the mutant allele if the normal locus is deleted or lost—as in Turner syndrome. When a girl manifests a disease usually seen only in males, it is wise to obtain a chromosome analysis to exclude the possibility of X chromosome deletion or X/autosome translocations. Yet, chromosome abnormalities are not the only reason for

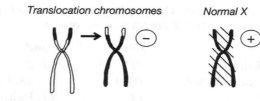

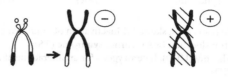

Figure 12-12. **X/autosome translocation causes Duchenne muscular dystrophy (DMD) in manifesting heterozygotes by eliminating cell mosaicism.** The + and − refer to wild-type and mutant *DMD* alleles, respectively. A: Breakpoint at the *DMD* locus (arrow) on Xp21 creates a *de novo DMD* mutation. Although a heterozygote, she manifests DMD because her normal allele is always silent on the inactive X (shaded). B: Having inherited inheriting a *DMD* mutation this heterozygote loses her mosaicism because of a coincidental X/autosome translocation with breakpoint in Xq25 (arrow). She has muscular dystrophy because her normal *DMD* allele is always silent on the inactive X. In both girls, the X involved in the translocation carries a mutant *DMD* allele. They both manifest DMD as their protective normal *DMD* alleles on the normal X are never expressed because of the X/autosome translocation.

manifesting heterozygotes. Anything that causes extreme skewing of X inactivation or loss of mosaicism will also cause heterozygotes to manifest the full-blown clinical disease. As a corollary, skewed X inactivation provides a powerful means of ascertaining mutations that influence cell proliferation. Lesch Nyhan heterozygotes who eliminate mutant blood cells may unmask another X-linked mutation (the *hitchhiker* allele) if it is on the same chromosome that is invariably expressed. If the hitchhiker mutation is relatively advantageous, then it might interfere with the elimination of HPRT-deficient blood cells. The potential interplay between alleles on the two X chromosomes is limitless.

One wonders if the 5–10% of normal women who are not mosaics (those with >90% skewing) lose cells because of stochastic events? Or is their skewing the result of the initial choice of active X—not associated with disease as they have no disease-producing mutations in protein-coding genes on their active X? It is clear that (1) the patterns of X inactivation greatly influence expression of the mutation, and (2) there are many reasons that females heterozygous for a mutation may manifest diseases usually found only in males. The point to remember is that females who manifest male-specific X-linked diseases are likely to have skewed X inactivation.

To complete this discussion of manifesting heterozygotes, here I briefly summarize the reasons for their existence, using examples of heterozygotes who manifest hemophilia (listed in table 12-5). I hope that enumerating the causes of female hemophilia will illustrate the complexity of some of the cellular and metabolic interactions taking place in mosaic females, and how they influence the phenotype of women carrying X-linked mutations.

Hemophilia A is a bleeding disorder caused by a deficiency in the activity of coagulation factor VIII (FVIII) encoded by the factor VIII gene (*F8*). In most hemophilia A heterozygotes, the levels of this clotting factor are about 50% of normal, and usually this amount of FVIII is not quite enough, because these heterozygotes have mildly decreased coagulability when tested. This mild clotting abnormality does not produce any clinical abnormalities, and in fact it provides some protection against fatal heart disease[9] caused by clots in the coronary arteries.

However, females can manifest hemophilia (hemorrhaging into their joints and muscles, bruising easily, and excessively bleeding from wounds). A few do because they inherit defective *F8* genes from both parents. Yet, some affected females are heterozygous for the *F8* mutation. Their bleeding disorder sometimes is due to an X chromosome abnormality such as Turner syndrome or an X/autosome translocation that unmasks an inherited *F8* mutation [374]. In other cases, the *F8* heterozygote is also heterozygous for a mutation in the von Willebrand factor (encoded by a gene on chromosome 12), another player in the clotting cascade [375]. The two mutations act additively to produce the bleeding disorder. Another unusual mechanism is that the manifesting female may have an *F8* mutation inherited from her father and a mutation in the incontinentia pigmenti (*NEMO*) gene inherited from her affected mother [376]. Although hemophilia mutations do not affect cell proliferation, the mutant *IP* allele is detrimental to cell growth. Therefore, the wild-type *IP* allele on the paternal X is favored, so her paternal X is always the active X. Because his mutant hemophilia gene resides on this chromosome, this girl expresses the mutant *F8* allele in all of her cells and therefore has a bleeding problem. Table 12-5 lists heterozygous interactions as an explanation for some manifesting heterozygotes; the interactions between alleles in two clotting factors or between *IP* and *F8* mutations are examples of interactions of this kind.

Other heterozygotes with hemophilia are monozygotic twin females heterozygous for a mutation in their paternal *F8* gene. The reason that both had a bleeding disorder was that both had skewed X inactivation, as is prone to happen with twins. In this case, the skewing happened to favor expression of their father's mutant allele. The most severely affected girl was no longer mosaic, because all her cells expressed her paternal allele, whereas her less severely affected twin had some cells expressing the mother's normal allele. The degree of skewing closely correlated with both the coagulation parameters and the clinical phenotype of the twins. These twins were not discordant, but in other MZ twins only one manifests

9. The risk of deaths from heart disease is 36% less than normal, but their risk of death from cranial hemorrhage was slightly increased.

hemophilia because the other has random X inactivation. And in the case of the three-generation family in which three females were affected with classic hemophilia A due to a heterozygous missense mutation in the *F8* gene, all three of them had completely skewed X inactivation with only the mutant allele expressed in all tissues analyzed, including leukocytes, skin fibroblasts, bladder epithelium, and buccal mucosa. The *XIST* allele shared by all three was never on an inactive X in this family (figure 12-7), suggesting that an alteration within the X-inactivation center on the chromosome carrying the *F8* mutation prevented it from being inactivated. It is likely that these *manifesting heterozygotes* have hemophilia because of primary skewing of X inactivation, linked to the *Xist* locus and the XIC.

It is clear that there are many ways to create manifesting heterozygotes. Yet, heterozygous females with bleeding disorders represent a very small number of the total group of heterozygotes carrying the *F8* mutation. As a rule, most women carrying deleterious X-linked mutations are protected by their mosaicism; it is the loss of mosaicism—no matter the reason—that leaves them defenseless.

12.7. SUMMARY AND SPECULATIONS

Under normal circumstances, the patterns of X inactivation are determined initially by the random choice of active X during early embryogenesis. The chromosome designated at that time will be the active X for the life of that cell. However, the interplay between the two different active X chromosomes in the mosaic female will determine the ultimate composition of her mosaic cell populations. It is only after the creation of the cellular mosaicism by *cis* inactivation that the influence of all the specific alleles on the two active X chromosomes comes into play. And the two populations of cells in the mosaic female—each one commanded by a different active X chromosome—compete for predominance. In most women, the result of the competition ends in a dead heat, any minor growth advantage conferred by genes on one X canceling out any minor selective advantage of genes on the other X chromosome, and both populations are fairly equally represented in every one of her tissues.

This is a good thing. The opportunity for females to carry two alleles at a locus simultaneously provides versatility not possible in the hemizygous male. Therefore, cellular mosaicism most often confers an extraordinary biological advantage. In most women with a single copy of a defective X-linked gene, the mosaicism mitigates the clinical abnormalities associated with the same mutation in males.

Yet, in a significant number of females the result of the competition produces a winner, and one cell population becomes preeminent in the tissues in which the more influential genes are expressed. This also is a good thing, because in most cases, the cellular selection mechanism weeds out the abnormal cells. Because of the rate at which mutations occur, all females may be heterozygous for several deleterious X-linked mutations. The fate of cells expressing these mutations is determined by the influence of the mutation on cell proliferation. Whether or not cell selection occurs is determined by multiple factors. These include the ability of the gene product to be transferred from wild-type to mutant cells and the degree to which it affects cell proliferation; skewing is most apparent when the product of the mutant gene is nontransferable and has a strong influence on cell proliferation. In addition, genes at all the loci on both X chromosomes can affect the result; even the strong influence of mutant alleles at one X-linked locus can be modified by those at another. Therefore, the outcome of the competition between the two cell populations not only may differ among heterozygotes with the same mutation, it may differ in the same female from one tissue to another, depending on expression patterns of relevant genes. Although some mutant alleles will influence cell proliferation no matter what other genes reside on the chromosome, the effect of most variant genes may be more subtle and subject to the influence of other genes.

Unfortunately, some women lose this biological advantage. Occasionally, the mutation confers a proliferative *advantage* rather than disadvantage, and this leads to cell selection favoring the mutant allele, for example, in adrenoleukodystrophy. Or chromosome abnormalities that eliminate the cellular mosaicism can unmask detrimental mutations on the consistently active X chromosome or mask normal alleles that are never expressed. If the competition between cell populations favors the cells expressing the mutation, then females may manifest diseases that are usually seen only in males.

Now what does this tell us about *sex-specific* diseases? One reason that some diseases are considered to affect only one of the sexes is because we do not always recognize the sex differences in the expression of diseases. The practice of defining disorders by their syndromic phenotypes has proven to be enormously misleading regarding the true cause of the disease. The OPD group was considered as four independent X diseases until the *filamin A* gene was identified and shown to be mutant in all of them. The differences in phenotype were due to the location of the mutation in the gene and the sex of the individual in whom it occurs. Rett syndrome affected only females until identification of *MECP2* showed that the same mutation often had different manifestations in males. It is likely that even diseases considered to occur exclusively in males have at least some minor manifestations in females if one knows what to look for.

Although there may be other gender differences in sex-specific manifestations of disease, many of them are the consequence of both sexes having a single working X chromosome. Diseases expressed mainly in males result from the defects in their only copy of an X-linked gene, whereas females have a normal copy in reserve. Mosaicism for her X chromosome proteome has a large role in determining how a female responds to mutations in her X-linked genes. Mosaicism is usually advantageous, mediating transfer of essential gene products from normal to mutant cells, or eliminating deleterious cells. While some females completely avoid medical manifestations of their mutations, others must pay some price for surviving when their male counterparts did not. In any case female-only diseases are most often less severe than the male manifestations of the same mutation. However, occasionally females may manifest male-only diseases, either because loss of the mosaicism exposes deleterious alleles or because the interactions have harmful effects.

It is tempting to consider the possibility of reversing inactivation of normal alleles in a cell expressing the mutant one as a means of ameliorating diseases in heterozygous females. The reality is that this would be difficult if not impossible to carry out, mainly because of the complexity of the interactions between cell populations, starting early in female development. The good thing is that the ultimate result of mammalian X dosage compensation in most females is cellular mosaicism, a unique form of gene therapy.

13

Epimutations, Chromatin Disorders, and Sex Differences in Phenotype

In previous chapters I have referred to X inactivation as an *epigenetic* process. Despite similar genetic content, the two X chromosomes in female cells have different activity states because their chromatin is not the same (see section 3.2, "Heterochromatin and Chromosome Silencing"). In fact, we have learned a great deal about epigenetics by comparing the chromatin of the mammalian active and inactive X chromosomes. The modifiers of the DNA sequence, such as the enzymes that methylate DNA or histones, or acetylate or deacetylate histones, as well as the noncoding RNAs like *Xist,* and other chromatin remodelers are referred to as *epigenetic* factors. *Epigenetic* is a term that literally means "on genes," reflecting the fact that epigenetic factors act upon genes by remodeling their chromatin. The modifications, which they induce are not normally part of the DNA sequence that is transmitted from an individual to its progeny. On one hand, we need epigenetic factors to ensure that chromatin is highly responsive, that is, able to remodel itself fast enough to carry out such dynamic processes as gene transcription, DNA replication, and repair. On the other hand, we need epigenetic factors to ensure that the chromatin configuration is stable enough to maintain the long-term silence of the genes and developmental programs that must remain repressed. Alone and in various combinations, these epigenetic "marks" serve as a code to tell the DNA polymerase and other transcription factors where to go, and when to go there, during the development and lifetime of an individual.

This chapter considers the disorders that occur when these epigenetic factors do not function properly. Such malfunctioning is usually attributable to mutations in the DNA of the affected gene. Yet, because the mutated gene is one that modulates the chromatin environment of many other genes, the loss of its function often badly affects the function of genes that are themselves structurally normal. DNA mutations that modify histone marks, or cause the loss of methylated CpG dinucleotides, affect gene expression by altering the activity state of chromatin. I will use the term *epimutation* to mean an error that is not present in the DNA of the affected gene, but nonetheless interferes with its function. You have seen how epigenetic factors inhibit transcription of the genes on the inactive X by modifying their chromatin environment. Aside from their role in X inactivation, such chromatin remodeling proteins not only silence genes that should not be expressed during specific developmental stages, or in specific tissues, but they also activate developmental programs in the embryo and modulate the levels of gene expression in all tissues.

13.1. EPIMUTATIONS USUALLY CAUSE SOMATIC DISEASES

Most of the genetic diseases that we know about result from mutations in the DNA coding sequence of the gene whose function is affected. Yet, a gene's functions can be just as effectively blocked by epigenetic modifications of its chromatin environment. DNA methylation serves as the major epigenetic mark during cell division where it transmits an activity state from one cell to all its progeny (see chapter 7.2, "Maintaining Inactivation by DNA Methylation of CpG Islands"). Because, unlike DNA mutations, the epigenetic modifications present in parents are usually erased in the fetus, most of them are not transmitted from parent to child. Therefore, the diseases caused by aberrant epigenetic modifications usually affect only somatic cells—for example, cancer cells. Inappropriate methylation of genes that should be expressed (tumor suppressor genes) and demethylation of genes that need to be repressed (oncogenes) are common features in the development of many malignant tumors.

Cancer progression is often initiated by DNA mutations that inappropriately wake up sleeping oncogenes or silence tumor repressor genes. Such tumor inducing genes along with others that promote transcription, replication, and chromatin remodeling are considered *candidate* genes for many tumors. Even if sequencing the tumor's DNA does not reveal a causative mutation these candidate genes in fact, may be malfunctional. They may have been silenced or impaired either by modifications in the underlying or neighboring chromatin, or by mutations in the transfactors required to effect their function. Recent searches for the genetic abnormalities that cause oncogenesis reveal that some of the oncogenes and tumor suppressor genes that drive the cancer's progression do not have DNA mutations; instead, they have epimutations that inappropriately silence or up-regulate their functions. Such epimutations are discovered most often by looking at methylation patterns of candidate genes. In one study of breast cancer, DNA mutations causing loss of function in susceptibility genes (*BRCA1*, *BRCA2*, and *RAD51C*), accounted for ~40% of hereditary breast and ovarian cancer, whereas epimutations that repress their function (specifically, highly methylated promoters in the same susceptibility genes), accounted for only ~2% of familial breast cancer [377]. However, the frequency of epimutations among sporadic tumors is considerably higher, as the *BRCA1* promoter is overmethylated in approximately 20% of sporadic breast cancer, and hypermethylation is frequently associated with functional loss of the second *BRCA1* gene [378]. In sporadic tumors, epigenetic abnormalities can act as initiating events serving as the first and/or second hit in

Knudson's model [379] of tumor development. Characteristically, such epimutations are encoded by one chromosome, but affect genes on one or more other chromosomes (see examples below).

13.2. EPIMUTATIONS IN PARENTAL IMPRINTING DISORDERS

Because epigenetic marks are erased during the development of the embryo,[1] we expect that many epimutations will not be inherited from one individual to another. Some exceptions to the rule are the diseases attributable to epigenetic changes in parentally imprinted genes, like the ones responsible for the Beckwith Wiedemann syndrome (see section 12.5, and *Appendix A*). As you remember, alleles are said to be imprinted when only one of the pair is expressed, and the choice of expressed allele is based on its parental origin (see section 10.3), Mutations that activate silent alleles, or silence alleles that should be active, are the usual culprits in these diseases. The outcome of mutations in parentally imprinted alleles depends on the sex of the parent who transmits the mutant allele, and the phenotypic effect of that mutant allele. All of the known human alleles that carry parental imprints are autosomal genes. You can imagine that isodisomy—that is, inheriting two of one parent's chromosomes and none of the other—would create a problem at *imprinted* loci, no matter whether mother's or father's chromosomes are lost. Often, having two copies of the active allele is just as deleterious as having none of them. At present, we know of about 100 mammalian genes that are reported as parentally imprinted, most of them from studies of mice. Genome-wide analysis of gene expression suggests that there may be many more loci where only a single allele is expressed; however, many of these alleles may not bear a parental imprint but are simply monoallelically expressed genes like olfactory receptors. In such genes, the choice of active allele is random in respect to parental origin.

The parentally imprinted genes, already identified, are not randomly distributed in the genome, but tend to occur in clusters. In humans, there are eight disorders[2] attributed to clustered imprinted genes on chromosomes 6, 7, 11, 14, 15, and 20. That they occur in clusters suggests that the control of imprinting is not at the

1. In mice, the first wave of genome-wide DNA demethylation takes place shortly after fertilization; the maternal genome is passively demethylated and the methylcytosine of the paternal genome is converted into hydroxymethylcytosine, which is passively eliminated. Imprinted (differentially methylated regions) are maintained despite this demethylation event. However, these imprints are removed in both male and female primordial germ cells by another wave of DNA demethylation that begins as the cells migrate toward the genital ridge [380].

2. Human imprinted disorders are Angelman syndrome (OMIM #105830), Prader-Willi syndrome (#176270), Beckwith-Wiedemann syndrome (#130650), Silver-Russell syndrome (#180860), maternal uniparental disomy 14 syndrome (no OMIM #), paternal uniparental disomy 14 syndrome (#608149), pseudohypoparathyroidism (#603233), and transient neonatal diabetes mellitus (#601410). Many of these disorders cause abnormal growth of the fetus.

level of single genes, but at the level of chromatin domains [381]. Several imprint-ing centers have been identified that carry methylation and histone marks, which differ on the two homologous chromosomes; such marks constitute the parental imprint. The imprinting centers serve as binding sites for regulatory factors and they control genes within the cluster *in cis*. A deletion in such an element typically affects the expression of most of the genes in the cluster. Such sex differences in the imprinting of father's and mother's alleles are established during spermato-genesis and oogenesis, respectively. As you might suspect the establishment and maintenance of these imprints are subject to errors, even though aberrant marks occur at a low rate.

Most familial cases of these imprinted gene disorders are due to abnormal chromosome segregation resulting in isodisomy, or deletions, or to point muta-tions in the DNA of the imprinted alleles that affect the deposition or erasure of the imprint. However, there are rare cases where it is not a DNA mutation, but an aberrant methylation mark that has persisted from one generation to the next [382]. Such imprinting defects usually are associated with sporadic occur-rence of the disorder, suggesting that they arise infrequently and are not present in all sperm or eggs. These rare imprinting defects are evidence that the parental methylation marks of imprinted genes are not always erased during embryonic development.

Environmental Insults to the Fetal Epigenome as a Cause of Adult Disease

Although rare imprinting errors occur, and are responsible for disease, they are usually not transmitted to more than one generation. Aside from the unique mouse agouti model, where environmental factors like starvation alter an unsta-ble (or metastable) *epiallele* by changing its methylation status, there are no com-pelling human examples of multigenerational transmission of acquired somatic mutations. On the other hand, there is abundant evidence that many adult dis-eases have their origins during fetal life, including obesity, cardiovascular disease, diabetes, and even schizophrenia. The roles of famine and intrauterine exposure of the fetus to endocrine disruptors in these diseases are well documented [383]. Diethylstilbestrol has been shown in a rat model to reprogram estrogen-respon-sive genes, making them more hormone sensitive, and prone to inducing tumors. The reprogrammed genes had changes in histone methylation and DNA methyla-tion [383].

Although exposure of male germ cells to agents that alter epigenetic factors could adversely influence the phenotype of his offspring, the protamines that replace histones in sperm should erase all the epigenetic modifications. The few histones that remain might be responsible for rare instances of transmission of aberrant parental imprints [384]. I refer you to the following reviews [380, 385] for further information about parental imprinting.

13.3. EPIGENETIC REGULATION OF AUTOSOMAL GENE EXPRESSION BY SEX CHROMOSOMES

Genome-wide transcription profiling in somatic tissues of mice reveals large-scale differences in the autosomal gene expression of males and females. Much of this can be attributed to differences in response to the sex hormones (estrogen and testosterone) because the sexual dimorphism in expression often correlates with differences at hormonal binding sites [386]. Yet, recent studies of mice that have been manipulated such that the sex chromosome complex is removed from gonadal function [387] suggest that some of the differential transcription is not hormone dependent. This has led some investigators to suggest that sex-specific regions of heterochromatin could exert effects on the epigenetic status of the rest of the genome. We are reminded that the Y chromosome in flies contains large regions of heterochromatin that alter the epigenetic balance of heterochromatin-euchromatin at autosomal loci, and regulate the expression of hundreds to thousands of autosomal and X genes. What is proposed as a mechanism is that the sex chromosomal heterochromatin can alter the epigenetic balance of factors such as DNA methyltransferases or histone-modifying enzymes, by serving as a "sink" for factors favoring the formation of heterochromatin [388–390]. These investigators suggest that the heterochromatic X chromosome in females and the predominantly heterochromatic Y chromosome in males could similarly alter epigenetic status genome-wide. And having a sink that removes epigenetic effectors from the rest of the genome would affect gene expression in regions deprived of these factors. What is assumed is that the epigenetic machinery is limited in abundance and under rigorous dosage control. This proposal would account for some sex differences in the expression of autosomal genes, and there is some preliminary evidence to support it: (1) Hypomethylation seems to be a feature of many polyploid cancer cells [391]; (2) methylation of CpG islands is correlated with hypomethylation in the body of the gene, and vice versa [392]; and (3) trisomic chromosomes are paradoxically less methylated than disomic ones [393]. These data suggest that there may be dosage compensation whenever chromosomes are added to (or subtracted from) the genome. In addition, the phenotypes associated with the so-called *chromatin disorders* (see below) suggest that some of the epigenetic factors, which seem overabundant and redundant in function, are unable to substitute for one another in cases where one of them is mutated.

13.4. DISORDERS OF THE EPIGENETIC MACHINERY

The number of documented cases of inheritance of aberrant methylation marks is small; yet, we are increasingly aware of inherited diseases that arise from DNA mutations in the genes encoding the epigenetic machinery. You might expect that mutations in genes encoding the DNA methyltransferases, methyl-binding proteins, histone acetylases and deacetylases, and histone methylases and demethylases, as well as other chromatin remodelers, might be lethal, contributing to the great loss of human embryos that occurs before the time that the fetus implants in the uterus. No doubt many are, but some mutations in such genes permit the fetus to survive gestation, and are indeed responsible for genetic diseases.

Wendy Bickmore [394, 395] was among the first to point out that inappropriate or altered chromatin structure can underlie some human genetic diseases. DNA mutations in some DNA methylases and DNA binding proteins are responsible for cases of ICF and Rett syndromes, respectively (Appendix A). In these cases, genes whose expression is affected are not always linked to the underlying mutation. Instead, they are innocent bystanders, affected by mutations in distant genes that can silence other genes by altering chromatin structure in their region. For example, Bickmore suggests that the DNA hypomethylation caused by a deficiency of the DNA methyltransferase DMT3B in the ICF syndrome leads to dysregulation of distant genes that perturb craniofacial, cerebral, and immunological development.

Mutations that compromise DNA methylation or create other chromatin modifications have a role in the parental imprinting disorders such as the autosomal syndromes of Beckwith-Wiedemann (Appendix A), Prader-Willi (OMIM #176270) and Angelmann (OMIM #105830). The DNA elements that control how the genes function are themselves controlled by epigenetic "marks." Clearly, severe deficiency of such factors would be lethal, but less severe deficiencies, or deficiencies affecting one gene in a family of genes with overlapping function, constitute a new class of diseases that can be considered chromatin diseases.

Some disorders encoded by genes on the X chromosome that affect chromatin are listed in table 13.1.

The 12 disorders listed in Table 13-1 are not exhaustive as new disorders are being identified at a fast rate. All of them are due to X chromosome mutations that affect chromatin structures and/or the process of transcription. Most of these mutations occur in the DNA. Like other X-linked genes, most of these defective genes are subject to X inactivation. Only JARID1C (KDM5C) and UTX (KDM6A) are expressed from both sex chromosomes. Yet, as all of these mutations, whether inherited or acquired de novo, affect genes that encode proteins important in transcription of all genes and their surrounding chromatin, they are poised to affect more cell processes than other genes do. For example, mutations in the genes encoding a DNA methylation-binding protein, or histone demethylase or histone acetylase, may affect the chromatin of other genes on the X chromosome, helping some of them to escape inactivation, and inhibiting the transcription of others just by interfering with their chromatin environment. Fortunately, there is a great deal of redundancy in carrying out such activities so that the effect of one defective gene may be somewhat limited. For example, there are five methylation-binding proteins, and many histone demethylases (OMIM lists at least two dozen of them). Surprisingly, few have enough overlapping functions to avoid the observed phenotypic abnormalities that are associated with their loss.

And, defective genes encoded on autosomes like the ones causing the ICF syndrome may also affect X-linked genes. The syndrome is attributable to a mutation

Table 13-1. X-Linked Chromatin Disorders[a]

Syndrome	Location on X	Gene Name	OMIM # Gene	Type of Protein / Function	Sex Affected	Reference[b]
ATRX	Xq21.1	ATRX	300032	SNF2-type helicase / *Chromatin remodeling*	Males	12, A & C
Coffin-Lowry	Xp22.1	RSK2	300075	Histone H3 kinase / *Cell cycle progression*	Males more severe	C
Kabuki 2	Xp11.3	UTX, KDM6A[c]	300128	Histone demethylase / *HOX gene regulation*	Males & females alike	A & C
Rett	Xq28	MECP2	300005	Methyl-CpG binding / *DNA methylation*	Females & mosaic males	12, A & C
XLMR[d]	Xp11.2	JARID1C, KDM5C[c]	314690	Histone demethylase / *Chromatin remodeling*	Males more severe	C
XLMR	Xp11.2	PHF8	300560	Histone demethylase / *Cell cycle progression*	Males	C
XLMR	Xq24	CUL4B	300304	E3 ubiquitin ligase / *DNA replication*	Males	12, A & C
XLMR	Xq24	UPF3B	300298	Nucleocytoplasmic shuttling / *Promotes nonsense-mediated decay*	Males	C
XLMR	Xp11.2	HUWE1	300697	E3 Ubiquitin ligase / *Ubiquitinates histone H1*	Males	C
XLMR	Xq21.1	BRWD3	300553	Bromo-domain protein. / *Chromatin regulation*	Males	C
XLMR	Xq13.1	HDAC8	300269	Histone deacetylase / *Chromatid cohesion ?*	Males more severe	C
XI skewing	Xq13.2	XIST[c]	314670	Long noncoding RNA / *X inactivation*	Females & Klinefelter males	12

[a] The list is not exhaustive, but illustrates points made in the text.

[b] 12 = chapter 12, A = *Appendix A*, C = *Appendix C*.

[c] *JARID1C* and *UTX* are genes that are expressed from the inactive X. *XIST* is expressed only from the inactive X.

[d] XLMR, Syndromic X-Linked Mental Retardation.

in the *de novo* DNA methyltransferase, *DMT3B* on chromosome 20, which sets up the initial methylation patterns for many genes, including some on the X chromosome. Deficiency of this methylase causes immunodeficiency, centromere instability, facial anomalies, and mild mental retardation due to defective methylation of DNA sequences throughout the genome; in the centromeric regions of chromosomes 1, 9, and 16, the hypomethylation induces chromosomal breakage and interchromosomal interchanges. In rare cases, these mutations lead to global DNA hypomethylation of a small proportion of the genome; most often this hypomethylation affects repetitive sequences in heterochromatin and imprinted genes. Yet studies of fibroblasts from a girl with the ICF syndrome revealed that the telomeric X-linked genes *G6PD* and *SYBL1* that are usually silent on the inactive X escape from X chromosome inactivation [396]. The promoter regions of many other genes, even though they remained silent, are undermethylated, and show an increased chromatin sensitivity to nuclease, indicating relaxation of the chromatin around these genes. The reason that most of these genes with hypomethylated promoters remain silent is that they remain late replicating; escape from silencing is seen only when replication advances to the timing characteristic of its homolog on the active X. All of the observed cases of ICF syndrome have only partial deficiency of the gene, which is the reason that they survive.

Imprinting epimutations that alter gene expression may activate a silent gene, whereas histone demethylases may either activate or inactivate genes. Therefore, the resulting phenotype depends on the function of the affected gene, the tissue in which it functions, when it is expressed, and amount of residual activity. Because epigenetic factors are usually expressed throughout development, the affected individuals tend to show effects of developmental insufficiencies. Many of them have congenital abnormalities that affect the growth and formation of skeletal and organ systems, the system affected depending on where the mutant gene should have been expressed during development. Unlike metabolic storage disorders these chromatin disorders do not seem to progress with age. Another unique feature is that the causative genes in these inborn errors of chromatin are frequently mutated in malignant tumors. Yet, those individuals born with the same germline mutations do not seem to be especially prone to such cancers. However, because such disorders have been recognized only recently, long-term follow up studies are not yet available.

13.5. SEX DIFFERENCES IN MANIFESTATIONS OF CHROMATIN DISORDERS

Table 13-1 shows that hemizygous males and heterozygous females may have different manifestations of some X-linked chromatin disorders, much the same as they do for other mutated X-linked genes. Males are the ones predominantly affected by mutations in the SWI-SNF2 helicase causing the ATRX syndrome (see Chapter 12 and *Appendixes A* and *C*). This helicase functions mainly in chromatin remodeling; it remains to be seen how this X-linked gene manages to regulate the transcription of the two loci, residing side by side on chromosome 16, that encode the alpha hemoglobin chains. The only clue is that ATRX RNA is enriched at G-rich telomeres and sub-telomeres, and these hemoglobin genes are located near the end of the short arm of chromosome 16. In this disorder, the mutated helicase represses the levels of RNA from both α-hemoglobin genes. ATRX mutations also produce severe developmental retardation and abnormalities of male sex differentiation. That more organ systems are not involved suggests that this helicase, a member of a large family of SNF2 helicases, has some tissue specificity. The females, heterozygous for the ATRX mutation, avoid the anemia, intellectual defects and abnormal facies seen in males, by eliminating mutant cells in expressing tissues during their embryonic development, such that they are essentially no longer mosaic, at least in those tissues. Studies of Atrx-deficient mice suggest that cell selection is restricted to specific stages of development and is not ongoing throughout the life of the animal [397].

Both males and females are affected by mutations in the RSK2 gene, which is important in cell cycle progression. These mutations cause Coffin-Lowry syndrome, a rare form of syndromic X-linked mental retardation. Males have the full manifestation, which in addition to cognitive problems, includes skeletal malformations, growth retardation, a hearing defect, and an abnormal gait; many females have some of the same symptoms but less severe. Studies of X inactivation in these affected carrier females in several kindred show moderate skewing of the inactivation pattern from the random distribution, with the *normal* allele favored [398, 399]. This suggests that half normal gene product is not sufficient for normality, so that females need to have more than half normal cells in order to be affected less severely than their brothers.

The Kabuki syndrome, whose manifestations include cognitive disability, postnatal dwarfism, and abnormal facial features affects males and females equally. This is not surprising because the majority of them have loss-of-function mutations in the autosomal *MLL2* gene on chromosome 12 that encodes a histone H3 lysine 4–specific methyl transferase (Kabuki syndrome 1). Several cases of chromosome abnormalities (X rings) with the same phenotype implicate the X chromosome in this disorder, but, only a handful of affected individuals have a documented mutation in the X-linked *KDM6A* gene (also called *UTX*) that demethylates lysine 27 of histone H3 (Kabuki Syndrome 2). The manifestations of both Kabuki syndromes are the same because they are caused by two genes acting in the same functional pathway: H3K4 methylation by *MLL2* and the demethylation of H3K27 through *KDM6A* both serve to open chromatin to make it more transcriptionally active; therefore, mutations in either of them would repress the function of promoters bearing these epigenetic marks.

One must ask why males and females are similarly affected by the X-linked *KDM6A* mutations. It seems that *KDM6A* is one of the rare pairs of XY genes that are still expressed to some extent from both sex chromosomes. The X locus escapes X inactivation, and the Y locus is also expressed. The Y paralog (called *UTY*) has 84% amino acid sequence similarity with *KDM6A* and might compensate for any decreased expression of *KDM6A* in males, despite the fact that its demethylase activity has yet to be demonstrated. Its effect may be mediated in a demethylase independent fashion as *KDM6A* also has a demethylase independent role in regulating chromatin structure in mesoderm [400, 401]. Knock out of the locus in male mouse ES cells results in a genome wide increase in H3K27me3 at all bivalent promoters, suggesting that Uty cannot compensate for the loss of Kdm6a [402]. However, the effect of knocking out both alleles in female mice is more severe than knocking out the single allele in males, so that *Uty* permits survival of the knockout males [402]. The germline is compromised in female but not male mice [402], because Kdm6A has a sex specific effect on the Rhox (reproductive homeobox) genes that influence female germ cell development and are highly expressed in ovary [400].

A sex difference in Kabuki disease expression has not been noted in humans, perhaps because of the low ascertainment of *KDM6A* mutations. Only six *KDM6A* mutations (3 deletions and 3 point mutations) have been identified so far, three in males and three in females Although *KDM6A* escapes X inactivation, Lederer et al. [401] found a skewed X-inactivation pattern in two girls (89:11 and 97:3), related to the presence of a large gene deletion because the deleted X chromosome was inactive in the majority of their cells. In contrast, the female with the 3-base-pair deletion had balanced X inactivation [403]. Neither pattern seemed to protect them much from the cognitive effects mediated by the deleted gene, although the females had less cardiac malformations than the males.

If two dosages of *KDM6A* are needed for a normal phenotype, one can understand why many 45,X Turner females have some features of the Kabuki syndrome, such as postnatal short stature and skeletal anomalies. There is a clear overlap between the congenital heart defects prevalent in male Kabuki patients (aortic coarctation and other left-sided obstructions) and those found in patients with monosomy X and ring (X) chromosomes. Yet, intellectual deficiency, a consistent feature of the Kabuki syndrome, is not a feature of Turner females who survive gestation. Perhaps the reason why most 45,X females do not have the complete Kabuki syndrome is because many of them may have been 45,X/46,XX mosaics, at least during their early embryonic development. Alternatively, expression of the gene from the single X chromosome in 45,X individuals might be greater than from a single X in individuals with two sex chromosomes, because of the kind of dosage compensation associated with adding or subtracting chromosomes [404]. Expression studies at the *KDM6A* locus in Turner females versus XY males might provide some answers.

The seven X-linked mental retardation syndromes (XLMR; table 12.1, OMIM #s 300354, 300676, 300534 300263, 300706, 300659, and 309585, and *Appendix C*) are often caused by relatively small *de novo* X deletions or duplications. Several of them map in Xp11.2, a region that seems prone to chromosome rearrangements. The males are the ones that are usually affected, whereas the heterozygotes, who are mainly asymptomatic, have severe skewing of X inactivation patterns. The severe skewing implies that much more than 50% normal activity is required to avoid the symptoms of the disorder. Whether cell selection disfavoring the X with the gene duplication, or the small deletions, has any role here remains to be seen. Whereas most of the other mutations result in loss of function, the mutations in the *HUWE1* gene are duplications, which increase the expression of the gene. One is struck by the number of X-linked mental retardation syndromes that are associated with histone methylases and demethylases, illuminating the role of histone modification and its modifiers in intellectual disability and congenital malformations.

The last X-linked disorder listed on Table 13-1 is primary skewing of X chromosome inactivation, the phenotype most often associated with mutations in the *XIST* gene. In both mouse and human females, *Xist* deletions that knock out the ability of the X chromosome to inactivate result in loss of one of the two cell populations in the mosaic female. The loss of mosaicism is a consequence of cell selection favoring the cell population in which the deleted locus is on the active X (normal *Xist* allele always on the inactive X; see figure 10-1). Therefore the same X chromosome is expressed in every cell of affected females, making her subject to the same health risks as normal males. Such females are ascertained only when they come to attention by manifesting some X-linked disease that is usually only seen in males. If the *XIST* locus is included in an extensive X chromosomal deletion that creates a minute X or small ring X chromosome, then the female will express two doses of some X-linked genes, which will cause severe phenotypes. Point mutations in the *XIST* promoter that result in less loss of function induce more modest skewing, such that the mutant allele less likely to be on the inactive X [135-137].

13.6. TREATMENT OF CHROMATIN DISORDERS

Epigenetic mechanisms are characterized by reversibility, and the fact that epigenetic marks can be changed offers possible therapeutic interventions for chromatin disorders. Studies of model organisms suggest that such disorders are treatable by agonists that will reverse the chromatin state [405]. Drugs such as the histone deacetylase inhibitor valproic acid that squeeze out more product from mutant genes are already being used to treat some genetic disorders, such as cystic fibrosis or Gaucher's disease—inherited disorders that arise from the misfolding of proteins. Studies of Gaucher's disease show that inhibiting histone deacetylases increases the acetylation of heat shock protein 90B, thereby reducing its affinity for, and prolonging the life span of, the mutant galactosidase protein [406]. A caveat is that most agonists like histone deacetylases and methylases inhibitors are not very specific and have the potential to be harmful. Nonetheless, as we learn more of the histone code, more specific therapies may be found.

13.7. SUMMARY AND SPECULATIONS

The discovery of chromatin disorders makes us further aware of the complexity of phenotypes attributable to mutations in single-copy genes. Perhaps it is surprising that the clinical disorders caused by mutations in the epigenetic machinery do not differ more from other X-linked disorders where the deficient gene product is part of a metabolic pathway. In both cases, the observed mutations often affect cognitive ability, and distort the normal growth patterns of the trunk, the limbs, the face, and the head of affected individuals. Even if disorders affecting epigenetic factors have a greater potential to influence the function of distant genes, one cannot easily predict the nature of the causative gene from the phenotype it produces. Yet, the common theme of profound intellectual deficit in males identifies this as a hallmark of chromatin disorders of the X-linked kind.

From the standpoint of X inactivation, mutations in the epigenetic machinery have the potential to affect imprinted alleles in heterochromatin. In some cases, this may lead to the inappropriate expression of silenced alleles on the inactive X in females. Knowing that as little as 5% of normal enzyme activity can provide enough gene product to avoid the dire consequences of many mutations, we can appreciate the effect of aberrant DNA methylation or histone deacetylase inhibitors that either increase or decrease gene expression. Chance activation of genes that should be silent could have deleterious effects; they may initiate abnormal cell proliferation, contribute a small effect to the development of common disorders, and in rare cases cause metabolic interference or induce autoimmune responses.

We can also appreciate the therapeutic opportunities that may be available not only to those who suffer from these disorders of the epigenetic machinery, but also from disorders of protein folding and no doubt other genetic disorders. Squeezing out just a little more gene product may ameliorate these diseases. Even if therapeutic agents cannot mitigate the phenotype, we are bound to learn a great deal about the regulation of our epigenome from studies of these patients.

14

Determinants of Female
Phenotypes

*As inheritors of the genetic experiments at meiosis we are each an individual
participant in the grand scheme of selection and evolution.*
                    —*Barton Childs,* Genetic Medicine [407]

The biology leading to the masculinization of the male fetus has been relatively
well worked out. We know a good deal about the complicated pathways induced
by the Y-linked *SRY* gene that triggers differentiation of the testes and the cascade of events needed to masculinize the XY fetus (reviewed in [408]). Whereas
quite a bit is known about the genetic program for maleness, considerably less
is known about the one for femaleness. Those who write about feminization
of the fetus usually say that it is the constitutive or default pathway to sexual
development—which has been the prevailing thought [409]. Although a functional testis is essential for the physical appearance characteristic of males, a
functional ovary is not needed for the phenotype of female body plan, at least
the appearance of one.

Even though genes specifically involved in ovarian development had not yet been
identified at the time of the first edition, I suggested that they must exist, as the
ovary is as structurally and functionally complex as other organs. Even if it develops
only when the testis pathway is absent or loses its command, there certainly must be
an active genetic pathway controlling its formation. In the interim, we have learned
a good deal about how ovaries develop. Considerable experimental evidence indicates that ovarian development is established by active repression of one or more
genes in the testicular pathway. Details of this ovarian pathway remain to be elucidated, but β-*catenin* is an important ovarian determinant and anti-testis gene. The
identification of *RSPO1*, the most upstream gene required for ovarian differentiation
by Giovanna Camerino and colleagues [410] not only shows that sex differentiation
is based on the antagonistic relationship between two different molecular pathways
(Sry/Sox9 versus Rspo1/β-catenin), but also sheds new light on the molecular basis
of what makes us a woman or a man. The ovary begins with the differentiation
of follicular cells. Future studies should help us to understand how genes involved

in specifying follicle cells act to repress testes determinants, and tip the balance in favor of ovary differentiation.

The female germ cells themselves are quite influential, because there is no ovary in their absence. And, the *Fox12* genes have been implicated in the maintenance of the ovary, perhaps by means of maintaining the integrity of germ cells [411].

As you can see, the elucidation of genes with unique functions in female development is a work in progress. Without doubt, X inactivation is one of the essential steps in the female developmental program. A single active X is absolutely required for female viability. Essential for their intrauterine survival, X inactivation also shapes their subsequent development by means of the mosaicism it creates. The influence of mosaicism is certainly dynamic, because the composition of cell populations in a female is unlikely to be the same in childhood, adolescence, and old age as it was at birth—or, for that matter, as it was at the onset of X inactivation before birth. In this, the final chapter, I tie together the various aspects of cellular mosaicism in a discussion of the factors that shape the female phenotype. I summarize the observations made in preceding chapters and continue the discussion of how her genetic makeup and chance experiences, along with these interactive cellular events, influence a woman's health and welfare.

14.1. THE DYNAMIC EFFECT OF INTERACTING CELL POPULATIONS ON THE HEALTH OF FEMALES

X Inactivation as a Determinant of Clinical Phenotype

There is little doubt that cellular mosaicism provides a remarkable biological advantage, but clearly, the outcome is never certain. It depends on many dynamic interactions, and these are influenced as much by chance events as by the blueprint for development. Table 14-1 provides a list of the factors that affect the clinical phenotype of females who carry detrimental mutations known to cause X-linked diseases. The repertoire of functional proteins (the functional proteome) of the heterozygous female has multiple determinants. Some have more to do with the nature of the mutation, and others with X inactivation, but both kinds of determinants are highly interconnected. The influence of mutations varies considerably depending on their effect on protein synthesis, and the chance presence of other factors affecting the expression of that mutation—because they ultimately affect the composition of her mosaic cell populations. Whether her heterozygous mutation has no effect or causes clinical disease depends on (1) how much of a specific protein is required for adequate function, (2) the amount of residual protein available to the cell, (3) whether the gene product is transferred between cells, and (4) whether the mutation influences the growth of the cells expressing it. In addition, the nature of the chromosome on which the mutant gene resides is also a factor affecting whether it will be expressed at all. Is it on a normal X chromosome, or an X/autosome translocation chromosome, or an X chromosome with a missing segment? Is it expressed from the active X chromosome? Is the locus silent or partially expressed from the inactive X?

Table 14-1. DETERMINANTS OF FEMALE PHENOTYPE

Mutation

- Is there a disease-related mutation on one parental X chromosome?
- Does the mutation produce a severe or mild deficiency of the encoded protein?
- Is the mutation "cell autonomous"? Or is there metabolic cooperation? Or cellular interference?
- Does the mutation influence the growth of mutant cells?
- Does the mutation reside on a normal X chromosome or one with a cytogenetic abnormality?
- Does the mutation have the potential to increase physiological diversity?
- Is the mutation in a gene that escapes inactivation?

X inactivation

- Is X inactivation random at onset? Or is there an XIC mutation?
- Is the female fetus a twin?
- Does the fetus have an X-autosome translocation or X deletion?
- Does the fetus have confined placental mosaicism?
- Is there cell selection? Does it favor mutant or normal cell?
- Is the locus on the inactive X partially expressed?

Other factors that influence outcomes have to do with chance skewing of X inactivation unrelated to the mutation. The randomness of the process is affected by mutations in the mechanism that initially chooses the active X in the embryo. It is also affected by random stochastic events that decrease the size of cell populations or have a bottleneck effect, such as twinning, and placental mosaicism for disomic and trisomic cells. No doubt the coincidence of two of these mechanisms within the same individual is quite rare. Yet, such coincidences do occur, and when they do, the end result is usually a manifesting heterozygote. Despite having one normal allele, such females have clinical manifestations very much like those of hemizygous males. The proximate reason for their illness is that the normal alleles either have been lost (as in the case of Turner syndrome) or have been permanently made inaccessible to the transcriptional machinery because they are always on the inactive X chromosome. Yet, one must keep in mind that the instances of disease manifestations due to skewing of X inactivation are relatively infrequent. In most cases, being able to express both alleles provides the means to ameliorate these diseases.

What I hope you will appreciate is that the physical and intellectual attributes of females—like males—are determined to a great extent by their X-linked genes. But, unlike males, whose development is influenced by whatever genes happen to be on their single X chromosomes, females have a little extra determinant, and this is the interaction between their mosaic cell populations that is not possible in nonmosaic XY males. Although the initial steps in X inactivation may be perilous ones—resulting in the demise of females before the stage when pregnancies are recognized—most often the mixed population of cells bestows a remarkable biological advantage, as well as a means to increase cellular diversity in our species.

X Inactivation as a Determinant of Normal Traits

The generally positive effects of interactions in mosaic cell populations are easiest to visualize in the case where one chromosome carries a deleterious mutation. After all, most of our knowledge of human biology has been acquired by viewing it through the window of disease or deleterious mutations. Yet, even in the absence of detrimental mutations, cellular mosaicism may be an advantage not only to the individual but also to her species. It is likely to contribute to some of the gender differences in behavior. There is little evidence of sex differences in cognition during infancy, and differences in performance on standardized tests undoubtedly reflect a complex mix of social, cultural, and biological factors [412]. Even though boys still do somewhat better on science and math tests in this country,[1] the gap is smaller and closing and may even close when women perceive that opportunities in the sciences are indeed sex-blind. But there are some differences in strategies used to solve the problems. Studies have shown that gender affects the way a person's brain responds to humor. Alan Reiss and colleagues [414] show that women viewing funny cartoons activate the parts of the brain involved in language processing and working memory more than do men and are more likely to activate with greater intensity the part of the brain that generates rewarding feelings in response to new experiences. Perhaps such examples are not attributable to native differences, but there are likely to be some. It does not seem far-fetched to me to think that cellular mosaicism has a role in some of these gender differences.

Some of the sex differences in physical traits between men and women may also be influenced by the inactivation status of a women's X-linked genes. By this I mean those genes on her inactive X chromosome that escape inactivation. Not the ones in the pseudoautosomal region PAR1, because such genes—transcribed from both X chromosomes in 46,XX females and from both X and Y in 46,XY males—are not differentially expressed. Instead, I mean the genes expressed to some extent from the unique regions of the inactive X—the ones that provide a little more normal X-linked gene products to XX females than to XY males. You may recall that such escapees can rescue the deleterious effects of some mutant X-linked genes (see "Orofaciodigital Syndrome Type 1" in section 12.5). Yet, even in absence of mutations, the additional expression from normal alleles on inactive X chromosomes may have an effect. The levels of expression are likely to vary, and some of the women with the highest expression levels may be at an increased (or decreased) risk of common diseases. Studies of mice have implicated such normal gene products in elevating the levels of lipids and insulin, which are risk factors

1. "In fact, girls outperformed boys in more countries in a science test given to 15-year-old students in 65 countries—but in the United States, boys led the girls" [413].

for obesity and diabetes, and may contribute to sex differences in body fat storage [415]. And more such cases are sure to come to light.

14.2. THE EFFECT OF X INACTIVATION ON NORMAL FEMALE PHENOTYPE AND CELL DIVERSITY

Even though some parameters are essential, the way development actually occurs is not determined by a rigid blueprint. There is a great deal of leeway for variation in the protein building blocks and gene regulatory pathways as long as the essential processes are not perturbed. Most of the variations that arise in our genomes may be neutral, having little influence on how we carry out the specific functions that they encode. Yet, some of these novel variations may be deleterious, affecting the viability of the cell, or even of the individual. Because we often have more cells of each kind than we need, the dysfunction of an occasional one because of mutations is of no import. It is only the ones that occur in the germline that have a dramatic effect. On the other hand, some of the heritable mutations may even be of value. Probably, there is little immediate advantage to the individual in whom such mutations arise, because our genes have gone through a long selection process, so the genes we possess at this time are probably the best adapted to the environment we are living in. On the other hand, should our environment drastically change, some of this variation may prove useful in adapting to such changes. Therefore, variation is most often a very good thing. In addition, it is likely to account for some of the more nuanced differences between the sexes.

Even in absence of detrimental mutant alleles, a female is the composite of two intermingling cells populations that share their X-linked gene products with each other. Meyer-Lindenberg and colleagues [416] have studied the impact of a common functional polymorphism in the promoter of the X-linked monoamine oxidase A (MAOA) gene on brain structure and function in a large sample of healthy human volunteers. In males the low-expression allele is associated with increased risk of violent behavior compared with the high-expression allele. The study identified differences in the circuitry for emotion regulation and cognitive control that may explain the association of MAOA with impulsive aggression in males, and the authors suggest that X inactivation in the human brain might be responsible for some of the findings observed in females (e.g., an intermediate level of emotional response in heterozygotes).

It is also likely that the mosaicism resulting from X inactivation contributes to the generation of cell diversity. Smallwood and colleagues [417] have pointed out that in the nervous system, cellular diversity is advantageous as a general strategy for enhancing the efficiency of signal processing and transmission. Their suggestion comes from their observations of color vision in New World monkeys. In these species, the single–X-linked pigment gene has three alleles, each encoding a pigment with a different spectral sensitivity. Males and homozygous females have dichromatic color vision, whereas heterozygous females have trichromatic color vision. Creating a mouse model (by *knocking in* a human allele), they observed a novel chromatic diversity among retinal ganglion cells in heterozygous females and enhanced chromatic discrimination. Their wider range of spectral sensitivities compared to males is due to the stochastic variation in the mosaic populations created by X inactivation [417]. Such mosaicism can generate cellular diversity for many physiological processes.

Smallwood et al. [417] suggested that functional mosaicism has the potential to create cellular diversity on an extremely rapid evolutionary time scale. The small size of X inactivation patches within the brain of heterozygotes ensures that virtually any structure of appreciable size within the brain will be mosaic (see figure 10-3D). The stochastic variation in the proportion of cells expressing each allele—could generate physiologic diversity that might be evolutionarily advantageous. New studies from this group show fine grain intermixing of inhibitory interneurons [432], suggesting that mosaicism for any X-linked gene affecting interneuron function will affect all cortical circuits. They remind us that a diversity-generating mechanism such as XCI, operating on all cells within the CNS at the level of local circuits, has the potential to introduce novel functions. The presence of mosaic cell populations, carrying functional alleles with different capacities to assemble and maintain synaptic transmissions, might influence how that signal is perceived. This would not be the case for autosomal genes, because even if the two alleles differed, the cells would be homogeneous for the blended expression pattern.

Despite behavioral differences between the sexes, surprisingly few anatomical differences have been identified in the brains of males and females. And RNA analysis has not found genes expressed solely in male or female neurons except for *Xist* and Y-linked genes. Richard Axel and colleagues [418] suggested that identification of more subtle differences is swamped by the vast majority of shared (autosomally encoded) circuits. Yet, mosaicism for X-linked genes involved in these circuits may contribute to some of these sex differences in behavior.

Just as the ability to express a variety of normal color vision alleles enhances the way that color is perceived, having cells that collaborate on the elaboration of a protein may result in novel molecules, that enhance the function being carried out. The diversity provided by expressing two alleles simultaneously but in different cells may lead to novel effects. Further, females have a greater repertoire of X-linked genes to transmit to the next generation.

14.3. EPILOGUE

Sexual reproduction evolved to ensure the survival of species by providing opportunities for new combinations of chromosomes in individuals. For this purpose, the X and Y chromosomes evolved to isolate the genes required for reproduction.

However, the bulk of the X chromosome consists of genes that have little to do with the reproductive attributes of individuals. Having the genetic determinants of being either male or female sets in motion a cascade of events, such as the need for dosage compensation. This in turn creates biological differences between the sexes that affect every aspect of their lives, not just the sexual ones.

Sex dosage compensation is largely a probability event, and so we should not be surprised that the outcome is highly variable. Although the ability to express two kinds of alleles affords a significant biological advantage to most females, the outcome is never certain. It depends on a multitude of complex interactions that are determined by the nature of mutations, their effect on cell growth, and the intercellular communication of gene products. The effect of "escape genes", and of chance chromosomal deletions and other rearrangements that skew patterns of X inactivation is also a part of the equation. Interacting cell populations in the mosaic female greatly influence the homeostasis of the individual and her ultimate health status. The interactions occur not only between the intermingling cells of a kind that express different X-linked alleles but also between other mosaic cells with different and sometimes conflicting tissue-specific functions. And how dynamic the process is: it is influenced by chance epigenetic events as well as variations in the normal genetic blueprint. One clearly sees that the results will never be the same for any two individuals, even monozygotic twins. We are all truly *individuals* in the grand scheme of selection and evolution.

Descriptions of Model X-linked and Related Diseases

The following X-linked or X-influenced diseases are listed with their disease name, their gene name, and their map locus (the location of the gene on the X chromosome), which can be ascertained from the banded X chromosome in figure 2-2. These data are followed by the protein that is deficient and then the OMIM number, which is the reference number for the disease in the Online Mendelian Inheritance in Man (OMIM) database (located at http://www.ncbi.nlm.nih.gov/Omim).

X-Linked Diseases

Adrenoleukodystrophy	*ALD*	Xq28
ABCD1	#300100	

The ALD protein (ABCD1) belongs to a family of transporter proteins that carry products across cell membranes. ABCD1 is found in the peroxisomes, which are membrane-bound bags containing the enzymes that oxidize fatty acids. Oxidation is a means to generate energy for the cell. Mutations in the *ABCD1* gene encoding this transporter protein lead to defective oxidation of fatty acids because the digestive enzymes cannot enter the peroxisomes. This results in an accumulation of very-long-chain fatty acids in all tissues of the body. Yet, this disorder, sometimes called "Lorenzo's oil disease," primarily affects the adrenal gland and the central nervous system, causing the loss of adrenal function and the progressive destruction of myelin—a protein that protects spinal cord nerves and the white matter of the brain. The loss of myelin from the brain is associated with rapid loss of the ability to walk, read, and understand language, and eventual death in childhood. However, the severity of disease is extremely variable depending on the degree of deficiency and other yet unknown factors. A remarkable feature of this disorder is that brothers—even twins—with the identical mutation may have different symptoms, somewhat related to the time when the first symptoms of the disease appear (age of onset). Males with early onset of their disease (before 10 years of age) usually have demyelinization of the brain, whereas often in those with later onset the demyelinization affects only the spinal cord. The cerebral form of the disease is referred to as adrenoleukodystrophy, whereas the spinal cord disease is called adrenomyeloneuropathy (AMN). Another unique feature is that many carrier females, as they age, develop a mild form of spinal cord disease, often diagnosed as AMN.

Alport Syndrome	*COL4A5*	Xq22.3
COL4A5 Collagen	#301050	

Alport syndrome, a group of hereditary diseases affecting the kidney, may also cause hearing loss and eye lesions. In the kidney, the basement membranes of both tubules and glomeruli often lack one of their type IV collagen components. Approximately 85% of Alport syndrome results from mutations in the X-linked COL4A5 collagen gene. Males with a COL4A5 deficiency almost always acquire end-stage renal disease, whereas females have a wide range of phenotypes ranging from asymptomatic to symptoms similar to that of males. As many as 25% of carrier females may have severe renal disease, but their disease usually begins later than in males.

Androgen Insensitivity Syndrome	*AR*	Xq11–12
Dihydrotestosterone receptor	#300068	

The male sex hormone testosterone is synthesized in the testes but must be transported to many tissues to carry out its function—that is, to masculinize the male fetus. However, for testosterone to function, it must first be transformed to its more active form, which is dihydrotestosterone (DHT). DHT is the androgenic hormone (androgen) needed for the development of the penis and scrotum. In turn, for DHT to be effective, it must be carried from the cytoplasm of the cell—the site of its synthesis—into the nucleus, where it turns on the genes encoding the proteins responsible for masculinization of these tissues. The carrier is a protein called the DHT receptor, or androgen receptor (AR). Mutations in the X-linked *androgen receptor AR* gene interfere with the cell's ability to transport DHT to the nucleus; hence, the fetus is said to be "insensitive" to the presence of this androgen. The XY fetus with androgen insensitivity cannot completely develop a penis and scrotum. The extent of masculinization is variable—depending on the severity of the AR deficiency. Affected males are often called male pseudo-hermaphrodites. Mutations in the *AR* gene usually have no effect in females. However, analysis of the methylation of the *AR* gene in females has provided a useful test for X inactivation (see chapter 5 & figure 12-7).

ATRX Syndrome	*ATRX*	Xq13
ATRX protein or XH2 (an SNF2–like helicase)	#301040	

The protein deficient in this α-thalassemia–mental retardation syndrome (ATRX) is thought to be a helicase belonging to a family of enzymes that are widely expressed during development and have a role in organizing chromatin. In human cells, ATRX protein associates with the ribosomal DNA genes. Usually only males are affected, and their strikingly uniform phenotype consists of severe mental retardation, microcephaly, characteristic facial features (wide-set eyes, epicanthus, a small, triangular upturned nose, and flat face), genital abnormalities, and an unusual, mild form of α-thalassemia called hemoglobin H disease. The low levels of RNA from both α-hemoglobin genes on chromosome 16 suggest that the mutation disrupts a *trans*-acting factor involved in regulating α-globin expression. The mental retardation is related to the loss of neurons, because ATRX is a critical mediator of cell survival during early neuronal differentiation. Some heterozygotes have rare blood cells containing hemoglobin H inclusions and mild mental retardation.

Barth Syndrome	*TAZ*	Xq28
Taffazin	#302060	

Barth syndrome (BTHS) is characterized by cardiomyopathy, skeletal myopathy, abnormal mitochondria, neutropenia, and an excess of 3-methylglutaconic acid. The lack of full-length tafazzin, a mitochondrial transacylase that remodels cardiolipin to its mature form, is responsible for deficient cardiolipin in mitochondria, especially those in cardiac and skeletal muscle. All affected individuals have been males; no female carriers have been reported with symptoms of the disease.

Borjeson-Forssman-Lehmann Syndrome	*PHF6*	Xq26.2
Zinc finger transcription factor 6	#301900	

The features include severe mental retardation, epilepsy, hypogonadism, low metabolism, marked obesity, swelling of facial tissue, and large but not deformed ears. Three carrier females had moderate mental retardation, in absence of other manifestations. The disease mechanisms are not known, but somatic mutations in the gene are associated with some cases of acute T-cell leukemia.

Bruton Agammaglobulinemia	*BTK*	Xq22.1
Tyrosine kinase	#300300	

Bruton tyrosine kinase is a key regulator of the development of the lymphocytes that originate in the bone marrow (B-cells). Mutations affecting this enzyme cause agammaglobulinemia, an X-linked immunodeficiency disorder characterized by the failure to produce mature B-cells. This leads to a deficiency of several immunoglobulins. In this disease, the immature B-cells (pre-B-cells) are present in the bone marrow but are unable to differentiate further, resulting in a lack of the circulating B-cells needed to fight infections. Therefore, males affected with this developmental arrest of B-cells are usually prone to severe bacterial infections. Protected by their mother's immunoglobulins during gestation, the infant males start to have infections at about 3 months of age. Their thymus-derived lymphocytes (T-cells) are not affected. Until the introduction of treatment with gamma globulin, these boys often succumbed to their infections. Carrier females have only normal circulating B-cells. Although the mutant pre-B-cell can be found in their bone marrow, they never mature.

CHILD Syndrome	*NSDHL*	Xq28
C4 demethylase	#308050	

CHILD syndrome is an acronym for an X-linked disorder characterized by Congenital Hemidysplasia with Ichthyosis and Limb Defects. Many organs are asymmetric with hypoplasia on the side of ichthyosis and limb malformation. Homologous to *Bare patch* mutations in mice, the mutated gene has a role in cholesterol biosynthesis. The affected individuals are usually female as the mutations are lethal in hemizygous males. Only mosaic males survive.

Chondrodysplasia Punctata 2	*EPB*	Xp11.23
Emopamil-binding protein	#302960	

This is the most well characterized of a genetically heterogeneous disorder characterized by punctiform calcification of the bones. Other features include skin defects (linear or whorled, and pigmented lesions and striated hyperkeratosis), coarse, lusterless hair and alopecia, cataracts, and skeletal abnormalities including short stature. Lethal in males, all the patients are female except for mosaic males who survive because of their population of wild-type cells.

Craniofrontonasal Syndrome	*EFNB1*	Xq12
Ephrin-B1	#304110	

Ephrin-B1 is a member of the ephrin family of transmembrane ligands for receptor tyrosine kinases. The prevailing thought is that ephrin-B1 plays a role in defining the position of the coronal suture of the skull and that it does this by mediating signals that repel cells from crossing the boundary between the frontal bone (neural crest cells) and the parietal bone (mesoderm cells), thus permitting the suture to remain open. Only the *EFNB1* mutations that completely incapacitate the protein cause craniofrontonasal syndrome. This syndrome is paradoxically more severe in carrier females than in mutant 46,XY males. In females and males mosaic for the mutation, the unprogrammed fusion of the coronal sutures produces craniosynostosis. Also, there is frontonasal dysplasia with wide-set eyes and a broad nose, and at times widening of the midline suture. In affected males, the only manifestations are abnormally wide-set eyes and an occasional cleft lip. The lack of ephrin-B1 protein in some but not all cells in females and mosaic males is thought to perturb the formation of the normal sharp neural crest/mesoderm tissue boundary at the future coronal suture, because the mixture of mutant and normal cells confuses the signaling process.

CUL4B-deficient XLMR   *CUL4B*   Xq24
Cullin-RING E3 Ubiquitin ligase   #300354

Cullins encode modules of one of the most abundant E3 ligase families. These scaffold proteins are crucial in a host of fundamental biochemical processes ranging from DNA replication and repair – to transcription and development. They are also important in the formation of heterochromatin. Missense and truncating mutations in CUL4B provide evidence that they have an important role in neuronal function and cognition. In addition to their intellectual deficit, affected males are short and obese, They have relative macrocephaly, abnormal gait, tremors, and hypogonadism. Carrier females are usually unaffected, and may have mild tremors.

Danon Disease   *LAMP2*   Xq24
Lysosome-associated membrane protein   #300257

This is one of three X-linked lysosomal disorders, and the only one not affecting a digestive enzyme. It results from a severe deficiency or complete absence of the LAMP2 glycoproteins, which make up a significant fraction of the glycoproteins in the lysosomal membranes. LAMP2 is thought to protect the lysosomal membrane from the digestive enzymes within the lysosomes, and to act as a receptor for proteins that are imported into lysosomes. Cardiac myocytes are ultrastructurally abnormal and heart contractility is severely reduced. Males suffer from cardiomyopathy, skeletal muscle weakness, and mental retardation starting in their first decade, whereas women, if affected, develop cardiomyopathy only as adults.

Dyskeratosis Congenita   *DKC1*   Xq28
Dyskerin   #305000

This premature aging syndrome is characterized by short telomeres. Diagnosis is based on the triad of abnormal skin pigmentation, nail dystrophy, and leukoplakia of the oral mucosa. Progressive bone marrow failure, which occurs in over 80% of cases, is the main cause of early mortality. Later mortality is due to pulmonary fibrosis, liver cirrhosis, and predisposition to malignancy. The ultimate cause of death is telomere shortening. Most of the patients are males. Female carriers have highly skewed X inactivation, which enables them to be disease free.

Epileptic Encephalopathy, Infantile, 9   *PCDH19*   Xq22
Protocadherin-19   #300088

The protocadherins are calcium-dependent cell-cell adhesion molecules. Found in the developing central nervous system, including the hippocampus and cortex, they are thought to have a role in cognitive function. *PCDH19* mutations cause a syndrome of female-restricted epilepsy of the early infantile type, and mental retardation. Similar mutations in males (who transmit the mutation to their affected daughters) do not cause ill effects. The mutations identified so far result in protein deficiency, or adversely affect the adhesiveness of PCDH19 by impairing calcium binding. It has been proposed that the disorder is attributable to mosaicism for this X-linked gene such that cell-to-cell signals are perturbed because of cellular interference. A related gene on the Y chromosome may confer some protection to mutant males (see "Cellular Interference" in section 12.3).

Fabry Disease	*GLA*	Xq22
Alpha-galactosidase A	#301500	

Alpha-galactosidase A is an enzyme found in lysosomes, the impermeable bags containing at least 60 digestive enzymes that are needed to degrade old cell proteins and recycle their components. Specifically, α-galactosidase A breaks down glycosphingolipids, which are components of most cell membranes. Mutations producing a deficiency of this protein lead to progressive accumulations of glycosphingolipids in the blood and lysosomes of most cells. The accumulation in blood vessels causes blockage and tissue damage, which in turn causes severe episodic pain (the earliest symptom) and eventually kidney and heart failure and cerebrovascular problems, leading to premature death. Most of the individuals with severe disease are males, who often require kidney transplants and enzyme replacement therapy. Female carriers may have disease manifestations; however, most affected girls and women have an attenuated form of the disease.

Fanconi Anemia	*FANCB*	Xp22.31
FANCB	#300514	

FANCB is one of several proteins that form a complex needed to repair damaged DNA, as a means of editing out some of the errors that occur during cell division. Mutations in any one of the FANC proteins produce anemia and platelet deficiency. Most of these proteins are encoded by autosomes, except for FANCB, which is encoded by the X chromosome. Fanconi anemia is characterized initially by congenital defects such as mental retardation and abnormal development of skin, kidney, and bone and later by progressive bone marrow failure. Usually males are the ones affected; they are growth retarded, and their cells are prone to apoptosis and chromosomal instability, which may result in malignancy. Most female carriers of the *FANCB* mutation are healthy with no signs of the mutation, because almost all of their cells function normally.

Fragile X Syndrome	*FMR1*	Xq27.3
FMR1 protein (FMRP)	#300624	

The *FMR1* gene encodes the FMR1 protein (called FMRP), whose role is still not well understood. The current view is that FMRP regulates messenger RNA transport and translation in a manner critical for the development of nerve cells. Mutations in this gene produce the common fragile X syndrome (occurring in

1 of 4,000 male births). The classic form of the disease is characterized by moderate to severe mental retardation associated with varying degrees of enlargement of the testes, ears, and jaw and high-pitched, animated speech. The mutation in most cases involves an expansion of a region where the trinucleotide CGG is highly repeated (i.e., CGGCGGCGGCGGCGG, etc.); the expansion is in the region of the gene that regulates its transcription. Normal individuals have <40 of these CGG repeats. Any trinucleotide that is repeated so many times may not always be copied accurately during DNA replication, and therefore, trinucleotide repeats are notoriously unstable in copy number, tending to gain or lose a number of the repeats. There are two degrees of mutation associated with this CGG repeat. One is a *premutation*—when the expansion is more than 50 but fewer than 200 repeats; the other is a *full mutation*—when there are more than 300 CGG repeats. Only the full mutation induces chromatin changes in the gene that give the appearance of a break in the chromosome, referred to as a "fragile site," which gives the name to the syndrome. Clinical abnormalities are associated with both premutation and full mutation, but they differ in nature as well as severity. In males, the premutation is associated with a tremor and abnormal gait in the sixth decade of age. Some carrier females have the same symptoms, and they also may show premature menopause. The full mutation in males is associated with the retardation syndrome, whereas carrier females usually have a milder form of retardation; some may be normal. Individuals with the full mutation have neither FMR1 RNA nor protein; their abnormalities are due to the deficiency of the FMR1 protein. On the other hand, the disorders associated with the premutation seem to be due to an excess of CGG-containing messenger RNA.

Hemolytic Anemia (X-linked)	*G6PD*	Xq28
Glucose-6–phosphate dehydrogenase	#305900	

Glucose-6–phosphate dehydrogenase (G6PD) is an enzyme in the hexose monophosphate pathway, which is the only means to generate ATP in red blood cells. Deficiency of this enzyme in red cells leads to chronic anemia, as well as acute anemias induced by some drugs. The deficiency of the enzyme is never complete, because such mutations would be lethal. Mutations leading to the enzyme deficiency are very common in populations of African origin or those living in other areas where malaria is prevalent because the deficiency has a protective effect against malarial infections. These common variants of G6PD (some associated with very mild enzyme deficiency) have been very useful as markers to identify one X chromosome from the other in heterozygous females for studies of gene mapping and disease associations. Carrier females usually are not anemic.

Hemophilia A	*F8*	Xq28
Factor VIII	#306700	

Coagulation factor VIII (FVIII) is one of many proteins that participate in the cascade of chemical reactions that enable the blood to clot after trauma—or when bleeding occurs. Mutations in the *F8* gene produce a bleeding disorder in males. The clinical features of hemophilia A all result from the lack of FVIII despite the presence of all the other coagulation factors and platelets. Affected individuals develop hemorrhages into joints and muscles, easy bruising, and prolonged bleeding from wounds—the severity depending on the extent of the deficiency of the clotting factor. Heterozygous females usually do not have bleeding problems.

Hemophilia B Christmas Disease	*F9*	Xq27
Factor IX	#306900	

Coagulation factor IX (FIX) is another of the many proteins that participate in the cascade of chemical reactions that enable the blood to clot and, like FVIII, it is encoded by the X chromosome. Mutations in the *F9* gene in males also produce a bleeding disorder. And like FVIII deficiency, affected individuals develop hemorrhages into joints and muscles, easy bruising, and prolonged bleeding from wounds—the severity depending on the extent of the deficiency of the clotting factor. Heterozygous females usually do not have bleeding problems.

Hunter Syndrome	*IDS*	Xq28
Iduronate sulfatase	#309900	

Iduronate sulfatase is another of the digestive enzymes packaged in the lysosomes and is the one needed to degrade the mucopolysaccharides chondroitin sulfate and heparin sulfate. In the absence of this enzyme's activity, large amounts of these mucopolysaccharides accumulate in tissues and urine. Although the severity depends on the degree of enzyme deficiency, affected males are often dwarfed because of bone abnormalities, with characteristic facial features, enlarged liver and spleen, and deafness. Deposits of these compounds in their blood vessels lead to heart disease and death in childhood or early in adulthood. Carrier females are usually unaffected but might have some accumulation of mucopolysaccharides with aging. Only rarely are females fully affected.

Hyperammonemia	*OTC*	Xp21.1
Ornithine transcarbamylase	#311250	

Ornithine transcarbamylase (OTC) is a key enzyme in the urea cycle, a metabolic pathway that prevents accumulation of toxic levels of ammonia. Elevated ammonia levels can interfere with brain function. Severe deficiency of OTC in males, due to mutations in essential structural or functional domains of the gene, results in intolerance to proteins in food and acute elevations in blood ammonia starting immediately after birth. If untreated, the disturbance in brain metabolism culminates in death during infancy. Carrier females have a milder form of the disease, exacerbated during pregnancy; they often eliminate meat from their diet because it makes them feel sick.

| Ichthyosis (X-linked) | *STS* | Xp22.31 |
| Steroid sulfatase | #308100 | |

Steroid sulfatase is an enzyme that removes a sulfate group from cholesterol and other steroid compounds. The deficiency of steroid sulfatase causes X-linked ichthyosis, a severe skin abnormality usually manifesting in affected males during the first year after birth. The epidermis of much of the body becomes dry and horny, like fish scales. The skin disorder is caused by the inability of cells to break down cholesterol sulfate, resulting in loss of water from the skin. Almost 90% of the mutations are extensive deletions of the gene caused by very small deletions of the X chromosome, because of its location close to the pairing region of the X and Y chromosomes. Some of these deletions may affect other genes in the region and cause a contiguous gene syndrome like Kallmans syndrome (#308700). Carrier females are usually normal, but delivery of a male infant may be associated with a delayed onset of labor because of steroid sulfatase deficiency in the fetal placental cells. The ability of the fetus to remove the sulfate from estrogen may have a role in the initiation of labor.

| Incontinentia Pigmenti | *NEMO* | Xq28 |
| IKK-gamma (NEMO) | #308300 | |

NEMO (NF-Kappa-B essential modulator) is a protein involved in a complex pathway that is needed for the development of teeth, skin, and brain. NEMO modulates the NF-Kappa-B signaling pathway, which protects against premature death of some skin cells (keratinocytes) during their differentiation. Mutations in the NEMO gene can produce an extreme susceptibility to cellular death in other tissues as well. Severe deficiency of NEMO protein causes incontinentia pigmenti, a disturbance of skin pigmentation often associated with variable degrees of malformation of the eye, teeth, skeleton, and brain. The disease is usually seen in females because most often it is lethal in fetal males. The rare male survivors have the abnormalities seen in females as well as severe immunodeficiencies that increase their susceptibility to infection. Manifestations in females are highly variable and include abnormal skin pigmentation, malformation of teeth and nails, and occasionally brain damage, evident from seizures, spasticity, and mental retardation. The skin shows swirling patterns of melanin pigment that starts as an inflammation shortly after birth. The swirls are due to death of those cells expressing the mutation and their replacement with cells expressing the normal gene. Most often, the mutation occurs during sperm production due to a common rearrangement of the father's X chromosome that creates a large deletion in the NEMO gene.

| Kabuki Syndrome 2 | *KDM6A (UTX)* | Xp11.3 |
| Lysine-specific demethylase 6A | #300867 | |

This is one of two congenital mental retardation syndromes characterized by postnatal dwarfism, skeletal abnormalities, and a peculiar facies reminiscent of the makeup of actors in the Japanese Kabuki theater. It is caused by mutations in the Jumonji C domain–containing *UTX* gene *(KDM6A)* that demethylates the trimethylated lysine 27 of histone 3 (H3K27), removing its *repressive* marks. This methylase associates with H3K4 methyltransferase MLL2, which deposes *activating* marks. It is thought that the two enzymes work together to coordinately regulate cellular differentiation. Mutations in MLL2, a gene on chromosome 12, cause the phenotypically similar Kabuki syndrome 1.

Because *KDM6A (UTX)* has a Y homolog (*UTY 309000*), it is partially expressed from the inactive X. It seems that more than one dose of *KDM6A* is needed for normal development in both sexes. To date, half the mutations in females have been microdeletions.

Kelley-Seegmiller Syndrome	*HPRT*	Xq26.2
Hypoxanthine phosporibosyltransferase	#300323	

Mutations that decrease HPRT activity to >1.5% of normal are responsible for the Lesch Nyhan Syndrome (#300322; see below). Those mutations that reduce the activity less (>3% but <8% residual enzyme activity) lead to an X-linked form of gouty arthritis and renal stones. Females are not affected. There is also enough enzyme produced in the mutant cells to obviate the cell selection that characterizes carriers of Lesch Nyhan syndrome.

Leri-Weill Dyschrondrosteosis	SHOX	Xp22.33
Homeobox containing transcription factor	#300582	

This disorder is characterized by short stature, with short extremities and arm deformities. It is due to heterozygous defects in the pseudoautosomal homeobox gene, SHOX, or by deletion of the SHOX downstream regulatory domain. Because the gene is in the pseudoautosomal region and is expressed by both Xs and the Y chromosomes, the inheritance follows an autosomal dominant pattern with both males and females affected but usually more severe in females. The homozygous deletion of the SHOX genes produces a more severe phenotype. *SHOX* overdosage, associated with extra sex chromosomes, leads to long limbs and tall stature. The *SHOX* locus is believed to be responsible for at least some part of the short stature associated with 45,X Turner syndrome.

Lesch Nyhan Syndrome	*HPRT*	Xq26.2
Hypoxanthine phosphoribosyltransferase	#300322	

The enzyme hypoxanthine phosphoribosyltransferase (HPRT) is needed, especially in the brain, for the reutilization of breakdown products of DNA, specifically for salvage of the purine bases (hypoxanthine and guanine). This enzyme adds a phosphate group to both molecules, and the small nucleotides that result (guanylic acid and inosinic acid) seem to be energy sources for the cell. A severe deficiency of the HPRT enzyme causes Lesch Nyhan syndrome, a disorder of purine metabolism. The features in affected males are mental retardation, dystonia due to a profound loss of dopamine in the basal ganglia, urinary stones, gout, and sometimes anemia. A unique feature that is also characteristic of this syndrome is the compulsive self-destructive biting of fingers and lips—evidence that a mutation in a single gene can cause abnormal compulsive behavior. Less severe mutations in this gene (Kelley-Seegmiller Syndrome) in males may produce only gout. Female carriers of the severe deficiency usually have no clinical abnormalities, not even gout.

Lowe Syndrome (Dent 2 Disease)	OCRL1	Xq26.1
Inositol 5-phosphatase	#309000	

The culprit in Lowe oculocerebrorenal syndrome is OCRL1, an X-linked gene encoding inositol 5-phosphatase enzyme (now called OCRL enzyme) that interacts with small GTPases during intracellular trafficking. Located in the Golgi complex, the protein is also found in the primary cilium of retinal pigment cells and in kidney tubular cells. The lack of OCRL enzyme causes cataracts, glaucoma, and mental retardation. The renal tubules lack the receptors that control the exchange of certain small molecules between the urine and the blood. Lowe syndrome is also called Dent 2 disease because the manifestations are similar to that of the milder Dent 1 disease (#300009). Females, heterozygous for such mutations do not usually manifest renal or ocular disease, but characteristically have corneal opacities, which are mostly benign, and provide a diagnostic test for carriers.

Monoamine Oxidase A Deficiency	MAOA	Xp11. 3
Monoamine Oxidase A	#300615	

Monoamine oxidase A (MAOA), along with monoamine oxidase B (MAOB), are the key enzymes that catabolize the monoamines such as serotonin. MAOA is the major clearing step for serotonin in the developing brain, whereas MAOB functions more after birth. Both enzymes are encoded by tandem X-linked genes that arose from the same ancestral gene. Mutations in the highly polymorphic MAOA gene, severe enough to result in undetectable enzyme activity, cause nondysmorphic mental retardation only in males. The affected males also may show aggressive and sometimes violent behavior; such behavior has also been observed with some polymorphic variations in the gene. The serotonergic system has been implicated in impulsivity and violent behavior in animal studies. Other population variants resulting in decreased expression of the gene have been associated with autism in males. A common functional polymorphism in the promoter of the MAOA gene (tandem repeats of variable number that affects the level of its expression) has been used to study the structure and function of the parts of the brain that are affected by the gene (i.e., cingulate gyrus, amygdala, insula, and hypothalamus) in normal males and females. Despite some controversy, the evidence indicates that MAOA is fully subject to X inactivation.

| Muscular Dystrophy, Duchenne Type | *DMD* | Xp21 |
| Dystrophin | #310200 | |

Dystrophin is one of a complex of structural proteins that stabilizes the muscle membrane and anchors it to the muscle fibers—in effect, mechanically supporting the membrane so that the muscle does not rupture when it contracts. These proteins were discovered only after the gene for dystrophin was found to be the cause of the most common fatal inherited childhood muscle disease, affecting 1 in 3,500 newborn males. Dystrophin deficiency produces accelerated muscle death, ranging from the severe muscular dystrophy, described by Duchenne, to the milder muscular dystrophy, described by Becker. Both result from mutations in the huge dystrophin gene that functions in muscle and brain. Mutations that completely eliminate the dystrophin protein cause the lethal childhood onset Duchenne dystrophy. Such boys are usually diagnosed by 5 years of age, wheelchair bound by age 12, and dead by 20. It is the progressive degeneration of the skeletal muscle fibers, with progressive weakness and the subsequent failure of respiratory muscles, that is ultimately fatal. The heart muscle is also affected, leading to fatal heart failure in at least 10% of affected males. Also, there may be mild mental retardation. Most carrier females are unaffected, but a few have milder disease. In males, the milder form of the disease (Becker muscular dystrophy) results from mutations that reduce the amount of the dystrophin protein.

| Muscular Dystrophy, Emery-Dreifuss Type | *EMD* | Xq28 |
| Emerin | #310300 | |

Emerin, the product of the *EMD* gene, is a ubiquitous protein that is on the nuclear membrane of many types of cells and interacts with many other proteins. It is thought that emerin is essential for proper signaling, during differentiation and regeneration of skeletal and cardiac muscle. Emerin deficiency results in a degenerative muscular dystrophy that is more benign than the Duchenne type Affected males have weakness and atrophy of their skeletal and cardiac muscles without involvement of the nervous system. This leads to deformities of the elbows and chest. However, the cardiac defect (atrial arrhythmias and atrioventricular block) is the most serious and life-threatening manifestation. Some female carriers have cardiac defects in the absence of any skeletal muscle abnormalities, suggesting that the predominant role of emerin is in cardiac conduction.

Neurodegeneration with Brain Iron	*WDR45*	Xp11.23
Accumulation (NBIA)		
WD40 Repeat Protein	# 300526	

WD40 repeat proteins are scaffold proteins, frequently defective in neurological disorders. They interfere with brain development or with the maintenance of normal brain function. The observed mutations in *WDR45*, an X-linked gene, which undergoes X inactivation, are unusual, as they are all *de novo,* and mostly females are affected, reminiscent of Rett syndrome. Yet, the rare affected males have the same phenotype as affected females. In all 20 reported cases (17 females, 3 males), the *de novo* mutation is predicted to make the protein non-functional [419]. The most likely explanation for the observations is that the mutation would normally be lethal even in heterozygotes. Therefore, survival requires that the mutation be rescued either by a preponderance of normal cells in the mosaic female, or by somatic mosaicism in the male. One of the three males was found to have two populations of WDR45 exon 23 amplicons in his blood DNA, consistent with a postzygotic mutation in a relatively small proportion of cells, which could explain the survival of rare males with this disorder. From these observations, we have an inkling of mutations that are usually lethal prior to implantation, if not for rare events (in this case, the right kind of cell mosaicism) that permit their survival.

| Orofaciodigital Syndrome Type I (OFDI) | CXORF5 | Xp22.2 |
| CXORF5 protein | #311200 | |

CXORF5 specifies a protein that regulates microtubules in a way yet to be elucidated. Mutations lead to defective cilia in humans and mice. The syndrome includes facial asymmetry, cleft lip and palate, malformations of the skull and hands, abnormal dentition, and often mental retardation. It can be distinguished from autosomal forms of OFD by polycystic kidney disease, which seems specific to type I. OFDI is seen only in females as the same mutations are lethal for males. Other mutations in *CXORF5* also cause some cases of Simpson-Golabi-Behmel syndrome type 2 and Joubert syndrome, which are also ciliopathies affecting only males. Of significance, *CXORF5* escapes X inactivation in humans but not in mice.

| Otopalatodigital Syndrome (OPD Group) | FLNA | Xq28 |
| Filamin A | #311300 | |

Filamin A is a widely expressed protein needed to remodel the shape of the cell and change its potential for migration. It regulates the organization of the cytoskeleton by binding to it and interacting with transmembrane receptor complexes and second messengers. Mutations in the *FLNA* gene can produce a variety of genetic disorders, depending on whether the mutation causes the loss of normal function or the acquisition of a novel one. Severe loss-of-function mutations in males are lethal *in utero,* and in females manifest as a localized disorder affecting migration of neurons called periventricular nodular heterotopia (PVNH1). Presumptive gain-of-function mutations cause bone diseases called skeletal dysplasias in males, with less severe manifestations in females. The OPD group consists of four syndromes—OPD1, OPD2, Melnick-Needles syndrome (MNS), and frontometaphyseal dysplasia (FMD)—that are all caused by mutations in the *FLNA* gene. MNS is a rare osteodysplasia, almost invariably leading to the intrauterine death of males; consequently, after birth the condition is limited to females. The symptoms in females are short stature, severe skeletal dysplasia, and genitourinary malformations (see table 12–3).

Rett Syndrome   *MECP2*   Xq28
Methyl CpG binding protein-2   #312750

Methyl CpG binding protein-2 (MeCP2) is a widely expressed nuclear protein that binds specifically to methylated CG dinucleotides in DNA. MeCP2 is thought to be a transcriptional repressor by virtue of its ability to modify chromatin. Because MeCP2 is abundant in some tissues, including brain, and barely detectable in others, it is likely that other proteins carry out its function in nonexpressing tissues. It is particularly well expressed in neurons at the time of neuronal maturation. MeCP2 has an affinity for methylated CpGs, associated with inactive genes, It also has an affinity for 5-hydroxymethylcytosine that is associated with active genes in neurons and other brain cells.

The prevailing thought is that critical genes are aberrantly expressed in its absence. Loss-of-function mutations in this protein cause Rett syndrome, a postnatal neurodevelopmental disorder that was initially considered to be limited to girls. Seemingly normal at birth, affected girls develop progressive developmental stagnation and rapid deterioration of intellectual function, ending in dementia, spasticity, and epilepsy. A unique feature is hand wringing, associated with a loss of purposeful hand movements. Identification of the molecular defect enabled a broader view of the disorder, which now includes girls with mild mental retardation as well as males with severe brain dysfunction. The syndrome in males is usually lethal in infancy (microcephaly, hypotonia, and breathing difficulties), whereas it has a later onset and is variable in females, even among sisters. Clearly, any specific mutation is more detrimental to males than to females. Some cases of Rett syndrome are caused by another X-linked gene (*CDKL5*) whose protein functions in the same metabolic pathway as MeCP2. Mutations resulting in *duplication* of the *MECP2* locus produce a characteristic syndrome in males (severe cognitive defects and progressive spasticity), whereas females usually are entirely unaffected.

Severe Combined Immunodeficiency Disease (SCIDX1)   *IL2RG*   Xq13.1
Interleukin-2 receptor gamma   #300400

The *interleukin-2 receptor gamma* (*IL2RG*) gene encodes the gamma subunit of the interleukin-2 receptor. Interleukin-2 (IL2 on chromosome 4; OMIM #147680) is essential for the growth and differentiation of lymphocytes derived from the thymus (T-cells), bone marrow (B-cells), and natural killer cells—functions that are mediated through the IL2 receptor. Therefore, mutations in *IL2RG* result in combined immunodeficiencies that range in severity, depending on the level of the deficiency. An autosomal form of combined immunodeficiency is caused by mutation in the *JAK3* gene (on chromosome 19p13), but *IL2RG* is by far the more common of the two mutations. The T-cells are most affected, and the B-cells are less mature than they should be. XSCID causes death in infancy because of susceptibility to viral, fungal, and bacterial infections. This disorder has been called the "Bubble Boy disease," referring to an affected male in Texas who lived in an isolation unit for a prolonged period. Attempts to transfer the essential gene to the T-cells of infants with the disease have been successful but have been complicated by the development of leukemia in some of the treated patients. Only males are affected, and carrier females have no symptoms of the disease.

Wiskott Aldrich Syndrome	*WAS*	Xp11.23
WAS protein	#301000	

T-cells mediate immunity against intracellular pathogenic organisms, such as viruses. For T-cells to carry out the immune response, they must interact with antigen-presenting cells (an immunological synapse). This requires that the cytoskeleton of the T-cell undergo reorganization. The WAS protein (WASP), named for the disease, functions in the complicated interactions involved in reorganizing the cytoskeleton. For this reason, the *WAS* gene is important in the differentiation of T-cells. For reasons yet unknown, it also has a role in the development of platelets. Mutations in the *WAS* gene in males lead to a life-threatening immunodeficiency characterized by a reduced number and size of platelets, extensive eczema, and recurrent infections. Unless cured by stem cell transplants, boys with the severe mutation die from bleeding and infection before 10 years of age. Less severe deficiency is associated with autoimmune disease and cancer. Females are usually not affected because they lack the mutant blood cell lineages (T-cells and platelets) and have only the normal lineages, possibly because WASP-deficient stem cells migrate less well than wild-type cells from their origin in the liver to the bone marrow.

Diseases Not X Linked but Influenced by X Inactivation

ICF Syndrome	*DMNT3B*	20q11.2
DNA methyltransferase 3B	#242860	

DNA methyltransferase 3B (DMNT3B) is one of the methyltransferase 3 proteins that act cooperatively to methylate CpG dinucleotides *de novo*. Deficiency of this enzyme is responsible for the ICF syndrome (immunodeficiency, centromere instability, and facial anomalies syndrome), characterized by defective methylation of DNA sequences in the centromeric regions of chromosomes 1, 9, and 16. This leads to defective stabilization of chromatin, which manifests cytologically as chromosomal breakage, undercondensation in the regions close to centromeres, and interchromosomal interchanges. Persons of both sexes with ICF syndrome also have mild mental retardation and facial anomalies such as widely spaced eyes, flat nasal bridge, low-set ears, and tongue protrusion. In addition, affected individuals have variable immunodeficiencies leading to recurrent infections. These abnormal features seem to be caused by a failure to establish normal patterns of DNA methylation during embryogenesis. Some genes up-regulated in ICF cells lose histone modifications characteristic of repressed chromatin and gain modifications characteristic of transcriptionally active chromatin. The chromosome defects that are unique to this syndrome suggest that the *DNMT3B* gene has a specific function in organizing chromatin. Some of the genes on the inactive X chromosome are not well inactivated, suggesting a role of this methylase in methylating the CpG islands on the inactive X that maintain the inactive state. However, because there are no gender-specific aspects to the syndrome, its role in maintaining X inactivation seems not to be a major problem. The mutations identified in ICF patients reduce but do not abolish the activity of DNMT3B. Deletion of the catalytic domain of the enzyme in mice invariably results in prenatal lethality.

| Beckwith-Wiedemann Syndrome | Complex imprinted region of 11p15.5 |
| Overexpression of IGF2 | #130650 |

Beckwith-Wiedemann syndrome (BWS) is a clinically heterogeneous disease involving excessive growth and an increased risk for developing embryonal tumors, especially of the kidney. The cardinal features of this disorder are defects of the abdominal wall, large tongue, low blood sugar, and overgrowth of the fetus. This condition is caused by a variety of genetic or epigenetic alterations within two domains of growth-regulating genes on human chromosome 11p15. The eight or more genes clustered in these domains are parentally imprinted and thought to be coordinately regulated. This regulation depends on the imprinted expression of *KCNQ1OT1*, which encodes an untranslated RNA. Most cases are sporadic; only 15% of cases are familial. About half of the familial cases have a germline mutation in a maternally imprinted tumor suppressor gene. However, most often, the disorder is due not to nucleotide mutations but to abnormal DNA methylation that causes inappropriate expression of one or another of these clustered genes. Duplications in this region are often involved in the pathogenesis.

The frequency of monozygotic twins—especially female twins—is higher than expected, and often only one of the twins is affected; the affected twin has loss of methylation in one of the imprinted genes in the cluster, resulting in the loss of imprint. It has been proposed that discordance for BWS in monozygotic twins is due to unequal splitting of the inner cell mass during twinning, thereby causing loss of imprinting. Alternatively, this region may be especially prone to losing its imprint because of faulty DNA methylation at a critical stage of pre-implantation development. This loss of imprinting may predispose to twinning as well as to discordance for BWS [364].

| Scleroderma | No known locus or gene |
| | #181750 (familial) |

Systemic scleroderma (SSc) is an autoimmune disease of connective tissue whose cause is unknown. Although the pathogenesis is poorly understood, the progression of the disease is known to involve the blood vessels, the immune system, and abnormal deposits in the extracellular matrix. The familial form of the disease has been mapped to chromosome 15q in the vicinity of the *FBN1* gene, but most cases are not familial. Because the disease is three to eight times more frequent in women than in men, the possibility that X chromosome inactivation has a role has been considered. Skewing of X inactivation was observed in blood cells of 64% of 55 informative patients compared with 8% of 124 informative controls. Extreme skewing (>90%) was observed in 27 patients (49%) and in only 3 controls (2.4%). However, X chromosome inactivation was random in all skin biopsy samples. Based on these studies, it is suggested that disturbances in X chromosome inactivation mosaicism may play a significant role in the pathogenesis of scleroderma in a subpopulation of females [367].

| Thyroiditis | No known locus or gene |
| | AITD, #608173 |

Thyroiditis is an inflammatory disease of the thyroid gland that is thought to be autoimmune in origin. The disease ultimately results in destruction of the thyroid gland and a deficiency of thyroid hormone that is essential for many metabolic functions. The autoimmune thyroid diseases (AITDs) include Hashimoto's thyroiditis and Graves disease. In both these diseases, thyroid-reactive T-cells are formed and infiltrate the thyroid gland. Together, the AITDs are the most common autoimmune disorders in the population, affecting between 2% and 4% of women and up to 1% of men. Graves disease and Hashimoto's thyroiditis are genetically heterogeneous—with only one locus in common to both diseases on chromosome 6, no gene has been identified. This locus was close to, but distinct from, the HLA region. Because of the excess of affected females, X inactivation has been considered as one of the potential causative factors, having to do with contributing to the failure of recognizing self-antigens, and there is evidence to support a role for skewed X inactivation [369].

Sex Chromosome Aneuploidy, Polyploidy, and Parthenogenetic Conceptuses

This table provides supplementary information about the various chromosome abnormalities discussed in chapter 11. When appropriate the name of the syndrome associated with the cytogenetic abnormality is given, and the range of karyotypes that are included in that condition is also given.

Monosomy X   Turner Syndrome
45,X; 46,X,i(X)(q10); 46,X,del(X)

In 1938, Henry Turner described the first patients with the syndrome that bears his name [310]; they were females who remained sexually infantile. However, only in 1959 was their lack of sexual development recognized as due to the loss of an X chromosome, or essential parts of it. Typically, the syndrome is characterized by infantile development of the external genitalia, uterus, and oviducts that are clearly differentiated along female lines. The body appearance is that of a prepubertal female with growth failure, resulting in short stature. The gonads, which look like normal ovaries at 3 months' gestation, lose oocytes before birth; this is followed by replacement of normal ovarian structure by connective tissue. Clinical abnormalities may or may not include multiple congenital malformations such as webbing of the neck, a broad, shieldlike chest with rudimentary nipples, and puffy swelling of the hands and feet. Some females have more serious abnormalities such as strictures of the aorta, limb deformities, and kidney malformations. The presence of a Barr body in some individuals, and its absence in others, suggested heterogeneity: Those without sex chromatin lack an entire X chromosome, whereas those with a Barr body have a single normal X and a second X that is abnormal, having either a short arm or long arm deletion, or a duplication of the entire long arm (short arm missing); this duplicated chromosome is called an isochromosome (i; see figure 11–2). They may also be mosaic with a mixture of cell lines—that is, 45,X/46,XX. As the condition can originate from loss of a Y as well as an X, some patients with Turner's syndrome may have 45,X/46,XY mosaicism, which increases the risk of gonadal tumors. In all cases, secondary sexual development can be induced by treatment with estrogen hormones.

Sex Chromosome Trisomy-1   Klinefelter Syndrome
47,XXY; 48,XXXY; 49,XXXXY

In 1942, Harry Klinefelter described nine adult males who came to his attention because of infertility and/or breast enlargement, starting at adolescence, associated with small testes and signs of testicular dysfunction. After puberty, their testes showed degenerative changes, ultimately resulting in loss of tubules and germ cells. The discovery of sex chromatin gave some insight into the cause: Unexpectedly (at the time), these males had at least one Barr body, and some had more than one. The number of Barr bodies correlated with the number of X chromosomes in their karyotypes. The strong male-determining properties of the Y chromosome are apparent because, even in the presence of four X chromosomes, the Y chromosome is able to induce a male appearance. However, the presence of more than one X chromosome in these males is associated with increased stature and infertility, and in some cases deformities of bones; with the greater number of X chromosomes comes mental retardation and more severe somatic abnormalities. Some with the syndrome may have 46XY/47XXY mosaicism, where the presence of some normal XY cells may ameliorate the phenotype. Other mosaics have been reported including rare individuals with 46XX/47XXY mosaicism.

Sex Chromosome Trisomy-2 (Y Disomy)   XYY Syndrome
47,XYY; 49,XYYYY

Men with additional Y chromosomes were first ascertained in a survey of inmates in maximum security hospitals. XYY males were initially depicted as having an increased likelihood of violent behavior. Although most are nonviolent, many have mild mental retardation and a tendency to come to the attention of police because of impulsive behavior. They are consistently taller than the average male. Based on limited studies, the fertility of XYY males does not seem to be impaired. Individuals with four Y chromosomes have additional somatic malformations. It is likely that the relatively normal phenotype associated with Y disomy is related to the fact that the Y chromosome is relatively bereft of genes, other than those coding for testicular function. However, the slight increase in mortality may be related to extra doses of Y-linked PAR1 genes.

Sex Chromosome Trisomy-3   Trisomy X
47,XXX; 48,XXXX; and 49,XXXXX

Females with 47,XXX are relatively common, occurring in 0.1% of liveborn female infants. Only a few of them have congenital malformations, so most do not come for medical care, and therefore relatively little is known about them. Yet, some 47,XXX females have mental or behavioral problems, and they tend to be taller than the average female. Some may have slightly greater morbidity and earlier mortality than 46,XX females. The fact that all the additional X chromosomes undergo X inactivation accounts for their relatively benign phenotype.

While some of them may have premature menopause, the majority seem to be fertile. The rare females with more than three X chromosomes are more severely affected with mental retardation and some somatic abnormalities.

Tiny Ring X Chromosomes
46,XXr; mosaic 45,X/46,X,Xr

Structural abnormalities of an X chromosome are usually associated with Turner syndrome. The abnormal X chromosome is usually the inactive X chromosome in each cell because of cell selection. However, there are individuals whose X chromosome is very small and has circularized in the process of repairing breaks occurring on both sides of its centromere. Because their ring chromosomes have lost the DNA sequences essential for X inactivation, and cannot inactivate, these females have two working copies of the genes located on the ring X chromosome. As a consequence, their clinical abnormalities are far more severe than those associated with Turner syndrome. These may include severe mental retardation and developmental delay, growth retardation at birth, and multiple congenital anomalies, including facial dysmorphism (coarse features, epicanthic folds, upturned nares, long philtrum, wide-set eyes), fusion of some fingers and toes, and increased frequency of heart defects. Each ring chromosome contains different segments of the chromosome—with the centromere being the only region present in all of them. Therefore, the phenotype is variable and depends on both the gene content and the nature of the specific alleles present on the X chromosome. Such ring chromosomes lack *XIST* function, explaining their failure to inactivate. The reason they are tiny is because larger chromosomes lacking *XIST* function are likely to be lethal before birth. Circular chromosomes such as these have problems replicating themselves, and they are often subject to additional breakage and may be lost from the cell. In this case, some cells will have only the normal X. This explains why most individuals with tiny ring X chromosomes are mosaic, also having a population of 45,X cells.

X/Autosome Translocations
46,X,t(X;A)

These are chromosomal rearrangements that involve simultaneous breakage in two chromosomes, one an X and the other an autosome (A). The broken segments of both chromosomes rejoin such that each repaired chromosome has a part of the autosome and part of the X chromosome. Any autosome can participate in such translocations. A reciprocal translocation usually produces what is called a balanced chromosome complement because no segment on either chromosome is lost from the genome or reduplicated. In many cases this is not the case as some rearrangement has occurred at or near the site of the breakpoint. However, even in absence of rearrangements, females carrying balanced translocations are at risk of offspring with unbalanced karyotypes—those that inherit only one of the translocation products. In balanced translocations, the normal X is always the inactive one, because cells in which the translocated chromosome was silenced do not survive. Inactivation of the normal X best maintains the genetic balance. As a consequence such females are no longer mosaics as they express the same X translocation chromosome in all of their cells. Usually, they have no clinical abnormalities, unless the breakpoint on the X chromosome perturbs the function of an X-linked gene, or loss of mosaicism in the female unmasks a mutation elsewhere on the translocated X. X/autosome translocations along with other X chromosome deletions that eliminate X mosaicism are frequently responsible for "'manifesting' heterozygotes" (see section 12.6).

Triploidy
69,XXX; 69,XXY; 69,XYY

Triploid zygotes usually arise from fertilization of an egg by two sperm or by fusion of the polar body with the egg nucleus. Almost none survive to birth, and it is rare for one that does to survive even a few days. Most have been ascertained as stillbirths and aborted products of conception. Triploid human embryos have three copies of each autosomal gene and three sex chromosomes, in all possible combinations, except that YYY is inviable, as it is never seen. They have multiple congenital abnormalities affecting many tissues. In triploids that survive until the third trimester, the phenotypes differ widely depending on the nature of the alleles that are triplicated. Some of the abnormal features are similar to those seen in fetuses with trisomy for an individual chromosome (malformations of the corpus callosum, small eyes, fusion of fingers and toes, low-set ears, cleft palate, and kidney anomalies commonly seen in trisomies 13 and 18 and simian creases, depressed nasal bridge, and heart malformations seen in trisomy 21). The gonads are appropriate for sex, but the genitalia may be abnormal in some male triploids [308]. Like diploid individuals, triploids undergo X inactivation, but unlike diploids, they may have more than one active X chromosome.

Parthenogenetic Conceptuses
46,XX (46,X^mX^m [ovarian teratomas] or 46,X^pX^p [hydatidiform moles])

These abnormal products of conception are tumors that result from the aberrant development caused when embryonic development is initiated parthenogenetically. Although it is not unusual in invertebrates to undergo embryonic development without fertilization, parthenogenetic development is highly unusual in mammals. The ovarian tumor originates when an unfertilized egg begins to undergo embryonic development, and so all the chromosomes are of maternal origin.

The male counterpart of the ovarian teratoma is the hydatidiform mole. This inviable product of conception has only the paternal set of chromosomes. The mole is an abnormal tumor of placental tissue that originates when a sperm fertilizes an egg that has lost its maternal complement of chromosomes. Therefore all its chromosomes are of sperm origin. These tumors tell us that maternal and paternal chromosomes are not identical, because they have different unique imprints, and that both parental genomes are essential for normal embryonic development. The absence of placental tissue in the ovarian tumor suggests that paternal genes are needed for placental development. Conversely, the absence of fetal tissue in the moles informs us that maternal genes are essential for development of the fetus. In both tumors, one of the pair of X chromosomes—even those that are replicate copies of one another—undergoes X inactivation, indicating that differences in parental origin or DNA content of the X chromosome are not required for inactivation to occur.

Effect of X Inactivation on Phenotype and Cell Selection in X-linked Disorders

The following X-linked diseases are examples of disorders where information is available about heterozygous females. They are listed with their disease name and their X map locus (the location of the gene on the X chromosome), which can be ascertained from the banded X chromosome in figure 2–2. These data are followed by the symbol for the mutant gene and then the OMIM number, which is the reference for the citation. Also given is the phenotype of males and females, whether or not the mutation leads to cell selection, the tissue that was assayed, and significant features, if any.

Abbreviations used include: MR, mental retardation; XLMR, X-linked mental retardation; WBC, white blood cells; T, T-cells; B, B-cells; AR, androgen receptor assay; G6PD, glucose-6- phosphate dehydrogenase, HPRT, hypoxanthine phosphoribosyl transferase; FMR1, fragile X; PGK, phosphoglycerate kinase; hets, heterozygotes; XI, X inactivation; PXI, paternal X inactivation; ND, not done.

Note:

1) The phenotype described is the one most often seen, unless otherwise indicated

2) Cell selection (skewing) favors the normal allele unless otherwise indicated.

3) In all cases chance skewing, unrelated to the mutation, influences the phenotype.

X-linked Disease	X Map	Gene	OMIM#	Phenotype MALES	Phenotype FEMALES	Cell Selection	Tissue	Assay
Adrenoleuko-dystrophy	Xq28	ABCD1	300100	Demyelinization of brain, spinal cord & adrenals. Often death in first decade.	Adreno- myelo neuropathy Spastic paraplegia with age	Yes, gradual. Favors mutant allele	WBC RBC, Skin fibroblast clones.	G6PD & fatty acids
Alport Syndrome	Xq22.3	COL4A5	301050	End stage renal disease	Milder renal disease	No	WBC Kidney glomeruli	HPRT & PGK. COL45A immuno-label
Androgen Insensitivity	Xq12	AR	300068	Feminization	None	ND		AR
ATRX Syndrome	Xq21.1	ATRX	301040	MR, Thalassemia	Hemoglobin H inclusions	Yes, severe	WBC Buccal	AR
Barth Syndrome	Xq28	TAZ	302060	Cardiomyopathy Methylglutaconic aciduria Abnormal mitochondria	None	Yes, severe	WBC Fibroblasts	AR in obligate heterozy-gotes

Borjeson-Forssman-Lehmann Syndrome	Xq26.2–3	*PHF6*	301900	MR, Obesity, Hypogonadism, Epilepsy	Mild MR	Yes, severe	WBC	FMR1, AR PGK1
Bruton Agamma-globulinemia	Xq22.1	*BTK*	300300	B cell deficiency	None	Yes, severe	B cells	AR
Charcot-Marie Tooth	Xq13.1	*CMTX1*	302800	Sensory & peripheral neuropathies	Milder	No	WBC	AR
CHILD Syndrome	Xq28	*NSDHL*	308050	Fetal lethal	Hemidysplasia Unilateral ichthyosis	Yes, (in mice)	Brain, skin, liver of *Bare Patches* mice	NSDHL activity
Chondrodysplasia Punctata 1	Xp22.23	*ARSE*	302950	MR, Bone defects Short stature Epiphiseal stippling	Milder symptoms	ND		
Chondrodysplasia Punctata 2 (Conradi-Hunermann Syndrome)	Xp11.23	*EPB*	302960	Fetal lethal Mosaic males survive	Bilateral ichthyosis Short stature Epiphiseal stippling Hair and skin defects	No	WBC	AR

(continued)

X-linked Disease	X Map	Gene	OMIM#	Phenotype MALES	Phenotype FEMALES	Cell Selection	Tissue	Assay
Chronic granulomatous disease	Xp11.4	CYBB	306400	Severe bacterial infections	Discoid lupus	No	WBC, Buccal	AR
Coffin-Lowry	Xp22.12	RSK2	303600	MR, Short stature, Abnormal facies, gait & fingers	Milder	No	WBC	AR
Craniofrontonasal Syndrome	Xq12	EFNB1	304110	Hypertelorism	Craniosynostosis Craniofacial asymmetry Skeletal abnormalities	No	Blood, Cranioperio-steum	AR Immuno-chemistry
Creatine Transporter Defect	Xq28	SLC6A8	300352	MR, Speech delay, Seizures	Milder	No	Skin fibroblasts Blood Hair roots	AR
Danon disease	Xq24	LAMP2	300257	MR, Cardiomyopathy, Skeletal muscle weakness	Later onset.	ND		
Dent disease1	Xp11.23	CLCN5	300009	Nephrolithiasis, Proteinurea	Less severe	ND		

Disease	Locus	Gene	OMIM	Clinical features			Tissue	mRNA
Dent disease 2	Xp11.23, Xq26.1	CLCN5, OCRL1 (digenic)	30009	Abnormal facies Ocular abnormalities Rickets Delayed growth	None	Yes, severe	WBC	mRNA
Diabetes Insipidus	Xq28	AVPR2	304800	Unresponsive to anti-diuretic hormone	None	No	WBC	AR
Dyskeratosis Congenita	Xq28	DKC1	305000	Defective telomeres, Premature aging, Bone marrow failure	None or milder	Yes, extreme	WBC Buccal	AR
Ectodermal Dysplasia, hypohydrotic with immune deficiency (HED)	Xq28	NEMO	300291	Fetal lethal or: Dysglobulinemia Recurrent infections Abnormal teeth	None	Yes, severe, with gradual elimination of mutant T cells	T cells	AR
Ectodermal Dysplasia	Xq13.1	ED1	305100	Defective skin, hair & nails	Variable severity	No	WBC	AR

(continued)

X-linked Disease	X Map	Gene	OMIM#	Phenotype MALES	Phenotype FEMALES	Cell Selection	Tissue	Assay
Epileptic encephalopathy early infantile 9	Xq22	PCDH19	300088	None	MR, Spasms Autism	ND ? metabolic interference		
Epileptic encephalopathy early infantile, 1	Xp21.3	ARX	308350	Spasms without brain malformations	Milder	ND		
Fabry disease	Xq22	GLA	301500	Progressive heart & kidney disease	Attenuated	No	Skin fibroblast clones	GLA
Fanconi Anemia	Xp22.31	FANCB	300514	Bone marrow failure, Predisposed to cancer	None	Yes, extreme	WBC	AR
Fragile X Syndrome	Xq27.3	FMR1	300624	XLMR, Congenital anomalies	Variable, milder	Yes, slight (full mutation)	WBC, Skin fibroblasts	FMR1 methylation

Disease	Location	Gene	OMIM	Phenotype	Heterozygote	Age variation	Tissue	Assay
Hemolytic Anemia	Xq28	G6PD	305900	Chronic anemia	None	Yes, slight with age	RBC, WBC	G6PD
Hemophilia A	Xq28	F8	306700	Bleeding disorder	None	No	Blood	50% F8 activity
Hemophilia B	Xq27	F9	306900	Bleeding disorder	None	No	Blood	Clotting activity
Hunter Syndrome	Xq28	IDS	309900	Mucopoly-saccharidosis	None	No	Skin fibroblast clones	IDS
Hyperammonemia	Xp21.1	OTC	311250	Males die if not treated	Affected hets have sporadic hyperammonemia	No	Liver	Histo-chemistry
Hypophos-phatemic Rickets	Xp22.1	PHEX	307800	Short stature Rickets, Bone deformities	None	ND		
Ichthyosis	Xp22.31	STS	308100	Extensive body ichthyosis, Corneal opacities	Late corneal opacities Expressed from XI	No, (Point mutation)	Skin fibroblast clones	STS & G6PD

(continued)

X-linked Disease	X Map	Gene	OMIM#	Phenotype MALES	Phenotype FEMALES	Cell Selection	Tissue	Assay
Incontinentia Pigmenti	Xq28	*NEMO*	308300	Fetal lethal	Cell death causes rash along Blaskos lines. Abnormal hair and teeth	Yes, severe	RBC, WBC Skin fibroblast clones	HPRT & G6PD
Kabuki Syndrome 2	Xp11.3	*KDM6A* or *UTX*	300867	MR, Dwarfism Kabuki faciés Skeletal abnormalities (UTY protects)	Like males	Yes	WBC	AR
Kelley-Seegmiller Syndrome	Xq26.2	*HPRT*	300323	Renal stones, Gout	None	No	Blood	HPRT
Lesch Nyhan Syndrome	Xq26.2	*HPRT*	300322	MR. Spastic cerebral palsy; Uric acid stones, Self-destructive biting	None	Yes, severe (blood). No, (skin)	RBC, WBC Skin fibroblast clones	HPRT, G6PD

Lowe Syndrome	Xq26.1	*OCRL1*	309000	MR, Cataracts, Rickets, Aminoaiduria	None	(100%) in one manifesting het unrelated to mutation	WBC	AR
Menkes Syndrome	Xq21.1	*ATP7A*	309400	Copper deficiency	None Mice die due to PXI	Yes, severe Caveat: 15 kb deletion	WBC, Lymphoblasts Skin fibroblasts	AR
Monamine Oxidase A deficiency (Brunner Syndrome)	Xp11.3	*MAOA*	300615	Mild MR. Aggressive impulsive behavior	None	ND		
Muscular dystrophy *Duchenne*	Xp21	*DMD*	310200	Muscular dystrophy Mild MR	Only when unrelated skew favors *mutant* cells	No	WBC	AR
Muscular Dystrophy *Emery-Dreifuss*	Xq28	*EMD*	310300	Muscular dystrophy Heart arrythmias	None	ND		

(continued)

X-linked Disease	X Map	Gene	OMIM#	Phenotype MALES	Phenotype FEMALES	Cell Selection	Tissue	Assay
Neurodegeneration with Brain Iron Accumulation (NBIA5)	Xp11.23	WDR45 (all de-novo)	300894	Fetal lethal, Mosaics survive to be affected	Parkinsonism, Dystonia, Dementia	? Only rare severely skewed females survive to manifest	WBC	AR
Orofaciodigital Syndrome	Xp22.2	CXORF5	311200	Fetal lethal	Malformations of face & digits Polycystic kidneys	No	WBC	AR
Oropalatodigital Syndrome 1	Xq28	FLNA	311300	OPD1	See Table 11–2	See Fig. 11–8	WBC	AR
Pelizaeus-Merzbacher	Xq22.2	PLP1 point mutation	312080	Myelin leukodystrophy	Milder	No	WBC, Lympho-blasts	AR
Rett Syndrome	Xq28	MECP2 point mutation	312750	Fetal lethal	MR, impaired speech, handwringing	No, Unless large deletion	WBC	AR

							T & B cells,	Cell count
SCIDX1	Xq13.1	IL2RG	300400	B & T cell immunodeficiency	None	Yes, extreme	T & B cells,	AR
CIDX1	Xq13.1	IL2RG	312863	Milder allele of SCIDS	None	Yes	Mostly affects T cells,	
Wiskott- Aldrich Syndrome	Xp11.23	WAS	301000	Deficiency of B & T cells, leukocyte & thrombocytes	None	Yes, severe	T, B cells & granulocytes	AR
XLMR Cullin Ring	Xq24	CUL4B	300354	MR, Short stature, Macrocephaly, Hypogonadism, Tremor, Abnormal gait	Rarely mild tremor, tics Mice die due to PXI	Yes, severe	WBC	AR
XLMR Claes-Jensen	Xp11.22	KDM5C/ JARID1C Also SMCX	300534	Short stature, Abnormal facies Developmental disability.	Milder	Yes, severe in 4 hets.	WBC	AR

(continued)

X-linked Disease	X Map	Gene	OMIM#	Phenotype MALES	Phenotype FEMALES	Cell Selection	Tissue	Assay
XLMR Siderius	Xp11.22	PHF8	300263	MR, Abnormal facies.	None	Yes, severe,	WBC	AR
XLMR Turner	Xp11.22	HUEW1 Micro-duplica-tions	300706	MR Assorted minor anomalies	None	Yes & No, severe in some females	WBC	AR
XLMR Wilson -Turner	Xq13.2	HDAC8 Point mutations	300269	MR, Microcephaly Craniofacial deformities	Milder	Yes, extreme	WBC	AR

Allele   One of two or more alternative forms of a gene. Each parent has two alleles but contributes only one of them to his or her offspring.

Aneuploidy   Loss or gain of individual chromosomes.

Annotation   Process of identifying genes from the DNA sequence using algorithms or other known characteristics of genes and information from databases.

Autosome   Any chromosome that is not a sex chromosome; most chromosomes.

Barr body   See **Sex chromatin.**

Blastocyst   Stage of embryogenesis when the embryo is a hollow ball made up of cells capable of giving rise to all tissues of an embryo. The outermost cells form the **trophectoderm,** which gives rise to the placenta, and the internal cells form the **inner cell mass,** which gives rise to the embryo proper.

Carrier   The term used to designate the heterozygote with two different alleles, when one of them has a mutation that interferes with its function. Carriers for X-linked mutations are almost always females.

Cell cycle   The stages in the growth and asexual (mitotic) reproduction of a cell; the time it takes to complete one cell generation, consisting of three major stages: (1) **interphase,** the stage when chromosomes replicate (synthesize their DNA) in preparation for cell division and the time when genes are transcribed into RNA; (2) **mitosis,** the stage when cell division occurs in somatic cells: the chromosomes that have replicated during interphase separate from one another and go to opposite poles for redistribution into daughter cells; and (3) **cytokinesis,** the stage when cleavage occurs to separate the daughter cells.

Cell memory   The ability of cells to pass on **epigenetic** marks, so that their daughter cells will bear similar marks.

Cell selection   A proliferative advantage or disadvantage favoring some cells and disfavoring others.

Centromere   The primary constriction of the chromosome that separates short (p) arms from long (q) arms; contains DNA sequences that direct movement of the chromosome to each pole.

Chimera   An individual created by the fusion of two different zygotes into a single embryo.

Chorion   The fetal part of the placenta derived from the **trophectoderm.**

Chromatin The nucleoprotein complex made up of protein (largely **histone** proteins) and embedded genes, which provides the structure for chromosomes. Chromatin is essential for compacting genomic DNA and plays a primary role in governing the expression status of genes. **Euchromatin** and **heterochromatin** are transcriptionally active and inert forms of chromatin, respectively.

Chromosomes The "packages" of condensed chromatin located in the nucleus of each cell. These packages facilitate the distribution of genes during cell division. Chromosomes move as independent units during **mitosis** and **meiosis**. They consist of a single DNA molecule before cell division and consist of two DNA molecules after replication. They occur in pairs, one from each parent.

Chromosome translocation The transfer of one chromosome segment to another chromosome—often nonhomologous—usually mediated by chromosome breakage and repair. If the exchange between chromosomes is reciprocal, the translocation is said to be balanced.

Cis Latin for "on the same side." Opposite of *trans*, which is Latin for across.

Cleavage The stage when the zygote becomes a multicellular embryo by dividing mitotically. Usually, the products of division stay attached to one another; occasionally they separate, forming twins.

Clone The cellular progeny of a single cell; a genetically identical group of cells, or an organism derived from a single individual by asexual means.

CpG island One of ~30,000 regions in the genome (500–2,000 base pairs long), consisting of dense clusters of cytosine–guanine (CpG) dinucleotides. They are often found within the regulatory regions of many mammalian genes and are usually unmethylated except on the inactive X. When the CpG island in the promoter region of a gene is methylated the gene usually is not transcribed.

Differentiation The process whereby descendants of one cell acquire permanent differences from the parent cell in structure and function.

Diploid Having two sets of chromosomes, one from each parent, characteristic of somatic cells, in contrast to haploid karyotypes of egg and sperm.

Disomic Having two copies of a specific chromosome, usually one from each parent.

DNA Deoxyribonucleic acid, a polymer of nucleic acids, found in the nucleus of all cells, often packaged in chromosomes. DNA is the basic hereditary material. It encodes the proteins responsible for the structure and function of all living organisms. DNA is made up of four paired molecules called bases (cytosine, guanine, adenine, and thymine), whose linear arrangement serves as the molecular code for proteins.

DNA methylation The **epigenetic** modification of cytosine that in the promoter of genes marks them for inactivation. Methylation in a CpG island marks the relevant gene as inactive, and enables the silence to be transmitted to the cells progeny.

DNA probe A labeled segment of DNA used to detect the presence of a homologous sequence by some form of molecular hybridization.

DNA replication The process taking place in interphase by which a DNA molecule is precisely reproduced in preparation for cell division. **DNA polymerase** is the enzyme that catalyzes DNA replication

DNA transfection Transfer of DNA from one individual into cells of another individual or species to enable it to make a novel product.

Dominance or **recessivity** Terms based on Morgan's rules for X-linked inheritance in flies; adapted for human genetics in the 1920s. *Dominant* was used to describe traits that are expressed in **heterozygotes,** whereas *recessive* described the traits expressed only in **homozygotes.** These definitions do not take into account cellular mosaicism or hemizygosity that characterizes linked inheritance and are too rigid to be useful in light of our present knowledge.

Dosage compensation The process by which the sex difference in numbers of X chromosomes is equalized. Many organisms have their own unique mechanism for accomplishing this, but usually regulation affects the process of transcription. Another kind of dosage compensation maintains the balance between the transcriptional output of X chromosomes with that of autosomes.

Embryo The term used to describe the conceptus during the stage of development when cells differentiate and organs form; in humans, the first eight weeks after conception.

Embryonic stem (ES) cells Cells derived from the inner cell mass of a **blastocyst** or **pre-implantation embryo** or from embryonic germ cells. These highly plastic cells with the potential for infinite self-renewal can be maintained in culture in their original undifferentiated state or can be induced to differentiate, forming many kinds of tissues.

Epiallele One of a pair of genetically identical alleles that are epigenetically distinct. See **Metastable epiallele.**

Epigenetics The study of changes in gene function that are mitotically heritable but do not entail a change in DNA sequence.

Epigenetic marks Modifications of histone proteins or DNA that reveal activity states of chromatin. For example: DNA methylation (repressive mark) and histone acetylation (activity mark), Such marks are the molecular means to inform the transcriptional mechanisms as to which genes to transcribe.

Euchromatin The kind of **chromatin** that contains genes with potential to be transcribed. In euchromatin, **histones** are usually acetylated—a modification that promotes an open structure accessible to transcription complexes.

Exons The regions of genes that encode the amino acids of protein, in contrast to **introns.**

Fertilization The union of egg and sperm to form the zygote.

Fetus The term used to describe the human conceptus during the last 32 weeks of gestation.

FISH Fluorescence *in situ* hybridization, the means of visualizing DNA or RNA sequences homologous to the DNA used as probe. The DNA probe is labeled with a fluorescent dye and hybridized to metaphase or interphase chromosomes that have been fixed on a microscopic slide.

Functional X disomy When two copies of some, or all, of the X-linked genes are being expressed.

Gain-of-function mutation A mutation resulting in novel functions of a protein that may perturb the physiological function.

Gametes The reproductive cells (ova in females and sperm in males).

Gastrula The stage of embryogenesis when the three germ layers (ectoderm, mesoderm, and endoderm) are being formed.

Gene The stretch of DNA that encodes all or part of a particular cellular protein; the hereditary unit of the DNA.

Genome The complete set of genes or chromosomes present in any individual or species.

Genotype   The genetic blueprint of the individual; the DNA sequence of one or more genes.

Gonad   Generic name for the organs (ovaries or testes) that manufacture the germ cells.

Hemizygote   An individual with only a single copy of a gene; usually used to refer to the hemizygous state of X-linked genes in males because males have only a single X chromosome.

Hermaphrodite   An individual with both male and female gonads.

Heterochromatin   A kind of **chromatin** that contains genes that cannot be transcribed. The structure of the chromatin is highly compacted, because the **histone** components of the chromatin have been modified to inhibit accessibility to transcription factors. Containing underacetylated histones and high levels of DNA methylation, heterochromatin remains condensed throughout most of the cell cycle and replicates at a later time than most **euchromatin**.

Heterozygote   An individual having two different alleles at a genetic **locus** on a homologous pair of chromosomes.

Histone   Proteins that provide the **nucleosome** structure for the DNA and the milieu that can modify the expression of the genes therein. The unit of **chromatin** structure is the **nucleosome**, which is composed of an octamer of histone proteins (two molecules each of histone H2A, H2B, H3, and H4) wrapped with two loops (140 base pairs each) of DNA (genes and regulatory DNA; see chapter 3 and figure 3-2).

Histone modification   Covalent histone modifications such as methylation, acetylation, and ubiquitination that regulate local chromosome structure and gene expression status. The modification involves adding a methyl, acetyl, or ubiquitin group to the tail of the histone. Such modifications can function as **epigenetic marks** identifying chromosome regions for the transcriptional machinery. They may serve as a signal for recognition by functionally relevant trans-acting factors, and one modification may operate synergistically in conjunction with another. **Histone acetylation** is the process by which a lysine is acetylated, and the **histone acetylases** are the enzymes that add the acetyl group to lysine.

Histone protein 1 (HP1)   HP1 is a key component of heterochromatin in diverse organisms. It binds to histone H3 that is methylated at the Lys9 position (H3K9me3).

Homologue   One member of a pair of chromosomes.

Homozygote   An individual having two copies of the same allele at a genetic **locus** on a pair of homologous chromosomes.

Hybrid cells   See **Mouse–human hybrids** and **Somatic cell hybridization**.

Hydatidiform mole   Placental tumor formed as a result of an X-bearing sperm fertilizing an egg that has lost its nucleus. The set of paternal chromosomes replicates itself so that the **karyotype** is always 46,X^PX^P, which precludes the development of the fetus because of parental **imprinting**. This is a good example of why both parental genomes are needed for the development of the zygote.

Imprinting   The term introduced by Crouse [421] to describe changes "in the state of a chromosome that occurs during one generation that allows it to be recognized as different in the next generation"; a form of epigenetic **cell memory**, often mediated by **DNA methylation** and/or **histone modification**.

Induced pluripotent stem cells   Adult cells that have been reprogrammed to express factors that induce and maintain cellular pluripotency.

Inner cell mass   The part of the **blastocyst** that becomes the embryo proper, in contrast to the **trophectoderm**, which gives rise to the placenta.

Introns   The intervening sequences in genes that separate the **exons**. They are eliminated from the final RNA transcript.

Inversion   A chromosomal segment that was deleted from a chromosome and reinserted in an end-to-end reverse position, or was inverted because of abnormal pairing of the chromosome during **meiosis**.

Karyotype   The chromosome constitution of an individual; for example, 46,XY of the male, 46,XX of the female, or 45,X/46,XX of a mosaic female with Turner syndrome. Also, a photograph of the chromosome contents of a single cell, arranged in order of size and morphology.

Locus   The chromosomal location of a gene, consisting of the DNA and chromatin of the gene itself and its regulatory elements. The various **alleles** of a gene all occupy the same locus.

Loss-of-function mutation   A mutation resulting in partial or complete loss of one or more functions of the protein.

Meiosis   The process of cell division that produces the **gametes**, reducing two sets of chromosomes to one set. In humans, 23 pairs of chromosomes are reduced to 23 singlets, the haploid set.

Meiotic sex chromosome inactivation (MSCI)   The epigenetic silencing of the X and Y chromosomes during early stages of spermatogenesis, reflected by the sex chromosome body. A special example of a more general mechanism called meiotic silencing of unsynapsed chromatin (MSUC), which silences unpaired chromosomes, as a meiotic checkpoint to protect against aneuploidy in subsequent generations. That MSUC does not take place during oogenesis no doubt accounts for the greater aneuploidy in oocytes than in sperm.

Metastable epiallele   Alleles that are variably expressed in genetically identical individuals due to epigenetic modifications established during early development. They are thought to be particularly vulnerable to environmental influences. The viable yellow (A(vy)) agouti allele, whose expression is correlated with DNA methylation, is a murine-metastable epiallele.

Methylation   The addition of a methyl group ($-CH_3$) to a DNA or histone molecule.

Mitosis   The process of cell division in somatic cells that produces daughter cells, needed for the growth and continual replacement of tissues.

Monosomic   Possessing or expressing only one copy of any chromosome.

Morula   A preimplantation embryo that consists of a ball of cleaving cells, before the **blastocyst** cavity is formed. In the mouse, the morula has 16–32 cells.

Mosaicism   The state of being composed of a mixture of cells having different genetic content, leading to differences in their function. In **chromosomal mosaicism**, the mixed populations of cells differ regarding the number of chromosomes—that is, X0/XX mosaicism. In **confined placental mosaicism**, the cells with different karyotypes occur only in the placenta and not in the embryo proper. In **X inactivation mosaicism**, the cells do not differ in content but differ regarding which X chromosome is expressed.

Mouse–human hybrids   Proliferating somatic cells that contain both mouse and human chromosomes within the same cultured cell. These cells were created from a human cell fused with a mouse cell by **somatic cell hybridization**.

Mutation   Any heritable change in the DNA sequence.

Nondisjunction   The failure of two members of a chromosome pair to segregate to different cells. As a result, one daughter cell receives both members of the pair, and the other gets neither of them.

Nucleosome   The basic unit of chromatin. A nucleosome is composed of an octamer of **histone** proteins, two each of H2A, H2B, H3, and H4 around which 146 base pairs of DNA wraps 1.7 times. Nucleosomes are assembled during DNA replication in two steps, by which histones H3 and H4 are first deposited onto DNA, and then histones H2A and H2B are added.

Ovarian teratoma   Tumor of the ovary in females that results from parthenogenetic induction of cleavage. Each cell has two copies of the maternal genome and no copy of the paternal one. These tumors differentiate into fetal tissues, but the absence of placental development precludes normal development of this nonfertilized zygote. The **karyotype** is always $46,X^mX^m$.

Painting probe   A probe designed for **FISH** analysis that consists of a mixture of unique DNA sequences from a specific chromosome. When this labeled probe is hybridized to **metaphase** or **interphase** chromosomes, it will detect the presence of sequences homologous to that chromosome—wherever they may be in the genome.

Parental imprinting   Parent-specific expression of only the maternal allele or only the paternal allele because of epigenetic marks or memory first acquired in the egg or sperm.

Parthenogenesis   Unusual form of reproduction where all the chromosomes in the conceptus come from only one parent. Also refers to the embryonic development that occurs in absence of fertilization that is seen in invertebrates and plants.

Paternal X inactivation   Imprinted form of X inactivation occurring in marsupials and rodent placental tissues. Paternal alleles are always inactive.

Phenotype   The observed characteristics (morphological, chemical, and behavioral) of an individual that are attributable to an interplay between his or her genes and their interaction with the environment.

Polymorphism   An variant allele or DNA sequence that occurs in the population with a frequency of >1%.

Polycomb group (PcG)   First discovered in flies, these protein complexes are essential epigenetic regulators of processes, such as cellular memory, cell proliferation, and genomic imprinting. Capable of long distance interactions, they exert their silencing functions by attracting and depositing repressive histone modifications, where they are needed. In many organisms, they mark the chromatin of their target genes by methylation at histone H3 lysine 27.

Position effect variegation   An epigenetic effect that occurs when a gene is brought abnormally close to heterochromatic repeats, leading to silencing of the gene in those cells

Promoter   The region of DNA at the beginning (in the 5' end) of a gene that initiates transcription by binding RNA polymerase.

Pseudoautosomal regions   Regions at the tips of X and Y chromosomes that resemble **autosomes** because they contain homologous XY genes that are exchanged freely during **meiosis**, therefore not behaving as if they were X- or Y-linked. Genes residing in these regions are expressed from X and Y chromosomes in males and both X chromosomes in females.

Random X inactivation   The kind of inactivation that occurs in most mammalian embryos characterized by an equal probability that maternal or paternal X is chosen the active X. In contrast to imprinted or **paternal X inactivation.**

Recombination   The exchange of DNA between homologous chromosomes during **meiosis,** which results in new combinations of genes so that the chromosome in the offspring differs from the one in the parents; contributes to diversity and individuality.

Remodeling of chromatin   Modifying chromatin to make it transcriptionally active or inactive.

Remodeling factor   A protein that alters the organization of **nucleosomes** to change the expression status of genes.

Repetitive DNA   DNA sequences that are present in multiple copies and in multiple places throughout the genome.

Ring chromosome   Chromosomes with two breaks (on either side of the **centromere**) that rejoin, resulting in a circular chromosome.

RNA   Ribonucleic acid, the intermediary by which DNA makes a protein. Using DNA as a template, RNA molecules are transcribed in the nucleus and find their way into the cytoplasm, where they are used for the synthesis of the protein specified by the gene. **RNA polymerase** is the enzyme that catalyses the formation of RNA, using DNA as the template. **Messenger RNA (mRNA)** is RNA that encodes and carries information from DNA to sites of protein synthesis for translation into a protein product. **Noncoding RNA** are RNA transcripts that do not encode proteins; some of them are involved in gene silencing and transcriptional modulation. **Splicing** is the process by which the introns are removed during processing of the transcripts. Sometimes pre-mRNA messages may be spliced in several different ways, allowing a single gene to encode multiple proteins. **Polyadenylation** is the mechanism by which most mRNA molecules are terminated at their 3′ ends. The poly(A) tail added to the transcript aids in mRNA stability, export of the mRNA from the nucleus, and translation.

Sex chromatin   The inactive X chromosome in a relatively condensed form observed in the nucleus of **interphase** cells; also called **Barr body.**

Sex chromosome body   Condensed **chromatin** of inactive X and Y chromosomes during spermatogenesis. See **XY inactivation** or **Meiotic sex chromosome inactivation (MSCI).**

Sex chromosomes   Special pair of chromosomes that are needed for sex determination; usually called X and Y, but in birds they are called Z and W.

Sex determination   The mechanism responsible for the male–female sexual dimorphism. Often, the sex determinants are carried by the sex chromosomes.

Sex linkage   Genes that reside on either X or Y chromosomes.

Sex-linked diseases   Diseases associated with mutations in genes on the sex chromosome. Practically all of them are on the X chromosome, with the exception of those affecting male sex determination or causing male sterility.

Skewed X inactivation   The number of cells with an active maternal X greatly differs from that with an active paternal X, such that the two mosaic cell populations are in no way equally represented. Paternal X inactivation represents an extreme case of skewed inactivation.

Somatic cell hybridization   Fusion of somatic cells of different kinds in cell culture to produce novel cells made of the two parental components; used to map genes, for genetic analysis, to determine the subunit structure of proteins and to separate one chromosome from its homologue in different hybrid cells.

Somatic cells All the cells of the body that are not germ cells.

Stochastic Governed by the laws of probability and chance.

Syndromes Set of anomalies, abnormalities, or symptoms that are (1) common manifestations of the same disease, although not necessarily limited to that disease; and (2) usually occur together and hence define the syndrome. Some well-recognized syndromes are Klinefelter, Lesch Nyhan, Rett, and Turner syndromes.

Telomere The specialized structures that mark both ends of the chromosome. Telomeres are needed to replicate the ends of the chromosomes, thus protecting the chromosomes from shortening.

Transcription The synthesis of a RNA using DNA as template. This RNA acts as a messenger to carry the code for a particular protein to the ribosomes, where proteins are made.

Transgenes Alien (i.e., not their own) genes present in an individual that arrived there by transfection.

Translation The synthesis of a protein subunit on ribosomes based on the coded information in the messenger RNA.

Triploid An individual with three copies of each chromosome and a total of 69 chromosomes.

Trisomic An individual having three copies of a single chromosome, with a total of 47 chromosomes.

Trophectoderm See **Blastocyst**.

X/autosome translocation An exchange between segments of X chromosomes with **autosomes**.

Xce X chromosome controlling element, mouse. This locus has not been fully identified but has been defined genetically because there are several alleles; each has a different effect (or strength), in determining the frequency its X is the inactive X in the cell. It is believed to modify *Xist* expression in some way. The effect of the known alleles is relatively subtle. The locus is missing from the human **XIC**.

X chromosome inactivation (XCI) The mammalian mechanism of **X dosage compensation**. See also **paternal X inactivation; random X inactivation; skewed X inactivation**

X inactivation center (XIC) The localized region of the X chromosome needed for *cis* inactivation, located in band Xq13.2 on the human X.

X inactivation spreading Extension of the inactivation signal from its source along the entire X chromosome, or into neighboring autosomal chromatin in the case of X-autosome translocations.

X inactive specific transcript (*XIST* in humans, *Xist* in other animals) Gene in the X inactivation center that initiates *cis* inactivation; noncoding RNA that coats all future inactive X chromosomes so as to initiate modification of the underlying chromatin that results in **heterochromatin**.

XY inactivation (XYI) In the developing sperm, the sex chromosomes form a unique sex or XY body. At this time in male **meiosis**, both X and Y are transcriptionally inactive, related to their being unable to pair properly in preparation for cell division. This is also called **meiotic sex chromosome inactivation (MSCI)**.

REFERENCES

1. Ohno S. *Sex Chromosomes and Sex-Linked Genes.* New York: Springer-Verlag; 1967.
2. Graunt J. Natural and political observations made upon the bills of mortality, London, 1662.
3. Dennerstein L. Gender, health and ill-health. *Women's Health Issues.* 1995;5:53–59.
4. Hassold T, Quillen SD, Yamane JA. Sex ratio in spontaneous abortion. *Ann Hum Genet.* 1983;47:39–47.
5. Griffin DK, Abruzzo MA, Millie EA, Feingold E, Hassold TJ. Sex ratio in normal and disomic sperm: evidence that the extra chromosome 21 preferentially segregates with the Y chromosome. *Am J Hum Genet.* 1996;59:1108–1113.
6. Jacobs PA, Hassold TJ, Henry A, Pettay D, Takaesu N. Trisomy 13 ascertained in a survey of spontaneous abortions. *J Med Genet.* 1987;24:721–724.
7. Hassold TJ, Jacobs PA, Leppert M, Sheldon M. Cytogenetic and molecular studies of trisomy 13. *J Med Genet.* 1987;24:725–732.
8. Rasmussen SA, Wong L-YC, Yang Q, May KM, Friedman JM. Population-based analyses of mortality in trisomy 13 and trisomy 18. *Pediatrics.* 2003;111:777–784.
9. Boklage CE. The epigenetic environment: secondary sex ratio depends on differential survival in embryogenesis. *Hum Reprod.* 2005;20:583–587.
10. Miller JF, Williamson E, Glue J, Gordon YB, Grudzinskas JG, Sykes A. Fetal loss after implantation. A prospective study. *Lancet.* 1980;2(8194):554–546.
11. Childs B. Genetic origin of some sex differences among human beings. *Pediatrics.* 1965;35:798–812.
12. Gissler M, Järvelin M-R, Louhiala P, Hemminki E. Boys have more health problems in childhood than girls: follow-up of the 1987 Finnish birth cohort. *Acta Paediatr.* 1999;88:310–314.
13. Cui W, Ma CX, Tang Y, et al. Sex differences in birth defects: a study of opposite-sex twins. *Birth Defects Res A Clin Mol Teratol.* 2005;73:876–880.
14. Nordenstrom A, Ahmed S, Jones J, et al. Female preponderance in congenital adrenal hyperplasia due to CYP21 deficiency in England: implications for neonatal screening. *Horm Res.* 2005;63:22–28.
15. Cartwright RA, Gurney K, Moorman AV. Sex ratios and the risks of haematological malignancies. *Br J Haematol.* 2002;118:1071–1077.
16. Shaffer LG, Tommerup N. *ISCN (2005): An International System for Human Cytogenetic Nomenclature.* Basel, Switzerland: Karger; 2005.

17. Veyrunes F, Waters PD, Miethke P, et al. Bird-like sex chromosomes of platypus imply recent origin of mammal sex chromosomes. *Genome Res.* 2008;18:965–973.

18. Lahn BT, Page DC. Four evolutionary strata on the human X chromosome. *Science.* 1999;286:964–967.

19. Rosen S, Skaletsky H, Marszalek JD, et al. Abundant gene conversion between arms of palindromes in human and ape Y chromosomes. *Nature.* 2003;423:873–876.

20. Glaser B, Myrtek D, Rumpler Y, et al. Transposition of SRY into the ancestral pseudoautosomal region creates a new pseudoautosomal boundary in a progenitor of simian primates. *Hum Mol Genet.* 1999;8: 2071–2078.

21. Ohno S, Becak W, Becak ML. X-autosome ratio and the behaviour pattern of individual X-chromosomes in placental mammals. *Chromosoma.* 1964;15:14–30.

22. Graves JAM. Mammals that break the rules: genetics of marsupials and monotremes. *Annu Rev Genet.* 1996;30:233–260.

23. Graves, JA. Sex chromosome specialization and degeneration in mammals. *Cell.* 2006;124: 901–914.

24. Graves JAM, Disteche CM, Toder R. Gene dosage in the evolution and function of mammalian X chromosomes. *Cytogenet Cell Genet.* 1998;80:94–103.

25. D'Esposito M, Ciccodicola A, Gianfrancesco F, et al. A synaptobrevin-like gene in the Xq28 pseudoautosomal region undergoes X inactivation. *Nat Genet.* 1996;13: 227–229.

26. Sarbajna S, Denniff M, Jeffreys AJ, et al. A major recombination hotspot in the XqYq pseudoautosomal region gives new insight into processing of human gene conversion events. *Hum Mol Genet.* 2012;21:2029–2038.

27. Lakich D, Kazazian H, Antonarakis S, Gitschier J. Inversions disrupting the factor VIII gene are a common cause of severe haemophilia A. *Nature Genetics.* 1993;5: 236–241.

28. Vermeesch JR, Petit P, Kermouni A, Renauld JC, Van Den Berghe H, Marynen P. The IL-9 receptor gene, located in the Xq/Yq pseudoautosomal region, has an autosomal origin, escapes X inactivation and is expressed from the Y. *Hum Mol Genet.* 1997; 6:1–8.

29. Muyle A, Zemp N, Deschamps C, Mousset S, Widmer A, Marais GA. Rapid de novo evolution of X chromosome dosage compensation in Silene latifolia, a plant with young sex chromosomes. *PLoS Biol.* 2012;10: e1001308.

30. Ross MT, Grafham DV, Coffey AJ, et al. The DNA sequence of the human X chromosome. *Nature.* 2005;434:325–337.

31. Muller HJ. Evidence of the precision of genetic adaptation. *Harvey Lectures.* 1947–48;43:165–229.

32. Park Y, Kuroda MI. Epigenetic aspects of X-chromosome dosage compensation. *Science.* 2001;293:1083–1085.

33. Deng X, Meller VH. Non-coding RNA in fly dosage compensation. *Trends Biochem Sci.* 2006;31:526–532.

34. Meyer BJ. Sex in the worm: counting and compensating X-chromosome dose. *Trends Genet.* 2000;16:247–253.

35. Vielle A, Lang J, Dong Y, et al. H4K20me1 contributes to downregulation of X-linked genes for C. elegans dosage compensation. *PLoS Genet.* 2012;8:e1002933.

36. Parkhurst SM, Meneely PM. Sex determination and dosage compensation: lessons from flies and worms. *Science.* 1994;264:924–932.

37. Jacob F. Evolution and tinkering. *Science.* 1977;196:1161–1166.

38. Conrad T, Akhtar A. Dosage compensation in Drosophila melanogaster: epigenetic fine-tuning of chromosome-wide transcription. *Nat Rev Genet.* 2011;13:123–134.

39. Meyer BJ. Targeting X chromosomes for repression. *Curr Opin Genet Dev.* 2010;20:179–189.

40. Kelley RL, Kuroda, MI. The Drosophila roX1 RNA gene can overcome silent chromatin by recruiting the male-specific lethal dosage compensation complex. *Genetics.* 2003;164:565–574.

41. Kuroda Y. Absence of Z-chromosome inactivation for five genes in male chickens. *Chromosome Res.* 2001;9:457–468.

42. Bisoni L, Batlle-Morera L, Bird AP, Susuki M, McQueen HA. Female-specific hyperacetylation of histone H4 in the chicken Z chromosome. *Chromosome Res.* 2005;13:205–214.

43. Grutzner F, Graves JAM. A platypus' eye view of the mammalian genome. *Curr Opin Genet Dev.* 2004;14:642–649.

44. Deakin JE, Chaumeil J, Hore TA, Marshall Graves JA. Unravelling the evolutionary origins of X chromosome inactivation in mammals: insights from marsupials and monotremes. *Chromosome Res.* 2009;17; 671–685.

45. Rens W, Wallduck MS, Lovell FL, Ferguson-Smith MA, Ferguson-Smith AC. Epigenetic modifications on X chromosomes in marsupial and monotreme mammals and implications for evolution of dosage compensation. *Proc Natl Acad Sci U S A.* 2010;107:17657–17662.

46. Lyon MF. Gene action in the X chromosome of the mouse. *Nature.* 1961;190: 372–373.

47. Russell LB. Genetics of mammalian sex chromosomes. *Science.* 1961;133: 1795–1803.

48. Beutler E, Yeh M, Fairbanks VF. The normal human female as a mosaic of X-chromosome activity: studies using the gene for G-6-PD deficiency as a marker. *Proc Natl Acad Sci USA.* 1962;48:9–16.

49. http://www.bioinfo.org.cn/book/Great%20Experments/great31.htm [accessed June 10, 2013].

50. Barr ML, Bertram EG. A morphological distinction between neurones of the male and female, and the behaviour of the nucleolar satellite during accelerated nucleoprotein synthesis. *Nature.* 1949;163:676–677.

51. Ohno S, Kaplan WD, Kinosita R. Formation of the sex chromatin by a single X-chromosome in liver cells of Rattus norvegius. *Exp Cell Res.* 1959;18:415–418.

52. Ohno S, Hauschka TS. Allocycly of the X-chromosome in tumors and normal tissues. *Cancer Res.* 1960;20:541–545.

53. Welshons WJ, Russell LB. The Y-chromosome as the bearer of male-determining factors in the mouse. *Proc Natl Acad Sci USA.* 1959;45:560–566.

54. Ford CE, Jones KW, Polani PE, De Almeida JC, Briggs JH. A sex-chromosome anomaly in a case of gonadal dysgenesis (Turner's syndrome). *Lancet.* 1959;7075:711–713.

55. Jacobs PA, Strong JA. A case of human intersexuality having a possible XXY sex-determining mechanism. *Nature.* 1959;183:302.

56. Lyon MF. Sex chromatin and gene action in the mammalian X-chromosome. *Am J Hum Genet.* 1962;14:135–148.

57. Davidson RG, Nitowsky HM, Childs B. Demonstration of two populations of cells in the human female heterozygous for glucose-6–phosphate dehydrogenase variants. *Proc Natl Acad Sci USA.* 1963;50:481–485.

58. Migeon BR, Jeppesen P, Torchia BS, et al. Lack of X inactivation associated with maternal X isodisomy: evidence for a counting mechanism prior to X inactivation during human embryogenesis. *Am J Hum Genet*. 1996;58:161–170.

59. Brown CJ, Willard HF. The human X inactivation centre is not required for maintenance of X-chromosome inactivation. *Nature*. 1994;368:154–156.

60. Hansen RS, Canfield TK, Gartler SM. Reverse replication timing for the XIST gene in human fibroblasts. *Hum Mol Genet*. 1995;4:813–820.

61. Migeon BR, Der Kaloustian VM, Nyhan WL, Young WJ, Childs B. X-linked hypoxanthine-guanine phosphoribosyl transferase deficiency: heterozygote has two clonal populations. *Science*. 1968;169:425–427.

62. Szybalski W. Use of the HPRT gene and the HAT selection technique in DNA-mediated transformation of mammalian cells: first steps toward developing hybridoma techniques and gene therapy. *Bioessays*. 1992;14(7):495–500.

63. Carrel L, Willard HF. X-inactivation profile reveals extensive variability in X-linked gene expression in females. *Nature*. 2005;434:400–404.

64. Brown CJ, Ballabio A, Rupert JL, et al. A gene from the region of the human X inactivation center expressed exclusively from the inactive X chromosome. *Nature*. 1991;349:38–44.

65. Migeon BR, Schmidt M, Axelman J, Ruta-Cullen C. Complete reactivation of X chromosomes from human chorionic villi with a switch to early DNA replication. *Proc Natl Acad Sci USA*. 1986;83:2182–2186.

66. Okamoto I, Patrat C, Thepot, D, et al. Eutherian mammals use diverse strategies to initiate X-chromosome inactivation during development. *Nature*. 2011;472(7343):370–374.

67. Migeon BR, Lee CH, Chowdhury AK, Carpenter H. Species differences in *TSIX/Tsix* reveal the roles of these genes in X chromosome inactivation. *Am J Hum Genet*. 2002;71:286–293.

68. Martin GR, Epstein CJ, Travis R, et al. X-chromosome inactivation during differentiation of female teratocarcinoma stem cells in vitro. *Nature*. 1978;271:329–333.

69. Lee JT, Strauss WM, Dausman JA, Jaenisch R. A 450 kb transgene displays properties of the mammalian X-inactivation center. *Cell*. 1996;86:83–94.

70. Migeon BR, Kazi E, Haisley-Royster C, et al. Human X inactivation center induces random X inactivation in male transgenic mice. *Genomics*. 1999;59:113–121.

71. Tchieu J, Kuoy E, Chin MH, et al. Female human iPSCs retain an inactive X chromosome. *Cell Stem Cell*. 2010;7:329–342.

72. Mekhoubad S, Bock C, de Boer AS, Kiskinis E, Meissner A, Eggan K. Erosion of dosage compensation impacts human iPSC disease modeling. *Cell Stem Cell*. 2012;10:595–609.

73. Walker CL, Cargile CB, Floy K, Delannoy M, Migeon BR. The Barr body is a looped X chromosome with telomere association. *Proc Natl Acad Sci USA*. 1991;88:6191–6195.

74. Chadwick BP, Willard HF. Multiple spatially distinct types of facultative heterochromatin on the human inactive X chromosome. *Proc Natl Acad Sci U S A*. 2004;101:17450–17455.

75. Morishima A, Grumbach MM, Taylor JH. Asynchronous duplication of human chromosomes and the origin of sex chromatin. *Proc Natl Acad Sci USA*. 1962;48:756–763.

76. German J. DNA synthesis in human chromosomes. *Trans NY Acad Sci.* 1962;24:395–407.

77. Yen ZC, Meyer IM, Karalic S, Brown CJ. A cross-species comparison of X-chromosome inactivation in Eutheria. *Genomics.* 2007;90:453–463.

78. Huynh KD, Lee JT. Imprinted X inactivation in eutherians: a model of gametic execution and zygotic relaxation. *Curr Opin Cell Biol.* 2001;13:690–697.

79. Sugawara O, Takagi N, Sasaki M. Correlation between X-chromosome inactivation and cell differentiation in female preimplantation mouse embryos. *Cytogenet Cell Genet.* 1985;39:210–219.

80. Epstein CJ, Smith S, Travis B, Tucker G. Both X-chromosomes function before visible X-chromosome inactivation in female mouse embryos. *Nature.* 1978;274:500–503.

81. Kratzer PG, Gartler SM. Hprt activity changes in preimplantation mouse embryos. *Nature.* 1978;274:503–504.

82. Gutierrez-Adan A, Oter M, Martinez-Madrid B, Pintado B, De La Fuente J. Differential expression of two genes located on the X chromosome between male and female in vitro-produced bovine embryos at the blastocyst stage. *Mol Reprod Dev.* 2000;55:146–151.

83. Taylor DM, Handyside AH, Ray PF, Dibb NJ, Winston RML, Ao A. Quantitative measurement of transcript levels throughout human preimplantation development: analysis of hypoxanthine phosporibosyl transferase. *Mol Hum Reprod.* 2001;7:147–154.

84. Singer-Sam J, Chapman V, LeBon JM, Riggs AD. Parental imprinting studied by allele-specific primer extension after PCR: paternal X chromosome-linked genes are transcribed prior to preferential paternal X chromosome inactivation. *Proc Natl Acad Sci USA.* 1992;89:10469–10473.

85. Chapman VM. X chromosome regulation in female mammals. In: Constantini F, Jaenisch R, eds. *Genetic Manipulation of the Early Embryo.* Cold Spring Harbor, NY: Cold Spring Harbor Laboratory; 1985:11–20.

86. Chapman VM. X chromosome regulation in oogenesis and early mammalian development. In: Rossant J, Pedersen R, eds. *Experimental Approaches to Mammalian Embryonic Development.* Cambridge: Cambridge University Press; 1986:365–398.

87. Chapman VM. Mechanisms of X chromosome regulation. *Annu Rev Genet.* 1988;22:199–233.

88. Huynh KD, Lee JT. Inheritance of a pre-inactivated paternal X chromosome in early mouse embryos. *Nature.* 2003;426:857–862.

89. Mak W, Nesterova TB, de Napoles M, et al. Reactivation of the paternal X chromosome in early mouse embryos. *Science.* 2004;303:666–669.

90. Khalil AM, Boyar FZ, Driscoll DJ. Dynamic histone modifications mark sex chromosome inactivation and reactivation during mammlian spermatogenesis. *Proc Natl Acad Sci USA.* 2004;101:16583–16587.

91. Wolpert L. *From Egg to Embryo: Determinative Events in Early Development.* Cambridge: Cambridge University Press; 1986:41.

92. Monk M, Harper MI. Sequential X chromosome inactivation coupled with cellular differentiation in early mouse embryos. *Nature.* 1979;281:311–313.

93. Tan SS, Williams EA, Tam PPL. X-chromosome inactivation occurs at different times in different tissues of the post-implantation mouse embryo. *Nat Genet.* 1993;3:170–174.

94. Wutz A, Jaenisch R. A shift from reversible to irreversible X inactivation is triggered during ES cell differentiation. *Mol Cell.* 2000;5:695–705.

95. Russell LB. Mammalian X-chromosome action: inactivation limited in spread and in region of origin. *Science.* 1963;140:976–978.

96. Russell LB, Montgomery CS. The use of X-autosome translocations in locating the X-chromosome inactivation center. *Genetics.* 1965;52:470–471.

97. Therman E, Sarto GE, Patau K. Center for Barr body condensation on the proximal part of the human Xq: a hypothesis. *Chromosoma.* 1974; 44:361–366.

98. Therman E, Sarto GE, Palmer CG, Kallio H, Denniston C. Position of the human X inactivation center on Xq. *Hum Genet.* 1979;50:59–64.

99. Cattanach BM. Control of chromosome inactivation. *Annu Rev Genet.* 1975;9:1–18.

100. Leppig KA, Brown CJ, Bressler SL, et al. Mapping the distal boundaries of the X-inactivation center in a rearranged X chromosome from a female expressing XIST. *Hum Mol Genet.* 1993;2:883–887.

101. Lee JT, Lu NF, Han Y. Genetic analysis of the mouse X-inactivation center reveals an 80kb multifunction domain. *Proc Natl Acad Sci USA.* 1999;96:3836–3841.

102. Heard E, Mongelard F, Arnaud D, Chureau C, Vourc'h C, Avner P. Human XIST yeast artificial transgenes show partial X inactivation center function in mouse embryonic stem cells. *Proc Natl Acad Sci USA.* 1999;96:6841–6846.

103. Chureau C, Prissette M, Bourdet A, et al. Comparative sequence analysis of the X inactivation center region in mouse, human, and bovine. *Genome Res.* 2002;12:894–908.

104. Brown CJ, Hendrich BD, Rupert JL, et al. The human XIST gene: analysis of a 17 kb inactive X-specific RNA that contains conserved repeats and is highly localized within the nucleus. *Cell.* 1992;71:527–542.

105. Brockdorff N, Ashworth A, Kay G, et al. The product of the mouse Xist gene is a 15 kb inactive X-specific transcript containing no conserved ORF and located in the nucleus. *Cell.* 1992;71:515–526.

106. Hendrich BD, Plenge RM, Willard HF. Identification and characterization of the human XIST gene promoter: implications for models of X chromosome inactivation. *Nucleic Acids Res.* 1997;25:2661–2671.

107. Nesterova TB, Slobodyanyuk SY, Elisaphenko EA, et al. Characterization of the genomic Xist locus in rodents reveals conservation of overall gene structure and tandem repeats but rapid evolution of unique sequence. *Genome Res.* 2001;11:833–849.

108. Orishchenko KE, Pavlova SV, Elisaphenko EA, et al. A regulatory potential of the Xist gene promoter in vole M. rossiaemeridionalis. *PLoS One* 7. 2012;e33994.

109. Duret L, Chureau C, Samain S, Weissenbach J, Avner P. The Xist RNA gene evolved in eutherians by pseudogenization of a protein-coding gene. *Science.* 2006;312:1653–1655.

110. Elisaphenko EA, Kolesnikov NN, Shevchenko AI, et al. A dual origin of the Xist gene from a protein-coding gene and a set of transposable elements. PLoS One. 2008;3:e2521.

111. Migeon BR, Winter H, Kazi E, et al. Low-copy-number human transgene is recognized as an X inactivation center in mouse ES cells, but fails to induce cis-inactivation in chimeric mice. *Genomics.* 2001;71:156–162.

112. Kay GF, Penny GD, Patel D, Ashworth A, Brockdorff N, Rastan S. Expression of Xist during mouse development suggests a role in the initiation of X chromosome inactivation. *Cell.* 1993;72:171–182.

113. Kay GF, Barton S, Surani MA, Rastan S. Imprinting and X chromosome counting mechanisms determine Xist expression in early mouse development. *Cell.* 1994;77:639–650.

114. Ray PF, Winston RML, Handyside AH. XIST expression from the maternal X chromosome in human male preimplantation embryos at the blastocyst stage. *Hum Mol Genet.* 1997;6:1323–1327.

115. Beckelmann J, Budik S, Bartel C, Aurich C. Evaluation of Xist expression in preattachment equine embryos. *Theriogenology.* 2012;78(7):1429–1436.

116. Ma M, Strauss WM. Analysis of the Xist RNA isoforms suggests two distinctly different forms of regulation. *Mamm Genome.* 2005;16:391–404.

117. Yildirim E, Kirby JE, Brown DE, et al. Xist RNA is a potent suppressor of hematologic cancer in mice. *Cell.* 2013;152:727–742.

118. Escamilla-Del-Arenal M, da Rocha ST, Heard E. Evolutionary diversity and developmental regulation of X-chromosome inactivation. *Hum Genet.* 2011;130:307–327.

119. Wutz A, Rasmussen RP, Jaenisch R. Chromosomal silencing and localization are mediated by different domains of Xist RNA. *Nat Genet.* 2002;30:167–174

120. Migeon BR, Luo S, Stasiowski BA, et al. Deficient transcription of XIST from tiny ring X chromosomes in females with severe phenotypes. *Proc Natl Acad Sci USA.* 1993;90:12025–12029.

121. Migeon BR, Luo S, Jani M, Jeppesen P. The severe phenotype of females with tiny ring X chromosomes is associated with inability of these chromosomes to undergo X inactivation. *Am J Hum Genet.* 1994;55:497–504.

122. Wolff DJ, Brown CJ, Schwartz S, Duncan AMV, Surti U, Willard HF. Small marker X chromosomes lack the X inactivation center: implications for karyotype/phenotype correlations. *Am J Hum Genet.* 1994;55:87–95.

123. Herzing LBK, Romer JT, Horn JM, Ashworth A. Xist has properties of the X-chromosome inactivation centre. *Nature.* 1997;386:272–275.

124. Lee JT, Jaenisch R. Long-range *cis* effects of ectopic X-inactivation centres on a mouse autosome. *Nature.* 1997;386:275–279.

125. Avner R, Wahrman J, Richler C, et al. X inactivation-specific transcript expression in mouse oocytes and zygotes. *Mol Hum Reprod.* 2000;6:591–594.

126. Panning B, Dausman J, Jaenisch R. X chromosome inactivation is mediated by Xist RNA stablization. *Cell.* 1997;90:907–916.

127. Ciaudo C, Bourdet A, Cohen-Tannoudji M, Dietz HC, Rougeulle C, Avner P. Nuclear mRNA degradation pathway(s) are implicated in Xist regulation and X chromosome inactivation. *PLoS Genet.* 2006;2:0874–0882.

128. Deuve JL, Avner P. The coupling of X-chromosome inactivation to pluripotency. *Annu Rev Cell Dev Biol.* 2011;27:611–629.

129. Barakat TS, Gunhanlar N, Pardo CG, et al. RNF12 activates Xist and is essential for X chromosome inactivation. *PLoS Genet.* 2011;7:e1002001.

130. Marahrens Y, Panning B, Dausman J, Strauss W, Jaenisch R. Xist-deficient mice are defective in dosage compensation but not spermatogenesis. *Genes Dev.* 1997;11:156–166.

131. Xu N, Tsai C-L, Lee JT. Transient homologous chromosome pairing marks the onset of X inactivation. *Science.* 2006;311:1107–1109.

132. Bacher CP, Guggiari M, Brors B, et al. Transient colocalization of X-inactivation centres accompanies the initiation of X inactivation. *Nat Cell Biol*. 2006;8:293–299.

133. Duszczyk MM, Wutz A, Rybin V, Sattler M. The Xist RNA A-repeat comprises a novel AUCG tetraloop fold and a platform for multimerization. *RNA*. 2011;17:1973–1982.

134. Duszczyk MM, Sattler M. (1)H, (1)(3)C, (1)(5)N and (3)(1)P chemical shift assignments of a human Xist RNA A-repeat tetraloop hairpin essential for X-chromosome inactivation. *Biomol NMR Assign*. 2012;6:75–77.

135. Plenge RM, Hendrich BD, Schwartz C, et al. A promoter mutation in the XIST gene in two unrelated families with skewed X-chromosome inactivation. *Nat Genet*. 1997;17:353–356.

136. Tomkins DJ, McDonald HL, Farrell SA, Brown CJ. Lack of espression of XIST from a small ring X chromosome containing the XIST locus in a girl with short stature, facial dysmophism and developmental delay. *Eur J Hum Genet*. 2002;10:44–51.

137. Pugacheva E, Tiwari VK, Abdullaev Z, et al. Familial cases of point mutations in the XIST promoter reveal a correlation between CTCF binding and pre-emptive choices of X chromosome inactivation. *Hum Mol Genet*. 2005;14:953–965.

138. Chao W, Huynh KD, Spencer RJ, Davidow LS, Lee JT. CTCF, a candidate transacting factor for X-inactivation. *Science*. 2002;295:345–347.

139. Hall LL, Byron M, Sakai K, Carrel L, Willard HF, Lawrence JB. An ectopic human XIST gene can induce chromosome inactivation in postdifferentiation human-HT-1080 cells. *Proc Natl Acad Sci USA*. 2002;99:8677–8682.

140. Lee J. Disruption of imprinted X inactivation by parent-of-origin-effects at Tsix. *Cell*. 2000;103:17–27.

141. Johnston PG, Cattanach BM. Controlling elements in the mouse. IV. Evidence of non-random X-inactivation. *Genet Res*. 1981;37:151–160.

142. Simmler M, Cattanach BM, Rasberry C, Rougeulle C, Avner P. Mapping the murine Xce locus with (CA)n repeats. *Mamm Genome*. 1993;4:523–530.

143. Thorvaldsen JL, Krapp C, Willard HF, Bartolomei MS. Nonrandom X chromosome inactivation is influenced by multiple regions on the murine X chromosome. *Genetics*. 2012;192:1095–1107.

144. Ogawa Y, Lee JT. Xite, X-inactivation intergenic transcription elements that regulate the probability of choice. *Mol Cell*. 2003;11:731–743.

145. Shevchenko AI, Malakhova AA, Elisaphenko EA, et al. Variability of sequence surrounding the Xist gene in rodents suggests taxon-specific regulation of X chromosome inactivation. *PLoS One*. 2011;6:e22771.

146. Lee JT, Davidow LS, Warshawsky D. Tsix, a gene antisense to Xist at the X-inactivation centre. *Nat Genet*. 1999;21:400–404.

147. Lee JT, Lu N. Targeted mutagenesis of Tsix leads to nonrandom inactivation. *Cell*. 1999;99:47–57.

148. Cohen DE, Lee JT. X-chromosome inactivation and the search for chromosome-wide silencers. *Curr Opin Genet Dev*. 2002;12:219–224.

149. Lee JT. Homozygous Tsix mutant mice reveal a sex-ratio distortion and revert to random X-inactivation. *Nat Genet*. 2002.

150. Stavropoulos N, Lu L, Lee JT. A functional role for Tsix transcription in blocking RNA accumulation but not in X-chromosomal choice. *Proc Natl Acad Sci USA*. 2001;98:10232–10237.

151. Lee JT. Regulation of X-chromosome counting by Tsix and Xite sequences. *Science.* 2005;309:768–771.

152. Navarro P, Pichard S, Sciaudo C, Avner P, Rougeulle C. Tsix transcription across the Xist gene alters chromatin conformation without affecting Xist transcription: implications for X-chromosome inactivation. *Genes Dev.* 2005;19:1474–1484.

153. Migeon BR, Chowdhury AK, Dunston JA, McIntosh I. Identification of TSIX encoding an RNA antisense to human XIST, reveals differences from its murine counterpart: implications for X inactivation. *Am J Hum Genet.* 2001;69:951–960.

154. Yang C, Chapman AG, Kelsey AD, Minks J, Cotton AM, Brown CJ. X-chromosome inactivation: molecular mechanisms from the human perspective. *Hum Genet.* 2011;130(2):175–185.

155. Migeon BR. The single active X in human cells: evolutionary tinkering personified. *Hum Genet.* 2011;130:281–293.

156. Lyon MF. X-chromosome inactivation and developmental patterns in mammals. *Biol Rev.* 1972;47:1–35.

157. Rastan SJ. Non-random X-chromosome inactivation in mouse X-autosome translocation embryos—location of the inactivation centre. *J Embryol Exp Morphol.* 1983;78:1–22.

158. Weaver D, Gartler S, Boue A, Boue JG. Evidence for two active X chromosomes in a human XXY triploid. *Hum Genet.* 1975;28:39–42.

159. Jacobs PA, Masuyama AM, Buchanan IM, Wilson C. Late replicating X chromosomes in human triploidy. *Am J Hum Genet.* 1979;31:446–457.

160. Migeon BR, Sprenkle JA, Do TT. Stability of the "two active X" phenotype in triploid cells. *Cell.* 1979;18:637–641.

161. Jacobs PA, Migeon BR. Studies of X-chromosome inactivation in trisomies. *Cytogenet Cell Genet.* 1989;50:75–77.

162. Migeon BR, Pappas K, Stetten G, Trunca C, Jacobs PA. X inactivation in triploidy and trisomy: the search for autosomal transfactors that choose the active X. *Eur J Hum Genet.* 2008;16:153–162.

163. Spilianakis CG, Lalioti MD, Town T, Lee GR, Flavell RA. Interchromosomal associations between alternatively expressed loci. *Nature.* 2005;435:637–645.

164. Lomvardas S, Barnea G, Pisapia DJ, Mendelsohn M, Kirkland J, Axel R. Interchromosomal interactions and olfactory receptor choice. *Cell.* 2006;126:403–413.

165. Carrel L, Willard HF. Counting on Xist. *Nat Genet.* 1998;19:211–212.

166. Clerc P, Avner P. Role of the region 3′ to Xist exon 6 in the counting process of X-chromosome inactivation. *Nat Genet.* 1998;19:249–253.

167. Avner P, Heard E. X chromosome inactivation: counting, choice and initiation. *Nat Rev Genet.* 2001;2:59–67.

168. Penny GD, Kay GF, Sheardown SA, Rastan S, Brockdorff N. Requirements for Xist in X chromosome inactivation. *Nature.* 1996;379:131–137.

169. Gilbert S. General principles of differentiation and morphogenesis. In: Epstein CJ, Erickson RP, Wynshaw-Boris A, eds. *Inborn Errors of Development.* New York: Oxford University Press; 2003:21–22.

170. Clemson CM, Hall LL B, M, McNeil J, Lawrence JB. The X chromosome is organized into a gene-rich outer rim and an internal core containing silenced nongenic sequences. *Proc Natl Acad Sci USA.* 2006.

171. Beletskii A, Hong Y-K, Pehrson J, Egholm M, Strauss WM. PNA interference mapping demonstrates functional domains in the noncoding RNA Xist. *Proc Natl Acad Sci USA*. 2001;98:9215–9220.

172. Jeon Y, Sarma K, Lee JT. New and Xisting regulatory mechanisms of X chromosome inactivation. *Curr Opin Genet Dev*. 2012;22:62–71.

173. Brown CJ, Baldry SE. Evidence that heteronuclear proteins interact with XIST RNA in vitro. *Somat Cell Mol Genet*. 1996;22:403–417.

174. Gartler SM, Riggs AD. Mammalian X-chromosome inactivation. *Annu Rev Genet*. 1983;17:155–190.

175. Chadwick BP, Willard HF. Chromatin of the Barr body: histone and nonhistone proteins assoicated with or excluded from the inactive X chromosome. *Hum Mol Genet*. 2003;12:2167–2178.

176. Umlauf D, Goto Y, Cao R, et al. Imprinting along the Kcnq1 domain on mouse chromosome 7 involves repressive histone methylation and recruitment of Polycomb group complexes. *Nat Genet*. 2004;36:1296–1300.

177. Silva J, Mak W, Zvetkova I, et al. Establishment of histone H3 methylation on the inactive X chromosome requires transient recruitment of Eed-Enx1 polycomb group complexes. *Dev Cell*. 2003;4:481–495.

178. Chaumeil J, Okamoto I, Guggiari M, Heard E. Integrated kinetics of X chromosome inactivation in differentiating embryonic stem cells. *Cytogenet Genome Res*. 2002;99:75–84.

179. Heard E. Recent advances in X-chromosome inactivation. *Curr Opin Cell Biol*. 2004;16:247–255.

180. Heard E. Delving into the diversity of facultative heterochromatin: the epigenetics of the inactive X chromosome. *Curr Opin Genet Dev*. 2005;15:482–489.

181. Chow JC, Heard E. Nuclear organization and dosage compensation. *Cold Spring Harb Perspect Biol*. 2010;2:a000604.

182. Lyon MF. X-chromosome inactivation spreads itself: effects in autosomes. *Am J Hum Genet*. 1998;63:17–19.

183. Riggs AD, Singer-Sam J, Keith DH. Methylation of the PGK promoter region and an enhancer way-station for X-chromosome inactivation. *Prog Clin Biol Res*. 1985;198:211–222.

184. Lyon MF. X-chromosome inactivation: a repeat hypothesis. *Cytogenet Cell Genet*. 1998;80:133–137.

185. Bailey JA, Carrel L, Chakravarti A, Eichler E. Molecular evidence for a relationship between LINE-1 elements and X chromosome inactivation: the Lyon repeat hypothesis. *Proc Natl Acad Sci USA*. 2000;97:6248–6249.

186. Cantrell MA, Carstens BC, Wichman HA. X chromosome inactivation and Xist evolution in a rodent lacking LINE-1 activity. *PLoS One*. 2009;4:e6252.

187. Chong S, Kontaraki J, Bonifer C, Riggs AD. A functional chromatin domain does not resist X chromosome inactivation: silencing of cLys correlates with methylation of a dual promoter-replication origin. *Mol Cell Biol*. 2002;13:4667–4676.

188. Popova BC, Tada T, Takagi N, Brockdorff N, Nesterova TB. Attenuated spread of X-inactivation in an X;autosome translocation. *Proc Natl Acad Sci USA*. 2006.

189. Sharp AJ, Spotswood HT, Robinson DO, Turner BM, Jacobs PA. Molecular and cytogenetic analysis of the spreading of X inactivation in X;autosome translocations. *Hum Mol Genet*. 2002;11:3145–3156.

190. Doi A, Park IH, Wen B, et al. Differential methylation of tissue- and cancer-specific CpG island shores distinguishes human induced pluripotent stem cells, embryonic stem cells and fibroblasts. Nat Genet. 2009;41:1350–1353.

191. Wolf SF, Migeon BR. Clusters of CpG dinucleotides implicated by nuclease hypersensitivity as control elements of housekeeping genes. Nature. 1985;314:467–469.

192. Ball MP, Li JB, Gao Y, et al. Targeted and genome-scale strategies reveal gene-body methylation signatures in human cells. Nat Biotechnol. 2009;27:361–368.

193. Cotton AM, Lam L, Affleck JG, et al. Chromosome-wide DNA methylation analysis predicts human tissue-specific X inactivation. Hum Genet. 2011;130;187–201.

194. Migeon BR, Holland MM, Driscoll DJ, Robinson JC. Programmed demethylation in CpG islands during human fetal development. Somat Cell Mol Genet. 1991;17:159–168.

195. Bestor TH. The DNA methyltransferases of mammals. Hum Mol Genet. 2000;9:2395–2402.

196. Hansen RS, Stoger R, Wijmenga C, et al. Escape from gene silencing in ICF syndrome: evidence for advanced replication time as a major determinant. Hum Mol Genet. 2000;9:2575–2587.

197. Chen Z, Riggs AD. Maintenance and regulation of DNA methylation patterns in mammals. Biochem Cell Biol. 2006;83:438–448.

198. Disteche CM. Escape from X inactivation in humans and mouse. Trends Genet. 1995;11:17–22.

199. Shapiro LJ, Mohandas T, Weiss R, Romeo G. Non-inactivation of an X-chromosome locus in man. Science. 1979;204:1224–1226.

200. Migeon BR, Shapiro LJ, Norum RA, Mohandas T, Axelman J, Dabora RL. Differential expression of steroid sulphatase locus on active and inactive human X chromosome. Nature. 1982;299:838–840.

201. Filippova GN, Cheng MK, Moore JM, et al. Boundaries between chromosomal domains of X inactivation and escape bind CTCF and lack CpG methylation during early development. Dev Cell. 2005;8:31–42.

202. Lingenfelter PA, Adler DA, Poslinski D, et al. Escape from X inactivation of Smcx is preceded by silencing during mouse development. Nat Genet. 1998;18:212–213.

203. Nesterova TB, Mermoud JE, Pehrson HK, Surani MA, McLaren A, Brockdorff N. Xist expression and macroH2A1.2 localisation in mouse primordial and pluripotent embryonic germ cells. Differentiation. 2002;69:216–225.

204. Gartler SM, Liskay RM, Gant N. Two functional X chromosomes in human fetal oocytes. Exp Cell Res. 1973;82:464–466.

205. Migeon BR, Jelalian K. Evidence for two active X chromosomes in germ cells of females before meiotic entry. Nature. 1977;269:242–243.

206. Driscoll DJ, Migeon BR. Sex difference in methylation of single-copy genes in human meiotic germ cells: implications for X chromosome inactivation, parental imprinting, and origin of CpG mutations. Somat Cell Mol Genet. 1990;16:267–282.

207. Abe M, Tsai SY, Jin SG, Pfeifer GP, Szabo PE. Sex-specific dynamics of global chromatin changes in fetal mouse germ cells. PLoS One. 2011;6:e23848.

208. Turner JM, Mahadevaiah SK, Elliott DJ, et al. Meiotic sex chromosome inactivation in male mice with targeted disruptions of Xist. J Cell Sci. 2002;115:4097–4105.

209. Turner JM, Aprelikova O, Xu X, et al. BRCA1, histone H2AX phosphorylation, and male meiotic sex chromosome inactivation. Curr Biol. 2004;14:2135–2142.

210. Turner JM, Mahadevaiah SK, Fernandez-Capetillo O, et al. Silencing of unsynapsed meiotic chromosomes in the mouse. *Nat Genet.* 2005;37:41–47.

211. Danshina PV, Geyer CB, Dai Q., et al. Phosphoglycerate kinase 2 (PGK2) is essential for sperm function and male fertility in mice. *Biol Reprod.* 2010;82:136–145.

212. Bao S, Miyoshi N, Okamoto I, Jenuwein T, Heard E, Azim Surani M. Initiation of epigenetic reprogramming of the X chromosome in somatic nuclei transplanted to a mouse oocyte. *EMBO Rep.* 2005;6:748–754.

213. Nolen LD, Gao S, Han Z, et al. X chromosome reactivation and regulation in cloned embryos. *Dev Biol.* 2005;279:525–540.

214. Kaslow DC, Migeon BR. DNA methylation stabilizes X chromosome inactivation in eutherians but not in marsupials: evidence for multi-step maintenance of mammalian X-dosage compensation. *Proc Natl Acad Sci USA.* 1987;84:6210–6214.

215. Migeon BR, Wolf SF, Axelman J, Kaslow DC, Schmidt M. Incomplete X dosage compensation in chorionic villi of human placenta. *Proc Natl Acad Sci USA.* 1985;82:3390–3394.

216. Mann MR, Lee SS, Doherty AS, et al. Selective loss of imprinting in the placenta following preimplantation development in culture. *Development.* 2004;131:3727–3735.

217. Wolf SF, Jolly DJ, Lunnen KD, Friedmann T, Migeon BR. Methylation of the HPRT locus on the human X: implications for X inactivation. *Proc Natl Acad Sci USA.* 1984;81:2806–2810.

218. Mohandas T, Sparkes RS, Shapiro LJ. Reactivation of an inactive human X chromosome; evidence for X inactivation by DNA methylation. *Science.* 1981;211:393–396.

219. Luo S, Torchia BS, Migeon BR. XIST expression is repressed when X inactivation is reversed in human placental cells: a model for study of XIST regulation. *Somat Cell Mol Genet.* 1995;21:51–60.

220. Migeon BR, Axelman J, Jeppesen P. Differential X reactivation in human placental cells: implications for reversal of X inactivation. *Am J Hum Genet.* 2005;77:355–364.

221. Takagi N, Sasaki M. Preferential inactivation of the paternally derived X chromosome in the extraembryonic membranes of the mouse. *Nature.* 1975;256:640–642.

222. Torchia BS, Call LM, Migeon BR. DNA replication analysis of FMR1, XIST and F8C loci by fluorescence in situ hybridization indicates non-transcribed X-linked genes replicate late. *Am J Hum Genet.* 1994;55:96–104.

223. Torchia BS, Migeon BR. The XIST locus replicates late on active X, and earlier on the inactive X based on FISH DNA replication analysis of somatic cell hybrids. *Somat Cell Mol Genet.* 1995;21:327–333.

224. Hansen RS, Canfield TK, Fjeld AD, Gartler SM. Role of late replication timing in the silencing of X-linked genes. *Hum Mol Genet.* 1996;5:1345–1353.

225. Gribnau J, Luikenhuis S, Hochedlinger K, Monkhorst K, Jaenisch R. X chromosome choice occurs independently of asynchronous replication timing. *J Cell Biol.* 2005;168:365–373.

226. Lande-Diner L, Cedar H. Silence of the genes—mechanisms of long-term repression. *Nat Rev Genet.* 2005;6:648–654.

227. Jacob F. Complexity and tinkering. *Ann NY Acad Sci.* 2001;929:71–73.

228. Grant J, Mahadevaiah SK, Khil P., et al. Rsx is a metatherian RNA with Xist-like properties in X-chromosome inactivation. *Nature.* 2012;487(7406):254–258.

229. Chang SC, Brown CJ. Identification of regulatory elements flanking human XIST reveals species differences. *BMC Mol Biol.* 2010;11:20.

230. Migeon BR. Is Tsix repression of Xist specific to mouse? *Nat Genet.* 2003;33: 337; author reply 337–338.

231. Tian D, Sun S, Lee, JT. The long noncoding RNA, Jpx, is a molecular switch for X chromosome inactivation. *Cell.* 2010;143:390–403.

232. Chureau C, Chantalat S, Romito A., et al. Ftx is a non-coding RNA which affects Xist expression and chromatin structure within the X-inactivation center region. *Hum Mol Genet.* 2010;20(4):705–718.

233. Clerc P, Avner P. Perspective: new lessons from random X-chromosome inactivation in the mouse. *J Mol Biol.* 2011.

234. Bach, I. Releasing the break on X chromosome inactivation: Rnf12/RLIM targets REX1 for degradation. *Cell Res.* 2012;22:1524–1526.

235. Vallot C, Huret C, Lesecque Y, et al. XACT, a long noncoding transcript coating the active X chromosome in human pluripotent cells. *Nat Genet.* 2013; 45(3):239–241.

236. Jegalian K, Page DC. A proposed path by which genes common to mammalian X and Y chromosomes evolve to become X inactivated. *Nature.* 1998;394:776–780.

237. Okamoto I, Arnaud D, Le Baccon P, et al. Evidence for de novo imprinted X-chromosome inactivation independent of meiotic inactivation in mice. *Nature.* 2005;438:369–373.

238. Migeon BR, Jan de Beur S, Axelman J. Frequent derepression of G6PD and HPRT on the marsupial X chromosome. *Exp Cell Res.* 1989;182:597–609.

239. Lock LF, Takagi N, Martin GR. Methylation of the HPRT gene on the inactive X occurs after chromosome inactivation. *Cell.* 1987;48:39–46.

240. Riggs AD. DNA methylation and cell memory. *Cell Biophys.* 1989;15:1–13.

241. Toniolo D, Martini G, Migeon BR, Dono R. Expression of the G6PD locus on the human X chromosome is associated with demethylation of three CpG clusters within 100 kb of DNA. *EMBO J.* 1988;7:401–406.

242. Loebel DA, Johnston PG. Methylation analysis of a marsupial X-linked CpG island by bisulfate genomic sequencing. *Genome Res.* 1996;6:114–123.

243. Luo S, Robinson JC, Reiss AL, Migeon BR. DNA methylation of the fragile X locus in somatic and germ cells during fetal development: relevance to the fragile X syndrome and X inactivation. *Somat Cell Mol Genet.* 1993;19:393–404.

244. McCarrey JR, Watson C, Atencio J, et al. X chromosome inactivation during spermatogenesis is regulated by Xist/Tsix-independent mechanism in the mouse. *Genesis.* 2002;34:257–266.

245. Goodfellow P, Mondello C, Darling S, Pym B, Little P, Goodfellow P. Absence of methylation of a CpG-rich region at the 5′ end of the MIC2 gene on the active X, the inactive X and the Y chromosome. *Proc Natl Acad Sci USA.* 1988;85:5605–5609.

246. Mondello C, Goodfellow PJ, Goodfellow PN. Analysis of methylation of a human X located gene which escapes X inactivation. *Nucleic Acids Res.* 1988;16:6813–6824.

247. Li XM, Alperin ES, Salido E, Gong Y, Yen P, Shapiro LJ. Characterization of the promoter region of human steroid sulfatase: a gene which excapes X inactivation. *Somat Cell Mol Genet.* 1996;22:105–117.

248. Ruta Cullen C, Hubberman P, Kaslow DC, Migeon BR. Comparison of Factor IX methylation on human active and inactive X chromosomes: implications for X inactivation and transcription of tissue-specific genes. *EMBO J.* 1986;5:2223–2229.

249. Berletch JB, Yang F, Xu J, Carrel L, Disteche CM. Genes that escape from X inactivation. *Hum Genet.* 2011;130:237–245.

250. Ke X, Collins A. CpG islands in human X-inactivation. *Ann Hum Genet.* 2003;67(pt 3):42–49.

251. Ciavatta D, Kalantry S, Magnuson T, Smithies O. A DNA insulator prevents repression of a targeted X-linked transgene but not its random or imprinted X inactivation. *Proc Natl Acad Sci USA.* 2006;103:9956–9963.

252. Percec I, Thorvaldsen JL, Plenge RM, et al. An N-ethyl-N-nitrosourea mutagenesis screen for epigenetic mutations in the mouse. *Genetics.* 2003;164:1481–1494.

253. Xue F, Tian C, Du F, et al. Aberrant patterns of X chromosome inactivation in bovine clones. *Nat Genet.* 2002;31:216–220.

254. Cooper DW, VandeBerg JL, Sharman GB, Poole WE. Phosphoglycerate kinase polymorphism in kangaroos provides further evidence for paternal X inactivation. *Nat New Biol.* 1971;230:155–157.

255. Ropers HH, Wolf G, Hitzeroth HW. Preferential X-inactivation in human placenta membranes: is the paternal X inactive in early embryonic development of female mammals? *Hum Genet.* 1978;43:265–273.

256. Harrison KB. X-chromosome inactivation in the human cytotrophoblast. *Cytogenet Cell Genet.* 1989;52:37–41.

257. Migeon BR, Do TT. In search of non-random X inactivation: studies of fetal membranes heterozygous for glucose-6–phosphate dehydrogenase. *Am J Hum Genet.* 1979;31:581–585.

258. van den Hurk JA, Hendriks W, van de Pol DJ, et al. Mouse choroideremia gene mutation causes photoreceptor cell degeneration and is not transmitted through the female germline. *Hum Mol Genet.* 1997;6:851–858.

259. Rodriguez TA, Sparrow DB, Scott AN, et al. Cited 1 is required in trophoblasts for placental development and for embryo growth and survival. *Mol Cell Biol.* 2004;24:228–244.

260. Willemsen R, Carola JM, Severijnen L-A, Oostra BA. Timing of the absence of FMR1 expression in full mutation chorionic villi. *Hum Genet.* 2002;110:601–605.

261. Wilkins JF, Haig D. Genomic imprinting of two antagonistic loci. *Proc Biol Sci.* 2001;268:1861–1867.

262. Fedoriw AM, Engel NI, Bartolomei MS. Genomic imprinting: antagonistic mechanisms in the germ line and early embryo. *Cold Spring Harb Symp Quant Biol.* 2004;69:39–45.

263. Bjornsson HT, Cui H, Gius D, Fallin MD, Feinberg AP. The new field of epigenomics: implications for cancer and other common disease research. *Cold Spring Harb Symp Quant Biol.* 2004;69:447–456.

264. Monk M, McLaren A. X-chromosome activitiy in foetal germ cells of the mouse. *J Embryol Exp Morphol.* 1981;63:75–84.

265. Wang PJ, Page DC, McCarrey JR. Differential expression of sex-linked and autosomal germ-cell-specific genes during spermatogenesis in the mouse. *Hum Mol Genet.* 2005;14:2911–2918.

266. Salido EC, Yen PH, Mohandas TK, Shapiro LJ. Expression of the X-inactivation associated gene XIST during spermatogenesis. *Nat Genet.* 1992;2:196–199.

267. Norris NP, Patel D, Kay GF, et al. Evidence that random and imprinted Xist expression is controlled by preemptive methylation. *Cell.* 1994;77:41–51.

268. Warshawsky D, Stavropoulos N, Lee JT. Further examination of the Xist promoter-switch hypothesis in X inactivation: evidence against the existence and function of a P0 promoter. *Proc Natl Acad Sci USA*. 1999;96:14424–14429.

269. Heard E, Clerc P, Avner P. X-chromosome inactivation in mammals. *Annu Rev Genet*. 1997;31:572–610.

270. Masui O, Bonnet I, Le Baccon P, et al. Live-cell chromosome dynamics and outcome of X chromosome pairing events during ES cell differentiation. *Cell*. 2011;145;447–458.

271. Lyon MF, Rastan S. Paternal source of chromosome imprinting and its relevance for X chromosome inactivation. *Differentiation*. 1984;26:63–67.

272. Tada T, Obata T, Tada M, et al. Imprint switching for non-random X-inactivation during mouse oocyte growth. *Development*. 2000;127:3101–3105.

273. Boumil RM, Lee JT. Forty years of decoding the silence in X-chromosome inactivation. *Hum Mol Genet*. 2001;10:2225–2232.

274. Chao W, Huynh KD, Spencer RJ, Davidow LS, Lee JT. CTCF, a candidate transacting factor for X-inactivation. *Science*. 2002;295:345–347.

275. Sado T, Hoki Y, Sasaki H. Tsix silences Xist through modification of chromatin structure. *Dev Cell*. 2005;9(1):159–165.

276. Ohhata T, Senner CE, Hemberger M, Wutz A. Lineage-specific function of the noncoding Tsix RNA for Xist repression and Xi reactivation in mice. *Genes Dev*. 2011;25:1702–1715.

277. Navarro P, Oldfield, A, Legoupi J, et al. Molecular coupling of Tsix regulation and pluripotency. *Nature*. 2010;468:457–460.

278. Wutz A, Smrzkat OW, Schweifert N, Schellanders K, Wagner EF, Barlow DP. Imprinted expression of the Ig2r gene depends on an intronic CpG island. *Nature*. 1997;389:743–749.

279. Onyango P, Miller W, Lehoczky J, et al. Sequence and comparative analysis of the mouse 1–Megabase region orthologous to the human 11p15 imprinted domain. *Genome Res*. 2000;10:1697–1710.

280. Migeon BR. Non-random X chromosome inactivation in mammalian cells. *Cytogenet Cell Genet*. 1998;80:142–148.

281. Farazmand A, Basur PK, Graphodatskaya G, Reyes ER, King WA. Expression of XIST sense and antisense in bovine fetal organs and cell cultures. *Chromosome Res*. 2004;12:275–283.

282. Lyon MF. Epigenetic inheritance in mammals. *Trends in Genetics*. 1993;9:123–128.

283. Tachibana M, Ma, H, Sparman, ML, et al. X-chromosome inactivation in monkey embryos and pluripotent stem cells. *Dev Biol*. 2012;371(2):146–155.

284. Johnston PG, Robinson ES. X chromosome inactivation in female embryos of a marsupial mouse (*Antechinus stuartii*). *Chromosoma*. 1987;95:419–423.

285. Hajkova P, Surani M. Programming the X chromosome. *Science*. 2004;303:633–634.

286. De La Fuente R, Hahnel N, Basrur PK, King WA. X inactive-specific transcript (Xist) expression and X chromosome inactivation in the preattachment bovine embryo. *Biol Reprod*. 1999;60:769–775.

287. Park WW. The occurrence of sex chromatin in early human and macaque embryos. *J Anat*. 1957;91:369–373.

288. O'Rahilly R. *Developmental Stages in Human Embryos. Part A: Embryos of the First Three Weeks (Stages 1 to 9).* Publication no. 631. Washington, DC: Carnegie Institution of Washington; 1973:167.

289. Migeon BR, Do TT. In search of nonrandom X inactivation: studies of the placenta from newborns heterozygous for glucose-6–phosphate dehydrogenase. In: Russell LB, ed. *Genetic Mosaics and Chimeras in Mammals.* New York: Plenum Publishing; 1978:379–391.

290. Adler DA, Rugarli EI, Lingenfelter PA, et al. Evidence of evolutionary up-regulation of the single active X chromosome in mammals based on Clc4 expression levels in Mus spretus and Mus musculus. *Proc Natl Acad Sci USA.* 1997;94:9244–9248.

291. Lyon MF. Mechanisms and evolutionary origins of variable X-chromosome activity in mammals. *Proc R Soc Lond B Biol Sci.* 1974;187:243–268.

292. Nguyen DK, Disteche CM. Dosage compensation of the active X chromosome in mammals. *Nat Genet.* 2005;38:47–53.

293. Deng X, Hiatt JB, Nguyen DK, et al. Evidence for compensatory upregulation of expressed X-linked genes in mammals, Caenorhabditis elegans and Drosophila melanogaster. *Nat Genet.* 2011;43;1179–1185.

294. Sybert VP. The adult patient with Turner syndrome. In: Albertsson-Wikland K, Ranke MB, eds. *Turner Syndrome in a Life Span Perspective: Research and Clinical Aspects.* Gothenburg, Sweden: Elsevier Science; 1995:205–218.

295. Jacobs PA, Betts PR, Cockwell AE, et al. A cytogenetic and molecular reappraisal of a series of patients with Turner's syndrome. *Ann Hum Genet.* 1990;54:209–223.

296. Skuse DH, James RS, Bishop DV, et al. Evidence from Turner's syndrome of an imprinted X-linked locus affecting cognitive function. *Nature.* 1997;387:705–708.

297. Clement-Jones M, Schiller S, Rao E, et al. The short stature homeobox gene SHOX is involved in skeletal abnormalities in Turner syndrome. *Hum Mol Genet.* 2000;9:695–702.

298. Twigg SR, Babbs C, van den Elzen ME, et al. Cellular interference in craniofrontonasal syndrome: males mosaic for mutations in the X-linked EFNB1 gene are more severely affected than true hemizygotes. *Hum Mol Genet.* 2013;22(8):1654–1662.

299. Urbach A, Benvenisty N. Studying early lethality of 45,X0 (Turner's syndrome) embryos using human embryonic stem cells. *PLoS One.* 2009;4:e4175.

300. Gropman A, Samango-Sprouse, CA. Neurocognitive variance and neurological underpinnings of the X and Y chromosomal variations. *Am J Med Genet C Semin Med Genet.* 2013;163(1):35–431.

301. Pennington B, Puck M, Robinson A. Language and cognitive development in 47,XXX females followed since birth. *Behav Genet.* 1980;10:31–41.

302. Ratcliffe S, Pan H, McKie M. The growth of XXX females: population-based studies. *Ann Hum Biol.* 1994;21:57–66.

303. Alvesalo L, Tammisalo E, Therman E. 47,XXX females, sex chromosomes, and tooth crown structure. *Hum Genet.* 1987;77:345–348.

304. Swerdlow AJ, Schoemaker MJ, Higgins CD, Wright AF, Jacobs PA. Mortality and cancer incidence in women with extra X chromosomes: a cohort study in Britain. *Hum Genet.* 2005;118:255–260.

305. Van Dyke DL, Witkor A, Palmer CG, et al. Ullrich-Turner syndrome with a small ring chromosome and presence of mental retardation. *Am J Med Genet.* 1992;43:996–1005.

306. Lachlan KL, Collinson MN, Sandford RO, van Zyl B, Jacobs PA, Thomas NS. Functional disomy resulting from duplications of distal Xq in four unrelated patients. *Hum Genet.* 2004;115:399–408.

307. Schmidt M, Du Sart D. Functional disomies of the X chromosome influence the cell selection and hence the X inactivation pattern in females with balanced X autosome translocations: a review of 122 cases. *Am J Med Genet.* 1992;42:161–169.

308. Doshi N, Surti U, Szulman AE. Morphologic anomalies in triploid liveborn fetuses. *Hum Pathol.* 1883;14:716–723.

309. Jacobs PA, Hassold T. The origin of numerical chromosome abnormalities. *Adv Genet.* 1995;33:101–133.

310. Turner HH. A syndrome of infantilism, congenital webbed neck and cubitus valgus. *Endocrinology.* 1938;23:566–574.

311. Dobyns WBF, Filauro A, Tomson BN, Chan AS, et al. Inheritance of most X-linked traits is not dominant or recessive, just X-linked. *Am J Med Genet.* 2004;129:136–143.

312. Harris H. *The Principles of Human Biochemical Genetics.* 3rd rev ed. Amsterdam: Elsevier/North Holland; 1980.

313. Gruneberg H. The molars of the tabby mouse, and a test of the "single-active X-chromosome" hypothesis. *J Embryol Exp Morphol.* 1966;5:223–244.

314. Mintz B. Gene control of mammalian pigmentary differentiation. I. Clonal origin of melanocytes. *Proc Natl Acad Sci USA.* 1967;58:344–351.

315. Happle R. X-chromosome inactivation: role in skin disease expression. *Acta Paediatr Suppl.* 2006;95:16–23.

316. Novelli M, Cossu A, Oukrif D, et al. X-inactivation patch size in human female tissue confounds the assessment of tumor clonality. *Proc Natl Acad Sci U S A.* 2003;100:3311–3314.

317. Migeon BR. X inactivation, female mosaicism, and sex differences in renal diseases. *J Am Soc Nephrol.* 2008;19:2052–2059.

318. Migeon BR. Selection and cell communication as determinants of female phenotype. In: Russell LB, ed. *Genetic Mosaics and Chimeras in Mammals.* New York: Plenum Publishing; 1978:417–432.

319. Mehta A, Ricci R, Widmer U, et al. Fabry disease defined: baseline clinical manifestations of 366 patients in the Fabry Outcome Survey. *Eur J Clin Invest.* 2004;34:236–242.

320. Wieland I, Jakubiczka S, Muschke P, et al. Mutations of the ephrin-B1 gene cause craniofrontonasal syndrome. *Am J Hum Genet.* 2004;74:1209–1215.

321. Twigg SRF, Kan R, Babbs C, et al. Mutations of ephrin-B1 (EFNB1), a marker of tissue boundary formation, cause craniofrontonasal syndrome. *Proc Natl Acad Sci USA.* 2004;101:8652–8657.

322. Davy A, Bush JO, Soriano P. Inhibition of gap junction communication at ectopic Eph/ephrin boundaries underlies craniofrontonasal syndrome. *PLoS Biol.* 2006;4:e315.

323. Dibbens LM, Tarpey PS, Hynes K, et al. X-linked protocadherin 19 mutations cause female-limited epilepsy and cognitive impairment. *Nat Genet.* 2008;40:776–781.

324. Depienne C, Bouteiller D, Keren B, et al. Sporadic infantile epileptic encephalopathy caused by mutations in PCDH19 resembles Dravet syndrome but mainly affects females. *PLoS Genet.* 2009;5:e1000381.

325. Bienzle U, Ayeni O, Lucas AO, Luzzatto L. Glucose-6-phosphate dehydrogenase and malaria. Greater resistance of females heterozygous for enzyme deficiency and of males with non-deficient variant. *Lancet.* 1972;1:107–110.

326. Luzzatto, L. G6PD deficiency and malaria selection. *Heredity (Edinb).* 2012; 108:456.

327. Usanga EA, Luzzatto L. Adaptation of Plasmodium falciparum to glucose 6–phosphate dehydrogenase-deficient host red cells by production of parasite-encoded enzyme. *Nature.* 1985;313:793–795.

328. Dewey MJ, Martin DJ, Martin G, Mintz B. Mosaic mice with teratocarcinoma-derived mutant cells deficient in hypoxanthine phosphoribosyltransferase. *Proc Natl Acad Sci USA.* 1977;74:5564–5568.

329. Migeon BR. Studies of skin fibroblasts from 10 families with HGPRT deficiency, with reference to X-chromosomal inactivation. *Am J Hum Genet.* 1971;23:199–210.

330. Belmont JW. Genetic control of X inactivation and processes leading to X-inactivation skewing. *Am J Hum Genet.* 1996;58:1101–1108.

331. Nyhan WL, Bakay B, Oconnor, J DO, Marks JF, Keele DK. Hemizygous expression of glucose-6-phosphate dehydrogenase in erythrocytes of heterozygotes for the Lesch-Nyhan syndrome. *Proc Natl Acad Sci USA.* 1970;65:214–218.

332. Bicocchi MP, Migeon BR, Pasino M, et al. Familial nonrandom inactivation linked to the X inactivation centre in heterozygotes manifesting haemophilia A. *Eur J Hum Genet.* 2005;13:635–640.

333. Allen RC, Zoghbi HY, Moseley AB, Rosenblatt HM, Belmont JW. Methylation of HpaII and HhaI sites near the polymorphic CAG repeat in the human androgen-receptor gene correlates with X chromosome inactivation. *Am J Hum Genet.* 1992;51:1229–1239.

334. Rozowsky J, Abyzov A, Wang J, et al. AlleleSeq: analysis of allele-specific expression and binding in a network framework. *Mol Syst Biol.* 2011;7:522.

335. Wang X, Soloway PD, Clark AG. Paternally biased X inactivation in mouse neonatal brain. *Genome Biol.* 2010;11:R79.

336. Plenge RM, Stevenson RA, Lubs HA, Schwartz CE, Willard HF. Skewed X-chromosome inactivation is a common feature of X-linked mental retardation disorders. *Am J Hum Genet.* 2002;71:168–173.

337. Nance WE. Do twin lyons have larger spots? *Am J Hum Genet.* 1990;46:646–648.

338. Puck JM. The timing of twinning: more insights from X inactivation. *Am J Hum Genet.* 1998;63:327–328.

339. Lau AW, Brown CJ, Penaherrera M, Langlois S, Kalousek D, Robinson WP. Skewed X-chromosome inactivation is common in fetuses or newborns associated with confined placental mosaicism. *Am J Hum Genet.* 1997;61:1353–1361.

340. Sharp A, Robinson D, Jacobs P. Age- and tissue-specific variation of X chromosome inactivation ratios in normal women. *Hum Genet.* 2000;107: 343–349.

341. Sandovici I, Naumova A, Leppert M, Linares Y, Sapienza C. A longitudinal study of X-inactivation ratio in human females. *Hum Genet.* 2004;115:387–392.

342. Kristiansen M, Knudsen GP, Bathum L, et al. Twin study of genetic and aging effects on X chromosome inactivation. *Eur J Hum Genet.* 2005;13:599–606.

343. Hatakeyama C, Anderson CL, Beever CL, Penaherrera MS, Brown CJ, Robinson WP. The dynamics of X-inactivation skewing as women age. *Clin Genet.* 2004;66:327–332.

344. Migeon BR, Axelman J, Jan de Beur, S, Valle D, Mitchell GA, Rosenbaum KN. Selection against lethal alleles in females heterozygous for incontinentia pigmenti. *Am J Hum Genet.* 1989;44:100–106.

345. Martinez-Pomar N, Munoz-Saa I, Heine-Suner D, Martin A, Smahi A, Matamoros N. A new mutation in exon 7 of NEMO gene: late skewed X-chromosome inactivation in an incontinentia pigmenti female patient with immunodeficiency. *Hum Genet.* 2005;118:458–465.

346. de Camargo Pinto LL, Maluf SW, Leistner-Segal S, et al. Are MPS II heterozygotes actually asymptomatic? A study based on clinical and biochemical data, X-inactivation analysis and imaging evaluations. *Am J Med Genet A.* 2011;155A:50–57.

347. Lin T, Lewis RA, Nussbaum RL. Molecular confirmation of carriers for Lowe syndrome. *Ophthalmology.* 1999;106:119–122.

348. Roschinger W, Muntau AC, Rudolph G, Roscher AA, Kammerer S. Carrier assessment in families with lowe oculocerebrorenal syndrome: novel mutations in the OCRL1 gene and correlation of direct DNA diagnosis with ocular examination. *Mol Genet Metab.* 2000;69:213–222.

349. Cau M, Addis M, Congiu R., et al. A locus for familial skewed X chromosome inactivation maps to chromosome Xq25 in a family with a female manifesting Lowe syndrome. *J Hum Genet.* 2006;51:1030–1036.

350. Seemann N., Selby, K., McAdam, L., et al. Symptomatic dystrophinopathies in female children. *Neuromuscul Disord.* 2011;21:172–177.

351. Mercier S, Toutain A, Toussaint A, et al. Genetic and clinical specificity of 26 symptomatic carriers for dystrophinopathies at pediatric age. *Eur J Hum Genet.* 2013. doi:10.1038/ejhg.2012.269.

352. Zou Y, Liu Q, Chen B, et al. Mutation in CUL4B, which encodes a member of cullin-RING ubiquitin ligase complex, causes X-linked mental retardation. *Am J Hum Genet.* 2007;80:561–566.

353. Jiang B, Zhao W, Yuan J, et al. Lack of cul4b, an e3 ubiquitin ligase component, leads to embryonic lethality and abnormal placental development. *PLoS One.* 2012;7:e37070.

354. Young JI, Zoghbi HY. X-chromosome inactivation patterns are unbalanced and affect the phenotypic outcome in a mouse model of Rett syndrome. *Am J Hum Genet.* 2004;74:511–520.

355. Thomas GH. High male:female ratio of germ-line mutations: an alternative explanation for postulated gestational lethality in males in X-linked dominant disorders. *Am J Hum Genet.* 1996;58:1364–1368.

356. Oostra BA, Willemsen R. The X chromosome and fragile X mental retardation. *Cytogenet Genome Res.* 2002;99:257–264.

357. Migeon BR, Moser HW, Moser AB, Sprenkle JA, Sillence D, Norum RA. Adrenoleukodystrophy: evidence for X-linkage, inactivation and selection favoring the mutant allele in heterozygous cells. *Proc Natl Acad Sci USA.* 1981;78:5066–5070.

358. Jangouk P, Zackowski KM, Naidu S, Raymond, GV. Adrenoleukodystrophy in female heterozygotes: underrecognized and undertreated. *Mol Genet Metab.* 2012;105:180–185.

359. Merrill AE, Bochukova EG, Brugger SM, et al. Cell mixing at a neural crest-mesoderm boundary and deficient ephrin-Eph signaling in the pathogenesis of craniosynostosis. *Hum Mol Genet.* 2006;15:1319–1328.

360. Robertson SP, Twigg SRF, Sutherland-Smith AJ, et al. Localized mutations in the gene encoding the cytoskeletal protein filamin A cause diverse malformations in humans. *Nat Genet.* 2003;33:487–491.

361. Ferrante MI, Giorgio G, Feather SA, et al. Identification of the gene for oral-facial-digital type I syndrome. *Am J Hum Genet.* 2001;68:569–576.

362. Thauvin-Robinet C, Cossee M, Cormier-Daire V, et al. Clinical, molecular, and genotype-phenotype correlation studies from 25 cases of oral-facial-digital syndrome type 1: a French and Belgian collaborative study. *J Med Genet.* 2006;43:54–61.

363. Weksberg R, Shuman C, Caluseriu O, et al. Discordant KCNQ1OT1 imprinting in sets of monozygotic twins discordant for Beckwith-Wiedemann syndrome. *Hum Mol Genet.* 2002;11:1317–1325.

364. Weksberg R, Shuman C, Smith AC. Beckwith-Wiedemann syndrome. *Am J Med Genet C Semin Med Genet.* 2005;137:12–23.

365. Butler MG, Theodoro MF, Bittel DC, Kuipers PJ, Driscoll DJ, Talebizadeh Z. X-chromosome inactivation patterns in females with Prader-Willi syndrome. *Am J Med Genet A.* 2006;143:469–475.

366. Stewart J. The female X-inactivation mosaic in systemic lupus erythematosus. *Immunol Today.* 1998;19:352–357.

367. Ozbalkan Z, Bagslar S, Kiraz S, et al. Skewed X-chromosome inactivation in blood cells of females with scleroderma. *Arthritis Rheum.* 2005;52:1564–1570.

368. Chitnis S, Monteiro J, Glass D, et al. The role of X-chromosome inactivation in female predisposition to autoimmunity. *Arthritis Res.* 2000;2:399–406.

369. Brix TH, Knudsen GP, Kristiansen M, Ohm KK, Orstavik KH, Hegedus L. High frequency of skewed X chromosome inactivation in females with autoimmune thyroid disease. A possible explanation for the female predisposition to thyroid autoimmunity. *J Clin Endocrinol Metab.* 2005;90:5949–5953.

370. Ozcelik T, Uz F, Akyerli CB, et al. Evidence from autoimmune thyroiditis of skewed X-chromosome inactivation in female predisposition to autoimmunity. *Eur J Hum Genet.* 2006;14:791–797.

371. Selmi C, Brunetta E, Raimondo MG, Meroni PL. The X chromosome and the sex ratio of autoimmunity. *Autoimmun Rev.* 2012;11:A531-A537.

372. Bianchi I, Lleo A, Gershwin ME, Invernizzi P. The X chromosome and immune associated genes. *J Autoimmun.* 2012;38:J187-J192.

373. Kunkel LM. 2004 William Allan Award address. Cloning of the DMD gene. *Am J Hum Genet.* 2005;76:205–214.

374. Migeon BR, McGinniss MJ, Antonarakis SE, et al. Severe hemophilia A in a female by cryptic translocation: order and orientation of factor VIII within Xq28. *Genomics.* 1993;16:20–25.

375. Mazurier C, Parquet-Gernez A, Gaucher C, Lavergne JM, Goudemand J. Factor VIII deficiency not induced by FBKKK gene mutation in a female first cousin of two brothers with haemophilia A. *Br J Haematol.* 2002;119:390–392.

376. Coleman R, Genet SA, Harper J, Wilke A. Interaction of incontinentia pigmenti and factor VIII mutations in a female with biased X inactivation, resulting in haemophilia. *J Med Genet.* 1993;30:497–500.

377. Hansmann T, Pliushch G, Leubner M, et al. Constitutive promoter methylation of BRCA1 and RAD51C in patients with familial ovarian cancer and early-onset sporadic breast cancer. *Hum Mol Genet.* 2012;21:4669–4679.

378. Esteller M, Silva JM, Dominguez G, et al. Promoter hypermethylation and BRCA1 inactivation in sporadic breast and ovarian tumors. *J Natl Cancer Inst.* 2000;92:564–569.

379. Knudson AG Jr. Mutation and cancer: statistical study of retinoblastoma. *Proc Natl Acad Sci U S A.* 1971;68:820–823.

380. Abramowitz LK, Bartolomei MS. Genomic imprinting: recognition and marking of imprinted loci. *Curr Opin Genet Dev.* 2012;22:72–78.

381. Horsthemke, B. Mechanisms of imprint dysregulation. *Am J Med Genet C Semin Med Genet.* 2010;154C:321–328.

382. Buiting K, Gross S, Lich C, Gillessen-Kaesbach G, el-Maarri O, Horsthemke B. Epimutations in Prader-Willi and Angelman syndromes: a molecular study of 136 patients with an imprinting defect. *Am J Hum Genet.* 2003;72:571–577.

383. Skinner MK. Environmental epigenomics and disease susceptibility. *EMBO Rep.* 2011;12:620–622.

384. Daxinger L, Whitelaw E. Transgenerational epigenetic inheritance: more questions than answers. *Genome Res.* 2010;20:1623–1628.

385. Bartolomei MS, Ferguson-Smith AC. Mammalian genomic imprinting. *Cold Spring Harb Perspect Biol.* 2011;3(7):a002592.

386. Yang X, Schadt EE, Wang S., et al. Tissue-specific expression and regulation of sexually dimorphic genes in mice. *Genome Res.* 2006;16:995–1004.

387. De Vries GJ, Rissman EF, Simerly RB, et al. A model system for study of sex chromosome effects on sexually dimorphic neural and behavioral traits. *J Neurosci.* 2002;22:9005–9014.

388. Wijchers PJ, Yandim C, Panousopoulou E., et al. Sexual dimorphism in mammalian autosomal gene regulation is determined not only by Sry but by sex chromosome complement as well. *Dev Cell.* 2010;19:477–484.

389. Wijchers PJ, Festenstein RJ. Epigenetic regulation of autosomal gene expression by sex chromosomes. *Trends Genet.* 2011;27:132–140.

390. Arnold AP. The end of gonad-centric sex determination in mammals. *Trends Genet.* 2012;28:55–61.

391. Davidsson J, Lilljebjorn H, Andersson A., et al. The DNA methylome of pediatric acute lymphoblastic leukemia. *Hum Mol Genet.* 2009;18:4054–4065.

392. Baylin SB, Jones PA. A decade of exploring the cancer epigenome—biological and translational implications. *Nat Rev Cancer.* 2011;11:726–734.

393. Kerkel K, Schupf N, Hatta K, et al. Altered DNA methylation in leukocytes with trisomy 21. *PLoS Genet.* 2010;6:e1001212.

394. Hendrich B, Bickmore W. Human diseases with underlying defects in chromatin structure and modification. *Hum Mol Genet.* 2001;10:2233–2242.

395. Bickmore WA, van der Maarel SM. Perturbations of chromatin structure in human genetic disease: recent advances. *Hum Mol Genet.* 2003;12(Suppl 2), R207-R213.

396. Hansen RS, Stoger R, Wijmenga C, et al. Escape from gene silencing in ICF syndrome: evidence for advanced replication time as a major determinant. *Hum Mol Genet.* 2000;9:2575–2587.

397. Muers MR, Sharpe JA, Garrick D, et al. Defining the cause of skewed X-chromosome inactivation in X-linked mental retardation by use of a mouse model. *Am J Hum Genet.* 2007;80:1138–1149.

398. Simensen RJ, Abidi F, Collins JS, Schwartz CE, Stevenson RE. Cognitive function in Coffin-Lowry syndrome. *Clin Genet.* 2002;61:299–304.

399. Wang Y, Martinez JE, Wilson GL, et al. A novel RSK2 (RPS6KA3) gene mutation associated with abnormal brain MRI findings in a family with Coffin-Lowry syndrome. *Am J Med Genet A.* 2006;140:1274–1279.

400. Berletch, J.B., Deng, X., Nguyen, D.K., and Disteche, C.M. Female bias in Rhox6 and 9 regulation by the histone demethylase KDM6A. PLOS Genetics . 2013:9(5):e1003489.

401. Lederer D, Grisart B, Digilio MC, et al. Deletion of KDM6A, a histone demethylase interacting with MLL2, in three patients with Kabuki syndrome. *Am J Hum Genet.* 2012;90:119–124.

402. Welstead, G.G., Creyghton, M.P., Bilodeau, S., Cheng, A.W., Markoulaki, S., Young, R.A., and Jaenisch, R. X-linked H3K27me3 demethylase Utx is required for embryonic development in a sex-specific manner. Proc Natl Acad Sci U S A 2012:109, 13004–13009.

403. Miyake N, Mizuno S, Okamoto N, et al. KDM6A point mutations cause Kabuki syndrome. *Hum Mutat.* 2012;34(1):108–110.

404. Veitia RA, Bottani S, Birchler JA. Cellular reactions to gene dosage imbalance: genomic, transcriptomic and proteomic effects. *Trends Genet.* 2008;24:390–397.

405. Berdasco M, Esteller M. Genetic syndromes caused by mutations in epigenetic genes. *Hum Genet.* 2013;132(4):359–383.

406. Yang C, Rahimpour S, Lu J, et al. Histone deacetylase inhibitors increase glucocerebrosidase activity in Gaucher disease by modulation of molecular chaperones. *Proc Natl Acad Sci U S A.* 2012;110(3):966–971.

407. Childs B. *Genetic Medicine.* Baltimore, MD: Johns Hopkins University Press; 1999.

408. Sekido R, Lovell-Badge R. Genetic control of testis development. *Sex Dev.* 2013; 7(1–3):21–32.

409. Hughes IA. Female development—all by default? *N Engl J Med.* 2004;351: 748–750.

410. Parma P, Radi O, Vidal V, et al. R-spondin1 is essential in sex determination, skin differentiation and malignancy. *Nat Genet.* 2006;38:1304–1309.

411. Yao HH-C. The pathway to femaleness: current knowledge on embryonic development of the ovary. *Mol Cell Endocrinol.* 2005;230:87–93.

412. Spelke ES. Sex differences in intrinsic aptitude for mathematics and science? A critical review. *Am Psychol.* 2005;60:950–958.

413. Fairfield H. Girls lead in science exam, but not in the United States. *New York Times,* February 4, 2012. http://www.nytimes.com/interactive/2013/02/04/science/girls-lead-in-science-exam-but-not-in-the-united-states.html. Accessed May 4, 2013.

414. Azim E, Mobbs D, Jo B, Menon V, Reiss AL. Sex differences in brain activation elicited by humor. *Proc Natl Acad Sci USA.* 2005;102:16496–16501.

415. Chen X, McClusky R, Chen J, et al. The number of X chromosomes causes sex differences in adiposity in mice. *PLoS Genet.* 2012;8:e1002709.

416. Meyer-Lindenberg A, Buckholtz JW, Kolachana B, et al. Neural mechanisms of genetic risk for impulsivity and violence in humans. *Proc Natl Acad Sci USA.* 2006;103:6269–6274.

417. Smallwood PM, Oveczky BP, Williams GL, et al. Genetically engineered mice with an additional class of cone photoreceptors: implications for the evolution of color vision. *Proc Natl Acad Sci USA.* 2003;100:11706–11711.

418. Shah NM, Pisapia DJ, Maniatis S, Mendelsohn MM, Nemes A, Axel R. Visualizing sexual dimorphism in the brain. *Neuron.* 2004;43:313–319.

419. Haack TB, Hogarth P, Kruer MC, et al. Exome sequencing reveals de novo WDR45 mutations causing a phenotypically distinct, X-linked dominant form of NBIA. *Am J Hum Genet.* 2012;91(6):1144–1149.

420. Migeon BR. X-chromosome inactivation: molecular mechanisms and genetic consequences. *Trends Genet.* 1994;10:230–235.

421. Crouse HV. The controlling element in sex chromosome behavior in *Sciara*. *Genetics.* 1960;45:1429–1443.

422. Kushnick T, Irons TG, Wiley JE, Gettis EA, Rao KW, Bowyer S. 45X/46/Xr(X) with syndactyly and severe mental retardation. *Am J Med Genet.* 1987;28:567–574.

423. Morrison H, Jeppesen J. Allele-specific underacetylation of histone H4 downstream from promoters is associated with X-inactivation in human cells. *Chromosome Res.* 2002;10:579–595.

424. Migeon B. Glucose-6–phosphate dehydrogenase as a probe for the study of X-chromosome inactivation in human females. *Gene Expression and Development.* New York: Alan R. Liss; 1983:189–200.

425. Clemson CM, McNeil JA, Willard H, Lawrence JB. RNA paints the inactive X chromosome at interphase: evidence for a novel RNA involved in nuclear/ chromosome structure. *J Cell Biol.* 1996;132:1–17.

426. Huynh KD, Lee JT. A continuity of X-chromosome silence from gamete to zygote. *Cold Spring Harb Symp Quant Biol.* 2004;69:103–112.

427. Cattanach B, Peters J, Searle T, eds. Special Issue of *Genetical Research* in honour of Mary Lyon. *Genet Res.* 1990;56:82.

428. Lyon MF. Attempts to test the inactive-X theory of dosage compensation in mammals. *Genet Res Camb.* 1963;4:93–103.

429. Gartler SM, Varadarajan KR, Luo P, Norwood TH, Canfield TK, Hansen RS. Abnormal X:autosome ratio, but normal X chromosome inactivation in human triploid cultures. *BMC Genet.* 2006 Jul 3;7(1):41.

430. Horvath, JE., Sheedy, CB, Merrett, SL, et al. Comparative analysis of the primate X-inactivation center region and reconstruction of the ancestral primate XIST locus. *Genome Res* 2011;21:850–862.

431. Jiang J, Jing Y, Cost GJ, et al. Translating dosage compensation to trisomy 21. *Nature.* 2013 Jul 17. doi: 10.1038/nature12394. [Epub ahead of print].

432. Wu H, Luo J, Yu H, et al. Cellular resolution maps of X-chromosome inactivation: implications for neural development, function, and disease. 2013 submitted.

433. Bondy C, Matura LA, Wooten N, Troendle J, Zinn AR, Bakalov VK. The physical phenotype of girls and women with Turner syndrome is not X-imprinted. *Hum Genet.* 2007;121:469–474.

Printed in the USA/Agawam, MA
February 15, 2023

805852.002